Broadening the Base of Addiction Mutual Support Groups

Mutual-help groups have proliferated, diversified and adapted to emerging substance-related trends over the past 75 years, and have been the focus of rigorous research for the past 30 years. This book reviews the history of mutual support groups for addiction that have arisen as adjuncts or alternatives to Twelve Step Programs, including secular mutual support groups like Secular Organization for Sobriety, Smart Recovery and Women for Sobriety, and faith-based mutual support groups like Celebrate Recovery. It also considers the mutual support groups attended by families and friends of addicts. These mutual support groups are examined in terms of their histories, theoretical underpinnings and intended communities.

The structures common in mutual support groups have influenced the rise of a new recovery advocacy movement and new recovery community institutions such as recovery ministries, recovery community centers, sober cafes, sober sports clubs and recovery-focused projects in music, theatre and the arts. This volume explores how collectively, these trends reflect the cultural and political awakening of people in recovery and growing recognition and celebration of multiple pathways of long-term addiction recovery.

This book was originally published as a special issue of the *Journal of Groups in Addiction and Recovery.*

Jeffrey D. Roth is Lecturer in the Department of Psychiatry at the University of Chicago, USA, and Editor of the *Journal of Groups in Addiction and Recovery* and the author of *Group Psychotherapy and Recovery from Addiction: Carrying the Message.* He is the Medical Director of Working Sobriety Chicago, an outpatient treatment program for addiction.

William L. White is Emeritus Senior Research Consultant at Chestnut Health Systems in the USA.

John F. Kelly is the Elizabeth R. Spallin Professor of Psychiatry in Addiction Medicine at Harvard Medical School, USA, and the Director of the Recovery Research Institute, Program Director of the Addiction Recovery Management Service, and the Associate Director of the Center for Addiction Medicine in the Department of Psychiatry at the Massachusetts General Hospital in Boston, Massachusetts, USA.

Broadening the Base of Addiction Mutual Support Groups

Bringing Theory and Science to Contemporary Trends

Edited by

Jeffrey D. Roth, William L. White
and John F. Kelly

Routledge
Taylor & Francis Group
LONDON AND NEW YORK

First published 2014
by Routledge
4 Park Square, Milton Park, Abingdon, Oxon, OX14 4RN

Simultaneously published in the USA and Canada
by Routledge
605 Third Avenue, New York, NY 10017

Routledge is an imprint of the Taylor & Francis Group, an informa business

British Library Cataloguing in Publication Data
A catalogue record for this book is available from the British Library

ISBN13: 978-0-415-83682-1 (hbk)

Typeset in Garamond
by Taylor & Francis Books

Publisher's Note
The publisher accepts responsibility for any inconsistencies that may have arisen during the conversion of this book from journal articles to book chapters, namely the possible inclusion of journal terminology.

Disclaimer
Every effort has been made to contact copyright holders for their permission to reprint material in this book. The publishers would be grateful to hear from any copyright holder who is not here acknowledged and will undertake to rectify any errors or omissions in future editions of this book.

Contents

Citation Information

The chapters in this book were originally published in the *Journal of Groups in Addiction and Recovery*, volume 7, issue 2–4 (April–December 2012). When citing this material, please use the original page numbering for each article, as follows:

Chapter 1
The Promise of Mutual Support
Jeffrey D. Roth
Journal of Groups in Addiction and Recovery, volume 7, issue 2–4 (April–December 2012) pp. 79–81

Chapter 2
Broadening the Base of Addiction Mutual-Help Organizations
John F. Kelly and William L. White
Journal of Groups in Addiction and Recovery, volume 7, issue 2–4 (April–December 2012) pp. 82–101

Chapter 3
SMART Recovery: Self-Empowering, Science-Based Addiction Recovery Support
A. Tom Horvath and Julie Yeterian
Journal of Groups in Addiction and Recovery, volume 7, issue 2–4 (April–December 2012) pp. 102–117

Chapter 4
Empowering Your Sober Self: The LifeRing Approach to Addiction Recovery
Martin Nicolaus
Journal of Groups in Addiction and Recovery, volume 7, issue 2–4 (April–December 2012) pp. 118–129

Chapter 5
Moderation Management: A Mutual-Help Organization for Problem Drinkers Who Are Not Alcohol-Dependent
Anna Lembke and Keith Humphreys
Journal of Groups in Addiction and Recovery, volume 7, issue 2–4 (April–December 2012) pp. 130–141

Chapter 6
Women for Sobriety: 35 Years of Challenges, Changes, and Continuity
Rebecca M. Fenner and Mary H. Gifford
Journal of Groups in Addiction and Recovery, volume 7, issue 2–4 (April–December 2012) pp. 142–170

Chapter 7
Ethnic-Specific Support Systems as a Method for Sustaining Long-Term Addiction Recovery
Arthur C. Evans, Jr, Ijeoma Achara-Abrahams, Roland Lamb, and William L. White
Journal of Groups in Addiction and Recovery, volume 7, issue 2–4 (April–December 2012) pp. 171–188

Chapter 8
Methadone Anonymous and Mutual Support for Medication-Assisted Recovery
Walter Ginter
Journal of Groups in Addiction and Recovery, volume 7, issue 2–4 (April–December 2012) pp. 189–201

Chapter 9
Mutual-Help Groups for People With Co-Occurring Disorders
Joan E. Zweben and Sarah Ashbrook
Journal of Groups in Addiction and Recovery, volume 7, issue 2–4 (April–December 2012) pp. 202–222

Chapter 10
Giving Back and Getting Something Back: The Role of Mutual-Aid Groups for Individuals in Recovery From Incarceration, Addiction, and Mental Illness
Chyrell D. Bellamy, Michael Rowe, Patricia Benedict, and Larry Davidson
Journal of Groups in Addiction and Recovery, volume 7, issue 2–4 (April–December 2012) pp. 223–236

Chapter 11
Use of Mutual Support to Counteract the Effects of Socially Constructed Stigma: Gender and Drug Addiction
Jolene M. Sanders
Journal of Groups in Addiction and Recovery, volume 7, issue 2–4 (April–December 2012) pp. 237–252

Chapter 12
Youth Participation in Mutual Support Groups: History, Current Knowledge, and Areas for Future Research
Lora L. Passetti, Susan H. Godley, and Mark D. Godley
Journal of Groups in Addiction and Recovery, volume 7, issue 2–4 (April–December 2012) pp. 253–278

Chapter 13
Al-Anon Family Groups: Origins, Conceptual Basis, Outcomes, and Research Opportunities
Christine Timko, L. Brendan Young, and Rudolf H. Moos

Journal of Groups in Addiction and Recovery, volume 7, issue 2–4 (April–December 2012) pp. 279–296

Chapter 14

New Addiction-Recovery Support Institutions: Mobilizing Support Beyond Professional Addiction Treatment and Recovery Mutual Aid
William L. White, John F. Kelly, and Jeffrey D. Roth
Journal of Groups in Addiction and Recovery, volume 7, issue 2–4 (April–December 2012) pp. 297–317

Please direct any queries you may have about the citations to
clsuk.permissions@cengage.com

Notes on Contributors

Ijeoma Achara-Abrahams, Philadelphia Department of Behavioral Health and Intellectual Disability Services, Philadelphia, Pennsylvania, USA.

Sarah Ashbrook, East Bay Community Recovery Project, Oakland, California, USA, and Private Practice, Berkeley, California, USA.

Chyrell D. Bellamy, Program for Recovery and Community Health, Department of Psychiatry, Yale University School of Medicine, New Haven, Connecticut, USA.

Patricia Benedict, Program for Recovery and Community Health, Department of Psychiatry, Yale University School of Medicine, New Haven, Connecticut, USA.

Larry Davidson, Program for Recovery and Community Health, Department of Psychiatry, Yale University School of Medicine, New Haven, Connecticut, USA.

Arthur C. Evans, Jr, Philadelphia Department of Behavioral Health and Intellectual Disability Services, Philadelphia, Pennsylvania, USA.

Rebecca M. Fenner, Women for Sobriety Inc., Quakertown, Pennsylvania, USA.

Mary H. Gifford, Women for Sobriety Inc., Quakertown, Pennsylvania, USA.

Walter Ginter, Medication-Assisted Recovery Support (MARS) Project, Port Morris Wellness Center, Bronx, New York, USA.

Mark D. Godley, Lighthouse Institute, Chestnut Health Systems, Normal, Illinois, USA.

Susan H. Godley, Lighthouse Institute, Chestnut Health Systems, Normal, Illinois, USA.

A. Tom Horvath, Practical Recovery, San Diego, California, USA, and SMART Recovery, Mentor, Ohio, USA.

Keith Humphreys, Department of Psychiatry and Behavioral Sciences, Stanford University, Stanford, California, USA, and Veterans Affairs Health Care System, Palo Alto, California, USA.

John F. Kelly, Harvard Medical School, Psychiatry, Massachusetts General Hospital-Harvard Center for Addiction Medicine, and Addiction Recovery Management Service, Psychiatry, Boston, Massachusetts, USA.

Roland Lamb, Office of Addiction Services, Philadelphia Department of Behavioral Health and Intellectual Disability Services, Pennsylvania, USA.

Anna Lembke, Department of Psychiatry and Behavioral Sciences, Stanford University, Stanford, California, USA.

Rudolf H. Moos, Center for Health Care Evaluation, Department of Veterans Affairs Health Care System, USA, and Department of Psychiatry and Behavioral Sciences, Stanford University Medical Center, Palo Alto, California, USA.

Martin Nicolaus, LifeRing Secular Recovery, Berkeley, California, USA.

Lora L. Passetti, Lighthouse Institute, Chestnut Health Systems, Normal, Illinois, USA.

Jeffrey D. Roth, Department of Psychiatry, University of Chicago, USA, and Working Sobriety, Chicago, USA.

Michael Rowe, Program for Recovery and Community Health, Department of Psychiatry, Yale University School of Medicine, New Haven, Connecticut, USA.

Jolene M. Sanders, Department of Sociology and Social Work, Hood College, Frederick, Maryland, USA.

Christine Timko, Center for Health Care Evaluation, Department of Veterans Affairs Health Care System, and Department of Psychiatry and Behavioral Sciences, Stanford University Medical Center, Palo Alto, California, USA.

William L. White, Research Division, Chestnut Health Systems, Punta Gorda, Florida, USA.

Julie Yeterian, Department of Psychiatry, Massachusetts General Hospital, Boston, Massachusetts, USA.

L. Brendan Young, Department of Communication Studies, The University of Iowa, Iowa City, Iowa, USA.

Joan E. Zweben, East Bay Community Recovery Project, Oakland, California, USA, and Department of Psychiatry, University of California, San Francisco, California, USA.

INTRODUCTION

The Promise of Mutual Support

From the inaugural issue of this journal, our interest in the use of groups in fostering recovery from addiction—both in professionally led therapy groups and mutual support groups—has brought together clinicians and researchers working to increase our understanding of these groups. These clinicians and researchers have served as reviewers and authors, have formed a readership for the journal, and have also become another kind of mutual support group. As the editor of the journal, I have the privilege of witnessing the functioning of this mutual support group, which usually "meets" in cyberspace through e-mail communication and "gathers" four times a year each time another issue of the journal appears.

As I described in my editorial for the inaugural issue, we are a diverse group and span a wide range of professions, theoretical orientations, and areas of interest within the field of recovery from addiction. That we function as well as we do is testimony to our willingness to keep our minds open to the views of others and to offer our time and energy in the service of writing about our work, in the process of reviewing the work of others and in the act of taking in the ideas of others in reading about their work. This spirit of open sharing has made possible this special issue on mutual support groups that have arisen outside of the framework of the best-studied mutual support group, Alcoholics Anonymous (AA).

I am deeply grateful to my coeditors, William White and John Kelly, for their willingness to join me in developing the concept of this special issue, for their work in recruiting colleagues to write the articles, for their sharing their wisdom in their own articles, and for their joining with me in practicing the principles of recovery in the production of this special issue. As has been the practice for this journal since its inception, each article is reviewed by a group of colleagues. The reviewers receive a copy of the manuscript without the author(s) identified, and the authors do not know who is reviewing their manuscript. Therefore, anonymity is respected, and principles are placed before personalities. The intent of the review process is inclusive and supportive. The reviewers are encouraged to be rigorously honest with their comments and feedback. Authors are invited to use the review process to learn about how a diverse audience has responded to their work, so that a revised article will more effectively reach their intended readers. For this special issue, the review process has included a group of our usual external reviewers with an additional internal reviewer to increase the unity of our message.

One of the many benefits of the growth of mutual support groups for recovery from addiction other than AA is that the most toxic myths about recovery mutual aid groups may be dispelled. With the availability of diverse mutual support groups, we enter into a potential for the scientific study of these groups without fear of sectarianism. Our hope as editors of this issue is that we offer a foundation for this kind of scientific study.

The introductory article, by Kelly and White, offers a model for comparing and contrasting the range of mutual support groups for recovery from addiction. Their article describes the similarities and differences among AA, SMART Recovery, Secular Organization for Sobriety, Moderation Management, LifeRing, and Women for Sobriety. This examination provides a context for the four articles in our first section, which provide a detailed description of SMART Recovery, Moderation Management, LifeRing, and Women for Sobriety. Accepting the utility and logic of having alternative, complementary structures in place to support recovery from addiction may help us to understand the need for the mutual support groups that have arisen for the more specific needs of other groups of recovering individuals. These other groups, described in four articles in the second section, include those with specific ethnicity, those who use medication alongside their mutual support-group involvement, those with co-occurring disorders, and those who have been involved in the criminal justice system. The third section moves our attention from the specific to the general. The article on the role of mutual support groups in addressing the stigma associated with addiction uses a sample of women recovering in Narcotics Anonymous to offer hypotheses that may be generalizable to other mutual support groups for recovery from addiction. The next article describes adolescent involvement in mutual support groups. Because this population stands at the position where addiction has just begun to fully form, the manner in which adolescents attach and engage in their mutual support groups may reveal insights into the utilization of diverse adult mutual support-group counterparts. In addition, many adolescents with substance use disorders have grown up in families with a complex intergenerational history of addiction. The next article examines the use of mutual support groups for recovery for families of alcoholics in Al-Anon. Our final article, by our three coeditors, offers a description of how the principles of recovery and mutual support are being practiced in a multiplicity of new recovery community institutions.

We invite you, now, to join in our mutual support group for the study of mutual support groups. Whether you are a reader being introduced to our group or a fellow traveler who has been studying mutual support groups for a long time, we wish that collectively we are able to offer each other our experience, strength, and hope. If you find inspiration in this special issue, please consider extending your own research by contributing to this journal.

Like all of the mutual support groups for recovery from addiction described in this special issue, this journal relies on its members to create progress among all who participate.

Jeffrey D. Roth, MD, FAGPA, FASAM
Editor-in-Chief

Broadening the Base of Addiction Mutual-Help Organizations

JOHN F. KELLY

Harvard Medical School, Psychiatry, Massachusetts General Hospital-Harvard Center for Addiction Medicine, and Addiction Recovery Management Service, Psychiatry, Boston, Massachusetts, USA

WILLIAM L. WHITE

Research Division, Chestnut Health Systems, Punta Gorda, Florida, USA

Peer-led mutual-help organizations addressing substance use disorder (SUD) and related problems have had a long history in the United States. The modern epoch of addiction mutual help began in the postprohibition era of the 1930s with the birth of Alcoholics Anonymous (AA). Growing from 2 members to 2 million members, AA's reach and influence has drawn much public health attention as well as increasingly rigorous scientific investigation into its benefits and mechanisms. In turn, AA's growth and success have spurred the development of myriad additional mutual-help organizations. These alternatives may confer similar benefits to those found in studies of AA but have received only peripheral attention. Due to the prodigious economic, social, and medical burden attributable to substance-related problems and the diverse experiences and preferences of those attempting to recover from SUD, there is potentially immense value in societies maintaining and supporting the growth of a diverse array of mutual-help options. This article presents a concise overview of the origins, size, and state of the science on several of the largest of these alternative additional mutual-help organizations in an attempt to raise further awareness and help broaden the base of addiction mutual help.

INTRODUCTION

At first glance, the notion of individuals with serious, objectively verifiable, cognitive and social impairments being able to facilitate life-saving changes in similarly impaired individuals may seem a little incongruous—from a derisory standpoint, a clear case of "the blind leading the blind." It is therefore striking to observe that peer-led mutual-help organizations composed of such individuals have been shown to facilitate the same kinds of salutary behavior changes as trained professionals (Humphreys & Moos, 2001, 2007; Moos & Moos, 2006; Timko, Moos, Finney, & Lesar, 2000; Timko, Sempel, & Moos, 2003). A potential reason for at least some of these mutual-help group benefits may lie in the humorous quip frequently expressed within recovery circles: "We may be sick, but we're not all sick on the same day."

In the addiction field, examples of mutual-help organizations have been well known, even synonymous with addiction recovery for more than 200 years (White, 1998). Alcoholics Anonymous (AA) is by far the largest and most recognized, and its size and impact have garnered much public health and research attention (Emrick, Tonigan, Montgomery, & Little, 1993; Kelly & Yeterian, 2012; Tonigan, Toscova, & Miller, 1996). However, many other mutual-help organizations have emerged since AA began, either inspired by, or in opposition to, it. These AA alternatives have received only limited attention, but due to their similar social orientation and group format, they may confer benefits comparable to those of AA. Given the diverse experiences and preferences of individuals seeking recovery from substance use disorder (SUD) and the valuable role that mutual-help organizations have been shown to play, raising the profile of a broader array of available mutual-help options may enhance the chances of recovery for more people. To this end, the purpose of this article is to describe six of the largest addiction recovery mutual-help AA alternatives: Self-Management and Recovery Training (SMART Recovery), Secular Organization for Sobriety (SOS), Moderation Management (MM), LifeRing, Women for Sobriety (WFS), and Celebrate Recovery (CR). We begin by providing a brief review of the growth and impact of AA followed by a summary of the origins, growth, size and reach, and state of the science on these alternative recovery mutual-help organizations.

ALCOHOLICS ANONYMOUS

AA experienced an inconspicuous beginning in Akron, OH, amid the post-prohibition era of the 1930s. AA has since grown from 2 members to more than 2 million members in 2011 and has been adapted and successfully assimilated into a variety of cultures globally (AA, 2001; Mäkela, 1996). Despite originating under the auspices of a quasireligious organization known as the Oxford Group (AA, 1957; Oxford Group, 1933) and operating at a grassroots community level, AA's language and concepts also have profoundly influenced our *professional* clinical approaches to addressing alcohol and other drug problems (McElrath, 1997; Roman & Blum, 1999; White, 1998), and its philosophy and concepts have imbued our broader language and culture (Travis, 2009).

AA's growing influence and purported success at facilitating long-term addiction recovery has garnered increasing public health and scientific scrutiny (Ferri, Amato, & Davoli, 2006; Institute of Medicine, 1990; McCrady & Miller, 1993). In terms of its verifiable impact, hundreds of published studies, many in top scientific journals, have supported the beneficial effects of AA in helping alleviate alcohol and other drug problems. This body of scientific literature has been summarized in narrative reviews as well as quantitatively, through rigorous meta-analyses (Emrick et al., 1993; Ferri et al.; Humphreys et al., 2004; Kaskutas, 2009; Kelly, 2003; Kownacki & Shadish, 1999; Tonigan et al., 1996; White, 2009). AA participation is associated with producing and maintaining salutary changes in alcohol and other drug use that are on par with professional interventions while simultaneously reducing reliance on professional services and thus lowering related health care costs (Humphreys & Moos, 2001; Humphreys & Moos, 2007; Humphreys et al.; Kelly & Yeterian, 2012). Despite some earlier concerns regarding AA's ability to cater effectively to women, young people, people of color, those with comorbid psychiatric illnesses, and non-religious/spiritual persons, research has found that AA confers similar benefits to women as men (Del Boca & Mattson, 2001; Kelly, Stout, Zywiak, & Schneider, 2006); to young people (Alford, Koehler, & Leonard, 1991; Chi, Kaskutas, Sterling, Campbell, & Weisner, 2009; Kelly, Brown, Abrantes, Kahler, & Myers, 2008; Kelly, Dow, Yeterian, & Kahler, 2010; Kelly, Myers, & Brown, 2000; Kennedy & Minami, 1993); to many (e.g., Ouimette et al., 2001; Timko, Sutkowi, Cronkite, Makin-Byrd, & Moos, 2011), but not all, persons with psychiatric conditions (e.g., those with severe social impairments and/or psychotic spectrum illness; Bogenschutz & Akin, 2000; Kelly, McKellar, & Moos, 2003; Noordsy, Schwab, Fox, & Drake, 1996; Tomasson & Vaglum, 1998); and to those individuals who are non-religious/spiritual or less religious/spiritual (Kelly et al., 2006; Winzelberg & Humphreys, 1999).

Additional anecdotal concerns have centered around AA's position on potentially helpful medications. In general, surveyed AA members have been found to be supportive of the use of psychotropic (e.g., antidepressants, antipsychotics) and relapse prevention medications (e.g., naltrexone, acamprosate, disulfiram), although there may be a vocal minority who oppose it (Meissen, Powell, Wituk, Girrens, & Arteaga, 1999; Rychtarik, Connors, Dermen, & Stasiewicz, 2000; Tonigan & Kelly, 2004). However, it is unclear whether this oppositional minority is specific to AA membership or is a more general facet of individuals attempting to recover; at least one study of alcohol-dependent individuals found that AA participation was unrelated to opposition to the use of medications (Tonigan & Kelly, 2004). Given the importance of this issue, however, AA itself has published a pamphlet on this matter in which it states that it is plainly wrong to deny any member the right to psychiatric medications (AA, 2001).

More rigorous evidence in support of AA emerging in the past 20 years, in particular, has moved AA from a peripheral status as a "nuisance variable" and potential obstacle to progress in the field, to playing a more central role in a recovery-oriented system of care (Kelly & White, 2011; Kelly & Yeterian, 2012; White, 2008). Stemming from these findings on AA's broad reach, effectiveness, and cost-effectiveness, professional interventions have been developed and tested, designed specifically to engage patients with these community mutual-help resources during and after treatment. These "Twelve-Step Facilitation" (TSF) interventions have been found to enhance patient outcomes in randomized controlled investigations (Kahler, Read, Stuart, Ramsey, McCrady & Brown, 2004; Kaskutas, 2009; Litt, Kadden, Kabela-Cormier, & Petry, 2009; Project MATCH Research Group, 1997; Sisson & Mallams, 1981; Timko & DeBenedetti, 2007; Timko, DeBenedetti, & Billow, 2006; Walitzer, Dermen, & Barrick, 2009), and consequently, TSF is now an "empirically supported treatment" as defined by the American Psychological Association and U.S. federal agencies.

With the emergence and increasing availability of illicit substances, addiction to drugs other than alcohol has become more prevalent. This led to adaptations of AA's formula to address the needs of individuals addicted to drugs other than alcohol. The largest among these is Narcotics Anonymous (NA) founded in 1953, which addresses all substances, but other 12-step based organizations soon emerged focusing on specific substances, such as Pot Smokers Anonymous (1968), Pills Anonymous (1975), Marijuana Anonymous (1989), Cocaine Anonymous (1982), Nicotine Anonymous (1985), and Crystal Meth Anonymous (1994). With the increased acknowledgement of the overlap between cormorbid psychiatric disorders and SUD (e.g., Regier, Narrow, & Rae, 1990), "dual-focused" mutual-help organizations have emerged providing support for both sets of problems simultaneously (e.g., Dual Disorders Anonymous [1982], Dual Recovery Anonymous [1989], and Double Trouble in Recovery [1993]). Family members, themselves gravely affected by addiction among loved ones, developed their own mutual-help groups based on the same 12-step and 12-tradition template as AA. The most notable among these were Al-Anon (1951), Alateen (1957), and Nar-Anon (1968).

All of the above organizations are based on AA's organizational template of the 12 steps and 12 traditions (AA, 1953). However, several other recovery organizations have emerged specifically to serve as secular and religious alternatives to AA and other 12-step programs. In the next section, we describe the origins, size and reach, and state of the science of several of the largest and earliest of these alternatives. Specifically, we describe: SMART Recovery, SOS, MM, LifeRing, WFS, and CR.

Self-Management and Recovery Training (SMART Recovery)

SMART Recovery began in 1994 as an offshoot of Rational Recovery (Horvath & Yeterian, this issue). The stated goals of SMART Recovery are to "support individuals who have chosen to abstain, or are considering abstinence from any type of addictive behavior (substances or activities), by teaching how to change self-defeating thinking, emotions, and actions; and to work towards long-term satisfactions and quality of life" (www.smartrecovery.org/intro/index.htm). It teaches self-empowerment and self-reliance and views addictions/compulsions as complex maladaptive behaviors with possible physiological factors. It teaches tools and techniques for self-directed change and encourages individuals to recover and live satisfying lives.

The SMART Recovery meetings have a contemporary cognitive-behavioral orientation, are educational, and include open discussions. It also explicitly advocates the appropriate use of prescribed medications and psychological treatments. It draws on evidence-based practices and "evolves as scientific knowledge of addiction recovery evolves" (www.smartrecovery.org/intro/index.htm). The main processes of recovery stated by SMART Recovery are enhancing and maintaining motivation to abstain, coping with urges, problem solving (e.g., managing thoughts, feelings, and behaviors), and lifestyle balance achieved and reinforced through meeting participation. Professionals and peers serve as volunteer facilitators of SMART Recovery meetings.

As of December 2011, SMART Recovery was reported to have more than 650 groups throughout the world, with most of them in the United States. The SMART Recovery Web site maintains a current listing of face-to-face meetings (which are available in most U.S. states) and daily online meetings (which offer either voice and/or text connection). In the most recent SMART Recovery participant survey (N = 513; http://www.surveymonkey.com/sr.aspx?sm=mYZaRq3wlN9vAaQhcXBXp4Aj82eJeDLX_ 2ftPftMvLLbI_3d), most SMART Recovery participants were Caucasian (93.2%), 42.7% were female, and the median age was approximately 50 years old. Slightly more than half (53.5%) of those surveyed reported being SMART Recovery members for less than 1 year. Despite SMART Recovery having a secular orientation and providing an alternative to 12-step organizations, 60.7% of members reported believing in some kind of god or higher power, and 85.2% reported attending AA or other 12-step organizations in addition to SMART Recovery. Thus, although there is a large overlap in 12-step participation among SMART members, it seems that SMART offers something potentially unique and appealing that is not offered in 12-step organizations.

Research on the effectiveness of SMART Recovery is limited. Two cross-sectional survey studies examined characteristics of SMART Recovery members (e.g., religiosity, locus of control) relative to members of other mutual-help organizations, such as AA (Atkins & Hawdon, 2007; Li, Feifer, & Strohm, 2000). One of these studies (Atkins & Hawdon) found a significant relationship between the duration of continuous abstinence and the extent of participation in mutual-help groups, which included SMART Recovery. This relationship did not differ by type of mutual-help organization. This suggests that the benefits from SMART Recovery participation may be similar to that of other mutual-help organizations (Horvath & Yeterian, this issue).

Although not a test of SMART Recovery as a mutual-help organization, a related study compared professionally led 12-step- and SMART Recovery-based intensive outpatient treatment programs for dually diagnosed patients (Brooks & Penn, 2003). Findings revealed SMART Recovery-based treatment was less effective at reducing alcohol use compared with the 12-step-based treatment, but it was more effective at improving participants' employment status and medical concerns. Several limitations were apparent in this study, however, including a high dropout rate and unequal treatment exposure across conditions. Also, as alluded to earlier, intensive outpatient treatment is not comparable to the context in which real-world SMART Recovery groups are run, and this study sample was composed of dually diagnosed individuals who may not be representative of most SMART Recovery members (Horvath & Yeterian, this issue).

SMART Recovery is beginning to make successful forays into other countries besides the United States. A small pilot study in Great Britain about participant ($N = 65$) perceptions of SMART Recovery (MacGregor & Herring, 2010) found that the majority of SMART Recovery attendees (79%) found groups to be very helpful and intended to continue attending within the next 3 months. Most had attended other mutual-help groups, such as AA, but reported SMART Recovery was more useful to them.

SMART Recovery is an interesting hybrid mutual-help organization in that it takes evidence-based motivational and cognitive-behavioral strategies evaluated in professional clinical settings and populations and implements these in a community mutual-help group context. It is growing nationally and internationally, and future research evaluation will reveal whether this translation of evidence-based clinical practice to a mutual-help context results in stronger engagement, retention, and recovery outcomes. Given the limited empirical literature on SMART Recovery, there are myriad research opportunities available to expand knowledge of its effectiveness, health care cost-offset potential, and potential for benefitting particular types of individuals, such as atheists and agnostics.

SECULAR ORGANIZATION FOR SOBRIETY

SOS was started in 1986 by James Christopher, a disaffected AA member looking to eradicate the spiritual/religious elements from the recovery mutual aid offered through 12-step fellowships. The organization refers to itself as "a self-empowerment approach to recovery" without any spiritual or religious involvement. Its therapeutic processes and general organizational principles are quite similar to AA however, and much of the organizational language is very similar to AA's 12 traditions. Meetings are typically 90 minutes in duration and each group is autonomous and self-supporting through its own voluntary contributions.

SOS does not possess a clear, sequential program of action, like AA, but does advocate honest sharing, association with others including other alcoholics, and a focused "Sobriety Priority" of abstaining from alcohol "no matter what." The organization's group meetings typically encourage self-admission of alcohol addiction, a daily reminder of this fact, the goal of enhanced quality of life ("the good life"), honest and confidential sharing with other affected individuals, and personal responsibility for recovery (Christopher, 1988). The course of action needed to achieve sobriety is largely left up to the individual to decide for himself or herself, but it is encouraged to be sought using the experience of those SOS members who have found it.

Despite its size and longevity, there has been very little research conducted on SOS to date. The largest survey of 158 members was published in 1996 by Connors and Dermen. The response rate was very low, however, ranging from somewhere between 15% and 29% (Connors & Dermen). Most of the members who responded were White (99%), male (73%), well educated (79.5% reported at least some college or more education), and about 40 years old on average. The majority (70%) reported no current religious affiliation, and 70% described themselves as atheist or agnostic and another 22% as spiritual but not religious. Respondents liked the lack of religious emphasis the best and found the interpersonal aspects of the organization the most helpful. The average number of years of sobriety was 6.3. About 30% were also attending AA meetings in addition to SOS. Average attendance frequency during the past year was about two to three times per month, and the total number of SOS meetings attended was 45.4 (Connors & Dermen).

With the limitation of the low response rate noted, it appears that in keeping with its goals and orientation, SOS tends to attract atheist/agnostic and nonreligious individuals, and the average meeting attendance figures suggest it is able to engage individuals for the long term. Although about one third of members also attended AA, the majority benefited from SOS, and much like in AA, which has 50% of its members with more than 5 years of sobriety, they appeared to find continued benefits despite an average of more than 6 years of sobriety. SOS's growth and staying power warrant further research on its member composition, effectiveness in helping individuals stay sober and improve quality of life, dropout rates, and mechanisms of change.

Moderation Management

MM, founded in 1994, is the only substance-focused mutual-help organization that explicitly advocates moderate, nonharmful use of alcohol and not complete abstinence. Given that the largest portion of the burden of disease, disability, and negative social and economic impact is attributable to this segment of hazardous/harmful drinking individuals, MM has immense public health potential.

MM embodies four major principles: self-management, balance, moderation, and personal responsibility. MM's main aim is to share strategies for successful moderation and the "restoration of balance," which include both changes in behavior and the management of emotions. Its main therapeutic process is through self-monitoring of drinking to keep within healthful limits. This is supported by MM group participation. A primary tool used in MM is "awareness." Daily drink charting is intended to bring an unconscious habit back to consciousness and within control. The very act of counting the number of drinks consumed each week is one of the key processes of therapeutic change. MM advocates nine steps (http://www.moderation.org/readings.shtml#9steps) that include an initial 30-day period of abstinence during which the member can assess how alcohol has affected them, set drinking limits, and begin to make lifestyle changes. MM members are asked to limit drinking to no more than 9 drinks per week, no more than 3 per day, for women; and to no more than 14 per week, no more than 4 per day for men. These limits are the same as those recommended by the U.S. National Institute on Alcohol Abuse and Alcoholism (NIAAA). Even after moderate drinking is begun within the context of MM, MM still recommends not drinking every day, but rather to abstain from alcohol completely on at least 3 to 4 days per week.

In terms of evidence for its beneficial effects, there have been no longitudinal studies or experimental efficacy studies. Two independent surveys have been conducted and show that MM appears to attract problem drinkers who are less severely dependent than those who seek to join AA and who possess greater social resources (Humphreys & Klaw, 2001; Kosok, 2006). These surveys have supported the notion that nondependent "problem drinkers" utilize MM and are mostly drinking in the harmful/hazardous range as opposed to the dependent range (Humphreys & Klaw; Kosok).

MM fills an important gap in the range of options for the large number of individuals who are nondependent drinkers but nevertheless are suffering from a range of alcohol-related problems. MM can therefore provide support and reduce harms attributable to alcohol without requiring abstinence. This is often an attractive option for many who do not see themselves needing to abstain completely. It can also provide an opportunity to gain support and structure while assessing, experientially, whether individuals can successfully moderate drinking behavior. The goal of a 30-day initial period of complete abstinence followed by a prescribed noncontinuous weekly drinking pattern and limiting quantity to within NIAAA guidelines is likely to quickly separate those individuals who will continue to benefit from MM from those for whom abstinence may be the easier and optimal goal. Typically in the course of alcohol dependence, sufferers possess a strong desire to be able to successfully regulate alcohol consumption. Although, MM's explicit focus is to cater to those wishing to continue to moderate over time, it may therefore also play an intermediate role by providing an opportunity for those dependent on alcohol to realize they are unable to stop or control their alcohol use in a supportive environment without criticism.

LIFERING

LifeRing for Secular Sobriety is a cognitive-behaviorally oriented support group that emphasizes a tradition of positive psychology rather than spirituality or religious ideas. Founded in 2001, it has grown to about 140 face-to-face meetings as well as online meetings with about 1,000 participants. It has already begun surveys of its membership (sample responded = 401) indicating 58% were male, the average age was 47.8 years old, more than 80% had attended some college, and 44% had a bachelors degree. The average length of sobriety was 2.74 years. In the past year, 40% reported attending a religious service of some kind. In keeping with LifeRing's goal of targeting any kind of substance dependence, survey respondents' primary substances covered a full range of substances of misuse including tobacco.

The LifeRing approach centers on empowerment of the "sober self" characterized by three major components: recognition, activation, and mastery. Recognition emphasizes insight and empowerment by realizing that the "sober self" is a part of who individuals are and has helped them access help and get to this point in their lives. Activation is about living in sobriety and facing the challenges of recovery, which is discussed in group meetings. Mastery is supported through empowering individual members to develop their own "Personal Recovery Program" (PRP). Individuals' PRPs can be allowed to occur naturally as things progress, or more strategically by working through the organization's *Recovery by Choice* workbook. This facilitates the formation of the PRP across nine different recovery-related domains.

The LifeRing approach is essentially a grassroots experientially based mutual-help group but is informed by the latest treatment and recovery research. Consequently, it incorporates ideas from cognitive-behavioral, motivational, humanistic, existential, and positive psychology areas. No studies have been conducted on LifeRing, but its continued expansion is evidence of its value to many individuals suffering a variety of substance addiction problems. Future research should focus on which individuals may be likely to engage with the organization and on its effectiveness in helping individuals maintain recovery.

WOMEN FOR SOBRIETY

WFS was established in 1975 by Jean Kirkpatrick, a woman in recovery, who found that AA did not meet all her needs. She believed that women needed their own groups, free from men and role expectations, in which to share their experiences and grow stronger. WFS has between 1,000 and 2,000 members in Canada and the United States and approximately 300 face-to-face meetings (Humphreys, 2004). Almost all these members are Caucasian, well educated, and middle class (Kaskutas, 1992). The WFS program "is an affirmation of the value and worth of each woman," as exemplified in its 13 Statements of Acceptance (Kirkpatrick, 1978). Kirkpatrick maintains that these statements can lead women to see themselves more positively, to increase their self-confidence, and to learn to see themselves as able to overcome their drinking and other problems. The changes they experience are reinforced by the group. WFS groups provide acceptance, nurturing, and a sense of belonging and are a place to release anxiety, share fears, and learn to trust.

A comprehensive survey of WFS membership (response rate = 73%, n = 600) was conducted by Kaskutas (1994). Respondents reported their reasons for attending WFS as well as AA and also reported their reasons for not attending AA. Study participants reported that they attended WFS for support and nurturance (54%), for a safe environment (26%), for sharing about women's specific issues (42%), and because of its positive emphasis (38%) and focus on self-esteem (39%). They reported attending AA primarily as insurance against relapse (28%), for its wide availability (25%), and for sharing (31%) and support (27%). Women who did not attend AA reported feeling as though they never fitted in to AA (20%), found AA too negative (18%), disliked the "drunkalogs" (14%) and the focus on the past (14%), and felt that AA was geared too much to men's needs (15%).

WFS is the only major organization specifically for women seeking recovery from alcohol addiction. It takes a positive and affirming stance through its focus on enhancing self-esteem, self-empowerment and self-acceptance, emotional growth, and spirituality: "Emotional growth is happiness; spiritual growth is peace. Together these create a competent, loving woman" (Kirkpatrick, 1978). Like SOS, AA, and others, WFS encourages continued involvement over the long haul, and similar to AA, WFS advocates a day-at-a-time approach. WFS has not grown rapidly in the United States or other countries since its beginning in the 1970s. Yet, its evident staying power and sizeable membership indicate that it plays an important role for alcohol-addicted women. Research is needed on its overall effectiveness and unique potential to engage women reluctant to attend AA.

CELEBRATE RECOVERY

In contrast to the other organizations mentioned previously, CR is an explicitly Christian-based religious recovery support organization functioning under the auspices of formal church organizations. CR was founded in 1991 at Saddleback Church in Lake Forest, CA. It was started by John Baker, an alcoholic who found recovery in AA, but who felt constricted in his ability to openly discuss his Christian beliefs within the AA context. He became inspired to begin a separate group where celebration of his addiction recovery along with his Christian values and beliefs could be expressed candidly. After obtaining the blessing and encouragement from his pastor (Rick Warren) from the Saddleback Church, he began the first CR meeting. This was initially based on AA's 12 steps but as things developed into the more formally known CR organization, 8 principles were derived based on the Beatitudes found in Christian Scripture (Matthew 5:1–12, King James Version). These principles describe a very similar sequential process and content as the 12 steps of AA (Baker, 2005; Headley, Olges, & Sickinger, n.d.). The organization does not focus exclusively on recovery from substance-related problems and instead allows anyone to attend who is having difficulty changing problematic and troubling patterns of behavior (i.e., it is open to those "healing from hurts, habits, and hang ups"; www.celebraterecovery.com). It is somewhat similar in this regard to SMART Recovery, which encourages membership for those suffering from substance or behavioral addiction problems.

CR meetings possess a similar format to 12-step meetings. However, the curriculum of CR is strictly monitored by the national organization (Headley et al., n.d.). To use the CR name and materials, a leader must agree to abide by the expectations listed in "The DNA of an Authentic Celebrate Recovery Meeting.," Typical CR meetings begin in a single, large group then break into smaller groups separated by gender and organized by content. Unlike AA but similar to other secular mutual-help organizations, members are discouraged from identifying themselves as their particular problem (e.g., "I'm Susan and I am an alcoholic"), and preference is given to self-identifying as "a Christian who is struggling with. . ." Similar to the AA model, CR encourages individual mentoring (like an AA sponsor), but in addition, has a small support network referred to as "accountability partners." In CR, sponsors fulfill largely the same role as an AA sponsor but more explicitly support spiritual growth through prayer and discussion of members' concerns and questions. The accountability partners are exclusive to CR and are described as a group of at least three to four people who are at a stage of recovery and who share the same challenge as the focal member. Such homogeneity in content and the recovery stage may enhance therapeutic cohesion and universality (Yalom & Leszcz, 2005). Accountability partners pray for each other and give and seek support through phone calls between face-to-face meetings (Headley, et al.).

CR has grown considerably since its beginning in 1991. According to the CR Web site (www.celebraterecovery.com), more than 170,000 individuals have completed the CR program, and there are approximately 17,000 CR group ministries operating around the world in approximately 50 countries. The structure of CR is noteworthy. Specifically, its broader focus on behavioral problems and concerns beyond substance use is likely to attract a larger number of potential members than would be the case if its sole focus was on substance-related problems alone. A potential downside of a broader focus, however, could be less group cohesion, universality, and mutual identification. That said, the meeting format of breaking into smaller subgroups with similar concerns and issues may help maintain and strengthen these therapeutic group elements. CR's rapid growth and popularity presents some evidence of its potential benefit. However, little is known about its ability to engage and retain members over time or whether it helps reduce relapse rates and enhances the odds of long-term recovery.

DISCUSSION AND CONCLUSIONS

Stemming from the rapid growth and influence of AA, a variety of secular, spiritual, and religious alternative mutual-help organizations have emerged during the past 40 years. This multitude of new groups reflects a reality of the diverse needs and preferences of individuals suffering from SUD. However, these alternatives, the largest of which are described herein, have experienced relatively slow growth and acceptance as the mutual-help landscape in the United States has been dominated largely by 12-step organizations such as AA and NA. There are several possible reasons for this slow growth and acceptance of these non-12-step alternatives in the United States. Some of these reasons may relate to differences in operational structure among the various organizations themselves; some may also relate to the degree of fit within the broader cultural context in which they have emerged; while others may pertain to a clinically driven "catch 22" scenario, whereby clinicians are reluctant to refer to smaller organizations or to organizations without a local presence, which in turn, continues to limit their growth. This, in turn, makes it difficult to conduct the kinds of research studies that have been conducted on larger organizations, such as AA, which have increased confidence in AA's effectiveness and thus led to more referrals. We discuss each of these reasons in the following paragraphs.

In terms of operational differences, one reason for the rapid growth of AA and other 12-step mutual-help organizations may be in part due to these organizations' decentralized and "horizontal" authority structure: There is no CEO, president, or leaders in the usual sense issuing top-down instructions—rather, there are only "trusted servants" who are elected by the group and encouraged to rotate regularly. Also, each group itself is completely autonomous and financially self-supporting and able to make its own decisions based on the democratically expressed collective "group conscience." It is merely suggested that 12-step groups adhere to the guidelines (the "12 traditions") outlined in the book, *Twelve Steps and Twelve Traditions* (AA, 1953). Consequently, anyone can start an AA meeting of any kind at any time provided the new group tries to adhere to these traditions. AA's co-founder, Bill W., himself described AA as a kind of "benign anarchy" because of this laissez-faire approach (AA, 1957). This policy of individual and group autonomy may be a major reason why AA and other similar organizations have grown so large. A possible downside of this approach, however, is that this "hands-off" policy affords no oversight, or "quality control," increasing potential variability in group dynamics, content, and any potential therapeutic benefit (Kelly, Stout, Magill, Tonigan, & Pagano, 2011; Tonigan, Miller, & Connors, 2001). AA membership growth may also be linked to its strong service ethic and its implicit expectation for prolonged, if not lifelong, participation (many of the alternatives profiled here expect participation only as long as needed and then encourage members to leave and get on with their lives). Indeed, almost half of the AA membership has 5 or more years of sobriety (AA, 2008).

In contrast, other organizations, such as SMART Recovery, possess a more typical centralized organizational structure, with a president, and require trained facilitators to run group meetings. Some other mutual-help organizations require certification for group leaders or otherwise possess a more "vertical" organizational structure that exerts elements of control of its groups. The consequence of these different policies may mean that the freedom inherent in 12-step organizations facilitates rapid growth, whereas growth may be constricted more by the barriers of consultation, training, and oversight that is often required in other mutual-help organizations.

The ultimate question, of course, may be one of "reach" versus "effectiveness" (Glasgow, Lichtenstein, & Marcus, 2003) or more commonly, "quantity versus quality." That is to say, does the greater oversight and centralized structure, designed to enhance model adherence and provide "quality control," actually result in sufficiently superior effectiveness and member benefit to justify the more tightly controlled approach, despite placing potential limitations on growth? Currently, there are no comparative effectiveness studies of mutual-help organizations to test this. In general, however, it may be that most recovery-focused mutual-help organizations confer broadly similar benefits. Generalizing from the results of comparative trials of professional treatments, this could well be the case (Morgenstern & Longabaugh, 2000), especially because all of the mutual-help organizations share common therapeutic elements, such as their social structure and group format (Humphreys, 2004; Yalom & Leszcz, 2005). These social components have been shown to be the major pathway through which AA confers its beneficial recovery effects (Kelly, Hoeppner, Stout, & Pagano, 2012). Renowned psychoanalyst, Carl Jung, asserted also that "the protective wall of human community" was one of the major general pathways to addiction recovery (AA Grapevine, 1968).

Another reason why AA and other 12-step organizations have grown so rapidly, particularly in the United States, may have to do with cultural fit and context. AA's emphasis on spirituality and its use of religious language may be particularly appealing in a country like the United States, where the majority of the population (85%) believes in some kind of deity or God (Kosmin & Keysar, 2009). As noted previously, even among some of the newer secular alternatives that have conducted membership surveys in the United States, almost half or more express religious beliefs and/or behaviors. Also, due to the disinhibiting effects of alcohol and other drugs, individuals suffering from SUD have often engaged in behaviors that run counter to their own values or moral code. Over time, this can lead to chronic self-denigration and self-blame. AA and similar 12-step organizations offer spiritual and quasireligious concepts that by their nature may provide an appealing and compassionate framework for self-forgiveness for those suffering from alcohol and other drug addiction that is not present in other mutual-help organizations (Kelly et al., 2011).

Finally, another possible reason why non-12-step mutual-help alternatives have not grown as rapidly as 12-step organizations may be due to a clinically related "catch 22" scenario: Clinicians are reluctant to refer patients to groups, such as WFS or LifeRing, because of the limited community availability of such groups; and fewer referrals, in turn, perpetuate this limited availability. Furthermore, smaller numbers of groups add to the difficulties of conducting research, positive findings from which could enhance confidence in their clinical utility and impact. The issue of conducting rigorous research on community organizations is not without challenges even under optimal conditions, particularly in conducting the gold standard of treatment research: the randomized controlled trial (RCT). The tightly controlled and highly insulated context of an RCT runs counter to the way real-world mutual-help groups are conducted. Nearly all are attended anonymously and (usually) voluntarily. No records are kept regarding who attends and what is said. Groups vary widely in their size and content. Because mutual-help groups are freely accessible in the community, it can be seen as unethical to randomly assign some RCT participants to attend and prohibit the attendance of others. These issues have led researchers to examine mutual-help groups mostly through other methods, such as through naturalistic, prospective effectiveness studies, but RCTs have been conducted on professionally delivered TSF interventions designed to engage individuals with these groups such as AA. These kinds of studies would be fairly straightforward to implement also with other mutual-help groups, such as SMART Recovery or LifeRing.

It is hoped that this "catch 22" trend can be reversed by greater clinical open-mindedness and willingness to take an extra step to learn more about the local availability of alternatives and therefore present patients with an informed choice that may ultimately increase the chances of some kind of engagement with a recovery resource (Kelly, Humphreys, & Yeterian, 2012).

The more recent non-12-step mutual-help alternatives may never grow as large as AA for some of the reasons outlined earlier. Nevertheless, they play a vital role in our society's overall response to the prodigious social, medical, and economic burden attributable to substance misuse by providing an array of potentially appealing alternatives. These alternatives merely reflect the demographic diversity and the varieties of addiction experiences and recovery preferences held by individuals suffering from SUD. Providing and supporting greater choice and more options will broaden the base of addiction mutual help. This, in turn, is very likely to enhance the chances of recovery for more individuals.

REFERENCES

Alcoholics Anonymous. (1953). *Twelve steps and twelve traditions.* New York, NY: Alcoholics Anonymous World Services.

Alcoholics Anonymous. (1957). *Alcoholics Anonymous comes of age.* New York, NY: Alcoholics Anonymous World Services.

Alcoholics Anonymous. (2001). *Alcoholics Anonymous: The story of how thousands of men and women have recovered from alcoholism* (4th ed.). New York, NY: Alcoholics Anonymous World Services.

Alcoholics Anonymous. (2008). *2007 membership survey: A snapshot of A.A. membership.* New York, NY: Alcoholics Anonymous World Services.

Alcoholics Anonymous Grapevine. (1968). *The Bill W.–Carl Jung letters.* New York, NY: Author.

Alford, G. S., Koehler, R. A., & Leonard, J. (1991). Alcoholics Anonymous–Narcotics Anonymous model inpatient treatment of chemically dependent adolescents: A 2-year outcome study. *Journal of Studies on Alcohol and Drugs, 52*(2), 118–126.

Atkins, R. G., Jr., & Hawdon, J. E. (2007). Religiosity and participation in mutual-aid support groups for addiction. *Journal of Substance Abuse Treatment, 33*(3), 321–331.

Baker, J. (2005). *Celebrate Recovery's updated leader's guide: A recovery program based on eight principles from the Beatitudes.* Grand Rapids, MI: Zondervan.

Bogenschutz, M. P., & Akin, S. J. (2000). 12-step participation and attitudes toward 12-step meetings in dual diagnosis patients. *Alcoholism Treatment Quarterly, 18*(4), 31–45.

Brooks, A. J., & Penn, P. E. (2003). Comparing treatments for dual diagnosis: Twelve-step and self-management and recovery training. *American Journal of Drug and Alcohol Abuse, 29*(2), 359–383.

Chi, F. W., Kaskutas, L. A., Sterling, S., Campbell, C. I., & Weisner, C. (2009). Twelve-Step affiliation and 3-year substance use outcomes among adolescents: Social support and religious service attendance as potential mediators. *Addiction, 104*(6), 927–939.

Christopher, J. (1988). *How to stay sober: Recovery without religion.* Buffalo, NY: Prometheus.

Connors, G. J., & Dermen, K. H. (1996). Characteristics of participants in Secular Organizations for Sobriety (SOS). *American Journal of Drug and Alcohol Abuse, 22*(2), 281–295.

Del Boca, F. K., & Mattson, M. E. (2001). The gender matching hypothesis. In R. Longabaugh & P. Wirtz (Eds.), *Project MATCH hypotheses: Results and causal chain analysis. Project MATCH Monograph Series* (Vol. 8). Bethesda, MD: National Institute on Alcohol Abuse and Alcoholism, 186–203.

Emrick, C. D., Tonigan, J. S., Montgomery, H., & Little, L. (1993). Alcoholics Anonymous: What is currently known? *Research on Alcoholics Anonymous: Opportunities and Alternatives* (pp. 41–76). Piscatawey, NJ: Rutgers Center for Alcohol Studies.

Ferri, M., Amato, L., & Davoli, M. (2006). Alcoholics Anonymous and other 12-step programmes for alcohol dependence. *Cochrane Database System Review, 3,* CD005032.

Glasgow, R. E., Lichtenstein, E., & Marcus, A. C. (2003). Why don't we see more translation of health promotion research to practice? Rethinking the efficacy-to-effectiveness transition. *American Journal of Public Health, 93*(8), 1261–1267.

Headley, K., Olges, D., & Sickinger, P. (n.d.). *Twelve-step referrals: A group counselor's guide to utilizing Alcoholics Anonymous and Celebrate Recovery.* Unpublished manuscript, Regent University: Virginia Beach, VA.

Horvath, A. T., & Yeterian, J. D. (2012). SMART Recovery: Self-empowering, science-based recovery support. *Journal of Groups in Addiction and Recovery, 7*(2–4), 102–117.

Humphreys, K. (2004). *Circles of recovery: Self-help organizations for addictions.* Cambridge, UK: Cambridge University Press.

Humphreys, K., & Klaw, E. (2001). Can targeting nondependent problem drinkers and providing Internet-based services expand access to assistance for alcohol problems? A study of the Moderation Management self-help/mutual aid organization. *Journal of Studies on Alcohol and Drugs, 62*(4), 528–532.

Humphreys, K., & Moos, R. (2001). Can encouraging substance abuse patients to participate in self-help groups reduce demand for health care? A quasi-experimental study. *Alcoholism: Clinical and Experimental Research, 25*(5), 711–716.

Humphreys, K., & Moos, R. H. (2007). Encouraging posttreatment self-help group involvement to reduce demand for continuing care services: Two-year clinical and utilization outcomes. *Alcoholism: Clinical and Experimental Research, 31*(1), 64–68.

Humphreys, K., Wing, S., McCarty, D., Chappel, J., Gallant, L., Haberle, B.,... & Weiss, R. (2004). Self-help organizations for alcohol and drug problems: Toward evidence-based practice and policy. *Journal of Substance Abuse Treatment, 26*(3), 151–158, 159–165.

Institute of Medicine. (1990). *Broadening the base of treatment for alcohol problems.* Washington, DC: National Academy Press.

Kahler, C. W., Read, J. P., Stuart, G. L., Ramsey, S. E., McCrady, B. S. & Brown, R. A. (2004). Motivational enhancement for 12-step involvement among patients undergoing alcohol detoxification. *Journal of Consulting and Clinical Psychology, 72*(4), 736–741.

Kaskutas, L. A. (1992). *An analysis of Women for Sobriety* (Unpublished doctoral dissertation). University of California, Berkeley, Berkeley, CA.

Kaskutas, L. A. (1994). What do women get out of self-help? Their reasons for attending Women for Sobriety and Alcoholics Anonymous. *Journal of Substance Abuse Treatment, 11*(3), 185–195.

Kaskutas, L. A. (2009). Alcoholics Anonymous effectiveness: Faith meets science. *Journal of Addictive Diseases, 28*(2), 145–157.

Kelly, J. F. (2003). Self-help for substance use disorders: History, effectiveness, knowledge gaps & research opportunities. *Clinical Psychology Review, 23*(5), 639–663.

Kelly, J. F., Brown, S. A., Abrantes, A., Kahler, C. W., & Myers, M. (2008). Social recovery model: An 8-year investigation of adolescent 12-step group involvement following inpatient treatment. *Alcoholism: Clinical and Experimental Research, 32*(8), 1468–1478.

Kelly, J. F., Dow, S. J., Yeterian, J. D., & Kahler, C. (2010). Can 12-step group participation strengthen and extend the benefits of adolescent addiction treatment? A prospective analysis. *Drug and Alcohol Dependence, 110*(1/2), 117–125.

Kelly, J. F., Hoeppner, B., Stout, R. L., & Pagano, M. (2012). Determining the relative importance of the mechanisms of behavior change within Alcoholics Anonymous: A multiple mediator analysis. *Addiction, 107*(2), 289–299.

Kelly, J. F., Humphreys, K., & Yeterian, J. D. (2012). Mutual aid groups. In S. Harrison & V. Carver (Eds.), *Alcohol and drug problems: A practical guide for counselors* (4th ed., pp. 169–197). Toronto, Ontario, Canada: Center for Addiction and Mental Health.

Kelly, J. F., McKellar, J. D., & Moos, R. (2003). Major depression in patients with substance use disorders: Relationship to 12-step self-help involvement and substance use outcomes. *Addiction, 98*(4), 499–508.

Kelly, J. F., Myers, M. G., & Brown, S. A. (2000). A multivariate process model of adolescent 12-step attendance and substance use outcome following inpatient treatment. *Psychology of Addictive Behaviors, 14*(4), 376–389.

Kelly, J. F., Stout, R. L., Magill, M., Tonigan, J. S., & Pagano, M. E. (2011). Spirituality in recovery: A lagged mediational analysis of Alcoholics Anonymous' principal theoretical mechanism of behavior change. *Alcoholism: Clinical and Experimental Research, 35*(3), 454–463.

Kelly, J. F., Stout, R., Zywiak, W., & Schneider, R. (2006). A 3-year study of addiction mutual-help group participation following intensive outpatient treatment. *Alcoholism: Clinical and Experimental Research, 30*(8), 1381–1392.

Kelly, J. F., & White, W. L. (Eds.). (2011). *Addiction recovery management*. New York, NY: Springer.

Kelly, J. F., & Yeterian, J. D. (2012). Empirical awakening: The new science on mutual help and implications for cost containment under health care reform. *Journal of Substance Abuse, 33*(2), 85–91.

Kennedy, B. P., & Minami, M. (1993). The Beech Hill Hospital/Outward Bound Adolescent Chemical Dependency Treatment Program. *Journal of Substance Abuse Treatment, 10*(4), 395–406.

Kirkpatrick, J. (1978). *Turnabout: Help for a new life*. New York, NY: Doubleday and Company.

Kosmin, B. A., & Keysar, A. (2009). *American Religious Identification Survey (ARIS)*. Hartford, CT: Trinity College.

Kosok, A. (2006). The Moderation Management programme in 2004: What type of drinker seeks controlled drinking? *International Journal of Drug Policy, 17*(4), 295–303.

Kownacki, R. J., & Shadish, W. R. (1999). Does Alcoholics Anonymous work? The results from a meta-analysis of controlled experiments. *Substance Use & Misuse, 34*(13), 1897–1916.

Li, E. C., Feifer, C., & Strohm, M. (2000). A pilot study: Locus of control and spiritual beliefs in Alcoholics Anonymous and SMART Recovery members. *Addictive Behaviors, 25*(4), 633–640.

Litt, M. D., Kadden, R. M., Kabela-Cormier, E., & Petry, N. M. (2009). Changing network support for drinking: Network Support Project 2-year follow-up. *Journal of Consulting and Clinical Psychology, 77*(2), 229–242.

MacGregor, S., & Herring, R. (2010). *The alcohol concern SMART Recovery pilot project final evaluation report*. London: Middlesex University Drug and Alcohol Research Group.

Mäkela, K. (1996). *Alcoholics Anonymous as a mutual-help movement: A study in eight societies*. Madison, WI: University of Wisconsin Press.

McCrady, B. S., & Miller, W. R. (1993). *Research on Alcoholics Anonymous: Opportunities and alternatives*. New Brunswick, NJ: Rutgers Center of Alcohol Studies.

McElrath, D. (1997). The Minnesota Model. *Journal of Psychoactive Drugs, 29*(2), 141–144.

Meissen, G., Powell, T. J., Wituk, S. A., Girrens, K., & Arteaga, S. (1999). Attitudes of AA contact persons toward group participation by persons with a mental illness. *Psychiatric Services, 50*(8), 1079–1081.

Moos, R. H., & Moos, B. S. (2006). Participation in treatment and Alcoholics Anonymous: A 16-year follow-up of initially untreated individuals. *Journal of Clinical Psychology, 62*(6), 735–750.

Morgenstern, J., & Longabaugh, R. (2000). Cognitive-behavioral treatment for alcohol dependence: A review of evidence for its hypothesized mechanisms of action. *Addiction, 95*(10), 1475–1490.

Noordsy, D. L., Schwab, B., Fox, L., & Drake, R. E. (1996). The role of self-help programs in the rehabilitation of persons with severe mental illness and substance use disorders. *Community Mental Health Journal, 32*(1), 71–81, 83–76.

Ouimette, P., Humphreys, K., Moos, R. H., Finney, J. W., Cronkite, R., & Federman, B. (2001). Self-help group participation among substance use disorder patients with posttraumatic stress disorder. *Journal of Substance Abuse Treatment, 20*(1), 25–32.

Oxford Group. (1933). *What is the Oxford Group?* London, UK: Oxford University Press.

Project MATCH Research Group. (1997). Matching alcoholism treatments to client heterogeneity: Project MATCH posttreatment drinking outcomes. *Journal of Studies on Alcohol, 58*(1), 7–29.

Regier, D. A., Narrow, W. E., & Rae, D. S. (1990). The epidemiology of anxiety disorders: The Epidemiologic Catchment Area (ECA) experience. *Journal of Psychiatric Research, 24*(Suppl. 2), 3–14.

Roman, P. M., & Blum, T. C. (1999). *National Treatment Center Study (Summary 3).* Athens, GA: University of Georgia.

Rychtarik, R. G., Connors, G. J., Dermen, K. H., & Stasiewicz, P. R. (2000). Alcoholics Anonymous and the use of medications to prevent relapse: An anonymous survey of member attitudes. *Journal of Studies on Alcohol and Drugs, 61*(1), 134–138.

Sisson, R. W., & Mallams, J. H. (1981). The use of systematic encouragement and community access procedures to increase attendance at Alcoholic Anonymous and Al-Anon meetings. *American Journal of Drug and Alcohol Abuse, 8*(3), 371–376.

Timko, C., & DeBenedetti, A. (2007). A randomized controlled trial of intensive referral to 12-step self-help groups: One-year outcomes. *Drug and Alcohol Dependence, 90*(2/3), 270–279.

Timko, C., Debenedetti, A., & Billow, R. (2006). Intensive referral to 12-step self-help groups and 6-month substance use disorder outcomes. *Addiction, 101*(5), 678–688.

Timko, C., Moos, R. H., Finney, J. W., & Lesar, M. D. (2000). Long-term outcomes of alcohol use disorders: Comparing untreated individuals with those in Alcoholics Anonymous and formal treatment. *Journal of Studies on Alcohol and Drugs, 61*(4), 529–540.

Timko, C., Sempel, J. M., & Moos, R. H. (2003). Models of standard and intensive outpatient care in substance abuse and psychiatric treatment. *Administration and Policy in Mental Health and Mental Health Services Research, 30*(5), 417–436.

Timko, C., Sutkowi, A., Cronkite, R. C., Makin-Byrd, K., & Moos, R. H. (2011). Intensive referral to 12-step dual-focused mutual-help groups. *Drug and Alcohol Dependence, 118*(2/3), 194–201.

Tomasson, K., & Vaglum, P. (1998). Psychiatric co-morbidity and aftercare among alcoholics: A prospective study of a nationwide representative sample. *Addiction, 93*(3), 423–431.

Tonigan, J. S., & Kelly, J. F. (2004). Beliefs about AA and the use of medications: A comparison of three groups of AA-exposed alcohol dependent persons. *Alcoholism Treatment Quarterly, 22*(2), 67–78.

Tonigan, J. S., Miller, W. R., & Connors, G. (2001). *Prior Alcoholics Anonymous involvement and treatment outcome.* Bethesda, MD: U.S. Department of Health and Human Services.

Tonigan, J. S., Toscova, R., & Miller, W. R. (1996). Meta-analysis of the literature on Alcoholics Anonymous: Sample and study characteristics moderate findings. *Journal of Studies on Alcohol and Drugs, 57*(1), 65–72.

Travis, T. (2009). *The language of the heart: A cultural history of the recovery movement.* Chapel Hill, NC: University of North Carolina.

Walitzer, K. S., Dermen, K. H., & Barrick, C. (2009). Facilitating involvement in Alcoholics Anonymous during out-patient treatment: A randomized clinical trial. *Addiction, 104*(3), 391–401.

White, W. L. (1998). *Slaying the dragon: The history of addiction treatment and recovery in America.* Bloomington, IL: Chestnut Health Systems.

White, W. L. (2008). *Recovery management and recovery-oriented systems of care: Scientific rationale and promising practices.* Pittsburg, PA: Northeast Addiction Technology Transfer Center, Chicago, IL: Great Lakes Addiction Technology Transfer Center, Philadelphia, PA: Philadelphia Department of Behavioral Health/Mental Retardation Services.

White, W. L. (2009). *Peer-based addiction recovery support: History, theory, practice, and scientific evaluation.* Chicago, IL: Great Lakes Addiction Technology Transfer Center and Philadelphia, PA: Philadelphia Department of Behavioral Health and Mental Retardation Services.

Winzelberg, A., & Humphreys, K. (1999). Should patients' religiosity influence clinicians' referral to 12-step self-help groups? Evidence from a study of 3,018 male substance abuse patients. *Journal of Consulting and Clinical Psychology, 67*(5), 790–794.

Yalom, I. D., & Leszcz, M. (2005). *The theory and practice of group psychotherapy* (5th ed.). New York, NY: Basic Books.

Part I: Mutual Support Groups Outside of Twelve Step Programs

SMART Recovery: Self-Empowering, Science-Based Addiction Recovery Support

A. TOM HORVATH
Practical Recovery, San Diego, California, USA; SMART Recovery, Mentor, Ohio, USA
JULIE YETERIAN
Department of Psychiatry, Massachusetts General Hospital, Boston, Massachusetts, USA

Self-Management and Recovery Training (SMART Recovery) is an international nonprofit organization that provides free, self-empowering, science-based mutual aid groups for abstaining from any substance or activity addiction. This article summarizes the development of the organization, the current status of face-to-face and online meetings, the characteristics of participants, the nature of the SMART Recovery approach to recovery (i.e., the intersection of what is self-empowering, evidence-based, and likely to be of use in a mutual aid group facilitated by a nonprofessional volunteer), the limited evidence of effectiveness currently available, and some of the prominent questions in need of investigation about SMART Recovery.

INTRODUCTION

Self-Management and Recovery Training (SMART Recovery) is an international nonprofit organization that offers free face-to-face and online mutual aid groups for individuals who are seeking to abstain, or who are considering abstinence, from one or more substance or activity addictions. Activity addictions, such as excessive gambling, spending, or video gaming, are also termed process or behavioral addictions. The SMART Recovery program of recovery is the intersection of what is self-empowering, evidence-based, and likely to be of use in a mutual aid group typically facilitated by a nonprofessional volunteer. Like the other "alternative" groups (Horvath, 2011), SMART Recovery offers a substantially different approach to recovery and a different meeting format than that of the 12-step spiritual fellowship, which is the dominant addiction mutual aid-group approach in the United States. These alternatives emerged out of frustration with the lack of diversity in addiction recovery support. Founded in 1994, SMART Recovery now appears likely to endure and to be of interest to individuals specifically seeking a science-based, self-empowering, and self-reliant approach to addiction recovery. This approach significantly differs from the powerlessness approach of the 12-step spiritual fellowships, or, except for Moderation Management, the generally less science-based approaches of the other alternatives. The SMART Recovery tools for recovery aim to increase the participant's capacity to maintain motivation, identify and cope with cravings, identify and modify irrational thinking and beliefs, and live with greater balance and attention to long-term goals in addition to short-term ones. Even at the beginning of the recovery process, these tools have face validity for individuals who prefer an active (vs. passive) coping style. The SMART Recovery slogan—"Discover the power of choice!"—appears to exemplify what these individuals are seeking from addiction recovery support.

ORIGINS AND HISTORICAL DEVELOPMENT

SMART Recovery was incorporated as a nonprofit U.S. organization in 1992. It began operating under the name SMART Recovery in 1994, before which it was named the Rational Recovery Self-Help Network and was affiliated with Rational Recovery Systems, Inc. (RRS), founded by Jack Trimpey in the 1980s. RRS originally contained a substantial component of rational emotive behavior therapy (REBT), developed by psychologist Albert Ellis. There continues to be no significant literature on REBT as an evidence-based addiction treatment. However, REBT was generally consistent with the emerging evidence base on cognitive-behavioral therapy (CBT) as an addiction treatment. Many professionals seeking to support or refer clients to a CBT-oriented addiction mutual aid group were drawn to RRS.

In February 1991, about 20 addiction professionals from around the United States gathered in Dallas, TX, at the invitation of Trimpey, to begin work on expanding the fledgling network of mutual aid groups Trimpey had created as he traveled around the United States promoting his work. The first author attended this meeting and has been continuously involved with SMART Recovery as a volunteer ever since.

This informal board met again in August 1992 in Sacramento and decided to pursue incorporation as a nonprofit. The nonprofit would promote the expansion of the mutual aid network, while Trimpey would operate his for-profit business. The nonprofit and the for-profit were to be mutually supportive. Incorporation was completed late in 1992. Galanter, Egelko, and Edwards (1993) conducted the first survey of RRS mutual aid participants in that year.

The next meeting, in Boston in 1993, established the nonprofit board of directors, with Joe Gerstein, M.D., as president. In 1994, the annual board meeting was held in San Diego, in conjunction with the annual meeting of the Association for Advancement of Behavior Therapy (now the Association for Behavioral and Cognitive Therapies). Increasing tension between Trimpey and the board culminated in the nonprofit changing its name and ending its affiliation with Trimpey.

This tension arose because the original intent of most board members was to establish a CBT-oriented group. Changes that Trimpey was making with RRS were taking that organization in other directions. The simplest resolution of the tension appeared to be for the organizations to end their affiliation. RRS continues to offer services and describes itself as "the exclusive, worldwide source of information, counseling, guidance, and direct instruction on independent recovery through planned, permanent abstinence, i.e., Addictive Voice Recognition Technique" (RRS, 2011).

Groups were informed of the change and offered the option of continuing their affiliation with the renamed nonprofit. For 2 months, the organization operated under the name Alcohol and Drug Abuse Self-Help Network, before choosing SMART Recovery as its operating name.

Without the leadership of Joe Gerstein from 1993 to 1995, SMART Recovery may not have survived. There was strong belief among board members and local affiliates that there was sufficient support for such an organization. SMART Recovery leaders were aware that Women for Sobriety and Secular Organizations for Sobriety already existed and were making progress despite the near monopoly of the 12-step spiritual fellowship. SMART Recovery garnered support because it was to be the first mutual aid group that explicitly looked to evidence-based addiction treatment for its approach, which would evolve as that evidence base evolved. However, even though conditions were promising, SMART Recovery might have dissipated without Gerstein's leadership, the multiple aspects of which are recorded by Allwood and White (2011). Gerstein's contributions have continued to the present time.

The board at that time consisted primarily of mental health professionals. Most localities had a professional advisor (later termed a volunteer advisor). The "peer professional partnership" model, although in operation from the beginning, would not be fully articulated until about 2008. For the first decade, as a solid base of recovering and longstanding volunteers emerged, SMART Recovery was governed primarily by professionals.

After its separation from RRS, SMART Recovery set about reestablishing itself. A central office was created in Beachwood (near Cleveland), OH, to coincide with the locations of the initial staff. Later, the office moved to Mentor, OH, also near Cleveland. Ultimately, Shari Allwood was appointed full-time executive director in 2005. Her history with SMART Recovery began in 1994. Without her administrative and interpersonal skills, the organization would likely not have prospered as it has.

The first decade of SMART Recovery included the following significant developments:

- 1994: A quarterly newsletter (*SMART Recovery News and Views*) began. A version of SMART Recovery was offered in the Danbury, CT, federal women's prison.
- 1995: The foundational document of SMART Recovery (*SMART Recovery Purposes and Methods*) was ratified. The first Web site (later moved to http://www.smartrecovery.org) was established.
- 1996: A training grant was received from the Robert Wood Johnson Foundation, leading to the annual conference, Internet listservs for internal communication, and a recommended reading list.
- 1997: SMART Recovery entered the Arizona state prison system.
- 1998: Online meetings, an online message board, and an international advisory council were established. Joe and Barbara Gerstein gave the first of many international presentations, in the United Kingdom.
- 1999: SMART Recovery was established in Australia (by Alex Wodak and Bronwyn Crosby). The SMART Recovery Tools for recovery were written. The National Institute on Drug Abuse (NIDA) mentioned SMART Recovery in the Principles of Drug Addiction Treatment (then inexplicably deleted this reference in the revised 2009 edition). A Small Business Innovative Research (SBIR) grant from the National Institutes of Health for creation of the SMART Recovery correctional (prison) program, InsideOut, was made to Inflexxion. The Board of Directors began seeking nominations for membership from meeting participants and volunteers.
- 2000: At the beginning of the year, RRS announced that it no longer sponsored mutual aid groups, ending any competition between the organizations. Monthly training by conference call for volunteers began. The practice, which had occurred since the organization's inception, that there is no requirement that a facilitator be in recovery, was expanded to include active outreach for nonrecovering facilitators. SMART Recovery was introduced into the Scottish prison system. By the end of the year, SMART Recovery had more than 300 meetings.
- 2001: Online facilitators and face-to-face facilitators held their first joint meeting.
- 2002: Bimonthly online trainings began.
- 2003: A half million dollar anonymous unrestricted donation was received. The board decided to spend this money as seed money rather than reserve it as endowment (a decision that might have bankrupted the organization, but was validated by later growth). Translations of basic SMART Recovery materials were completed in Spanish, Portuguese, and Russian. The

Substance Abuse and Mental Health Services Administration awarded a training grant, which funded a conference and the development of several training videos.

- 2004: The SMART Recovery Handbook was published to replace the Member's Manual. The Australian organization received a grant for $250,000 for basic operations. Linda Sobell conducted a motivational interviewing workshop as part of the 10th anniversary celebration at the annual conference in Phoenix. The board held its first strategic planning meeting and established the following five goals: marketing, facilitator development and support, enhancing the Internet presence, fundraising, and the development of SMART Recovery Therapy (the last goal was dropped several years later).

In SMART Recovery's second decade, most of the established directions of the organization continued. There have been additional licensing agreements with organizations in other countries and increasing emphasis on international operations, translation of the handbook into eight languages, publication of additional written works and videos, presentations to outside groups and other marketing efforts, the award to Reid Hester of a second SMART Recovery-related SBIR grant for the development of a SMART Recovery Web course, the establishment of an annual participant survey, and the offering of advertising opportunities (taken up thus far only by treatment centers) to generate additional revenue. The Web site (http://www.smartrecovery.org) and its activities continued as a central focus of the organization. The first non-English online meeting (in Mandarin Chinese) occurred in Spring 2012.

The organization also established policy positions with respect to medications (that appropriate use of prescribed medications was acceptable) and the disease concept (that participants could believe whatever they believed about addiction as a disease, because that concept was irrelevant to the SMART Recovery approach to recovery). The disease concept position reflected an update from an original position that addiction was a complex maladaptive behavior rather than a disease. The new position paralleled the position taken from the beginning about belief in a higher power, that such a belief or lack of it was a personal matter for each participant and not relevant to SMART Recovery participation.

At present, funding comes from three primary sources: publication sales, advertising, and donations (individual donors and pass-the-hat contributions at meetings). The organization is operationally frugal, with fewer than three full-time-equivalent administrative staff in the United States and some additional contract workers for the Web site. As a further example of frugality, members of the board pay for their own travel expenses for annual meetings and are expected to donate themselves or help the organization raise funds.

The context in which SMART Recovery emerged was one of increasing frustration with the lack of diversity in addiction recovery. As CBT and other non-12-step approaches to treatment and recovery were emerging in the scientific literature, evidence-based practitioners observed that the treatment industry was adopting these developments very slowly or not at all. With the establishment of the National Institute on Alcohol Abuse and Alcoholism and the NIDA in the 1970s, there has been substantial funding for both research and training in addiction treatment.

In addition to professional frustration in the United States with the lack of alternatives to 12-step recovery, atheists and agnostics and their organizations object to the higher-power belief proposed by the 12 steps. Advocates of the separation of church and state, as required by the First Amendment of the US Constitution, have objected to the government, typically via a judge or probation officer, ordering individuals to attend 12-step groups, which can be viewed as having a religious aspect. A full discussion of the religious aspect of the 12-step spiritual fellowship goes beyond the scope of this article. However, a significant factor in the growth of non-12-step mutual aid groups has been the set of judicial decisions that prohibit the government from ordering individuals to attend 12-step groups because of their religious aspect. Although 12-step groups are often viewed as "spiritual but not religious," between 1996 and 2007, five U.S. federal circuit courts of appeal have rejected that distinction. It remains the government's option to order someone to attend a mutual aid group or treatment, provided that a nonreligious option is available. The SMART Recovery Web site maintains an updated list of relevant court decisions (SMART Recovery, 2011).

For SMART Recovery long-term volunteers (some affiliated for more than 20 years), perhaps the most noteworthy frustration has been the slow growth of the organization given the large need for it. Long-term volunteers appear to maintain their motivation by savoring the immediate feedback from newcomers, who describe how happy they are to find an alternative to the 12-step spiritual fellowship, and from ongoing participants, who often credit their recovery to involvement with SMART Recovery. Volunteers also hope that a "tipping point" is approaching, after which SMART Recovery and other non-12-step groups will be widely viewed as being of equal value to 12-step groups and will be equally available.

MEMBERSHIP

As of May 2012, SMART Recovery had more than 690 groups throughout the world, including multiple daily online meetings (S. Allwood, personal communication, May 31, 2012). Most face-to-face meetings occur in the United States, where they are available in most states. Significant meeting concentrations also exist in Australia and the United Kingdom. The SMART Recovery

Web site maintains a current listing of all meetings. Online meetings provide either voice or text communication. Although many addiction professionals have been generally frustrated by the lack of diversity in addiction recovery, many SMART Recovery participants seek out the organization because of quite specific frustrations. They seek a recovery approach that does not, for instance, involve a higher power, or powerlessness, or the labels "addict" or "alcoholic," or belief in addiction as disease, or lifetime attendance (Horvath & Sokoloff, 2011).

Data on SMART Recovery's membership are available, as are data on its precursor, RRS. The earliest of these studies is a national survey of 433 RRS attendees (Galanter et al., 1993), which found that respondents were mostly college-educated males in their 40s who were seeking help for an alcohol problem. A much smaller study of SMART Recovery found a very similar member profile (67% male; $M_{age} = 46$; 82% had a college or graduate degree; Li, Feifer, & Strohm, 2000). The 2010 SMART Recovery participant survey ($N = 444$) also found that two thirds of participants were male. This survey found that while more than half of respondents were relatively new to SMART Recovery (i.e., had been attending for less than 6 months), most respondents were regular attendees at meetings, with 68% of the total sample attending at least one face-to-face meeting per week. A survey of 154 SMART Recovery Online users revealed that 58% of respondents were women, 95% were White, and 69% were between the ages of 40 and 59 (von Breton, 2009). A UK study found that among the 65 people who attended the SMART Recovery groups created by the Alcohol Concern Project, 32% were women, the average age was 47, and 77% were seeking help for an alcohol problem (with an additional 11% seeking help for alcohol and drugs and 9% for drugs only). One quarter of attendees had at least 1 year of abstinence at the time they were surveyed.

THEORETICAL BASIS OF SMART RECOVERY

It might be stated that SMART Recovery does not have a theoretical basis. SMART Recovery teaches tools for recovery that are based on what has been shown to be efficacious in the addiction treatment literature and on what is otherwise known about addiction recovery. These tools could be drawn from any evidence-based approach, or any other finding about recovery, provided that two additional criteria are met: (1) Is the tool self-empowering? And (2) would the tool be suitable in a mutual aid group facilitated by a nonprofessional volunteer? Even though these three elements (evidence, self-empowerment, suitability in a mutual aid group) were not fully articulated until SMART Recovery's second decade, they have provided an ongoing and largely unchanged foundation for the organization's approach to recovery. On that foundation, the specific tools for recovery taught in a SMART

Recovery meeting will evolve as the scientific evidence about addiction and recovery evolves.

There is preliminary evidence that internal locus of control is predictive of participation in SMART Recovery (Li et al., 2000). When such individuals look to their futures, they perceive addictive behavior as an issue they can manage by learning new ideas and techniques and practicing them sufficiently until the goal is accomplished. In contrast, the external locus-of-control individual looks to the future and believes that life will be largely shaped by what happens to the individual, with the individual having much less capacity to change outcomes. These individuals appear to be more suitable for the 12-step approach, which is oriented around powerlessness and acceptance.

A description of this difference between internal and external locus of control can be based on the Serenity Prayer, by Reinhold Niebhur. This prayer is widely used in 12-step groups: "God, grant me serenity to accept the things I cannot change, courage to change the things I can, and wisdom to know the difference." If this prayer were used in SMART Recovery, it might be transformed into the Courage Intention: "I intend to have courage to change the things I can, serenity to accept the things I cannot, and wisdom to know the difference."

Recovery as well as life appears to require a mixture of both serenity (acceptance) and courage (effort). Internal locus-of-control individuals favor active and courageous solutions, whereas external locus-of-control individuals favor acceptance. These individuals may view themselves, at least with respect to addiction, as powerless.

For example, an acceptance approach to coping with craving might emphasize the inevitability of cravings, the impossibility of coping directly with them, and the need for reliance on outside support to get past them safely. An active and courageous approach might emphasize: (1) exposure and response prevention for eliminating over time or at least greatly reducing the intensity, frequency, and duration of cravings; (2) memory practice for recalling fundamental aspects of craving (craving is time-limited, does not harm one, and cannot force one to use) to outlast each craving; and (3) relapse prevention or recovery maintenance techniques for managing the environment to reduce the occurrence of cravings and to reduce the risk in high-risk situations.

SMART Recovery emphasizes this courageous and active approach to recovery, while recognizing that some courage and activity are likely necessary in any approach to recovery, and that acceptance of powerlessness over some aspects of life, such as aging and death, is necessary if one is to remain in contact with reality.

The SMART Recovery approach is therefore based on ideas, tools, and techniques arising from the addiction treatment and recovery literature that empower the individual to gain control over the antecedents of addictive behavior. At present, evidence-based treatment approaches can be broadly divided into the following categories: CBT (including relapse prevention), motivational interviewing, behavioral couples, contingency management, addiction medication (e.g., methadone, buprenorphine, disulfiram), chemical counter-conditioning, and 12-step facilitation (Manuel, Hagedorn, & Finney, 2011). SMART Recovery tools draw inspiration primarily from CBT and motivational interviewing.

In addition to being self-empowering, the SMART Recovery approach needs to be workable in the mutual aid group environment, as facilitated by a nonprofessional volunteer. Therefore, many elements of the evidence-based addiction treatments just mentioned would not be applicable in SMART Recovery, even though they are self-empowering (e.g., couples sessions, the application of contingency management, medication management, and counter-conditioning procedures).

A last source of inspiration for the SMART Recovery approach is the accumulated wisdom about what might work in any mutual aid group. Meetings are structured enough to provide a sense of order. There are multiple opportunities for individuals to participate, but no requirement to do so. Social learning is facilitated by an emphasis on discussion rather than on monologue. In the 12-step spiritual fellowship, social learning is also facilitated by discussions with a sponsor, but there are no sponsors in SMART Recovery. Discussions are kept focused on the SMART Recovery approach as it might apply to the participants by a facilitator who is trained to be clearly in charge of the meeting. At least one SMART Recovery tool, brainstorming, arises from the need to maintain a cohesive group experience rather than from the addiction treatment literature.

REBT, developed by Albert Ellis, has also been a substantial influence on SMART Recovery, even though REBT itself is not an evidence-based treatment for addiction. However, REBT can be considered the pioneering form of CBT, which has clear empirical support. REBT includes a self-empowering philosophy of living and offers a wide range of literature that may be useful to participants. The ABC, a basic REBT technique (Activating event, underlying Belief, emotional or behavior Consequence), is one way to implement the core idea of CBT: It is not events but our interpretations of events that gives rise to our deliberate behavior. As Shakespeare has Hamlet state, "There is nothing either good or bad but thinking makes it so" (Act II, Scene 2).

SMART Recovery will continue to evolve as the scientific findings about addiction treatment and recovery evolve. It is conceivable that the SMART Recovery 4-Point Program might also evolve. For the present, these 4 points appear to provide an adequate framework for organizing the SMART Recovery approach, which supports participants in: (1) building and maintaining motivation, (2) coping with urges, (3) managing thoughts, feelings, and behaviors, and (4) living a balanced life. At present, these 4 points are implemented using a primary set of recovery tools, as shown in Table 1. The

TABLE 1 SMART Recovery Tools

Stages of Change: How ready am I to change?
Change Plan Worksheet: What do I want to change? Why? How much? How will I do it? What might get in the way?
Cost–Benefit Analysis: What are the costs and benefits of addiction, and of recovery? What conclusions do I draw after listing and comparing them?
ABC of REBT for Urge Coping: When I have a craving, what irrational beliefs do I typically have (e.g., craving makes me use, I can't stand having a craving so I need to use)?
ABC of REBT for Emotional Upsets: What irrational beliefs do I have about myself, others, or life and the world in general? Can I perceive how these beliefs lead to unnecessary emotional upset?
Destructive Imagery and Self-Talk Awareness and Refusal Method): I can expose the faulty thinking and misleading images that give rise to my cravings and vigorously counter-attack with an assertion of thoughts and images consistent with my long-term interests.
Brainstorming: In a meeting, all participants freely express any idea about a particular issue. Only after ideas are collected does discussion and evaluation of the ideas begin.
Role-Playing and Rehearsing: In a meeting, an expected difficult encounter is re-created for a participant to allow for practicing a constructive response.
Hierarchy of Values: What do I say is most important to me? Based on how I behave, what in fact appears to be most important to me? How different is what I say and what I do? What do I want to do about any discrepancies?

SMART Recovery Web site includes detailed descriptions about how to use each of these tools, as well as worksheets, exercises, coping statements, and information on additional tools. The tools will look familiar to professionals knowledgeable about CBT and motivational enhancement addiction treatment techniques. The tools will also appear to be "common sense" and thus have face validity to many participants unfamiliar with addiction treatment or the recovery literature.

The 4 points are not steps to be accomplished in a specific order, but tasks common to most individuals intending to maintain recovery. At different times in the course of recovery, different points may be more salient for specific individuals. Points 3 and 4 are ongoing challenges for all human beings. The tools are not a curriculum for recovery. They are presented as options for helping participants accomplish the 4 points. Most participants are likely to use only a few tools on a regular basis. The ABC and the CBA are the most commonly used tools.

A SMART Recovery meeting has the following sections: Welcome, Check-In, Agenda Setting, Discussion, Pass the Hat/Pass the Brochure and Announcements, Check-Out and Closing. The Welcome typically mentions that there is no charge for the meeting but donations are requested, that no one is required to participate, that the discussion should flow freely and interactively without monologues, that maintaining confidentiality after the meeting is expected, and that if anyone does not like how the meeting is unfolding, concern should be stated. In the around-the-room Check-In, participants may mention anything relevant to their recovery, except that criticism of other recovery approaches is discouraged. The Check-In gives the facilitator a general sense of what might make for a good discussion with this particular group of participants. Which tool or tools to apply is at the discretion of the facilitator, although groups with experienced participants may collaborate with the facilitator during Agenda Setting to decide how Discussion time will be used. A participant may request Discussion time to address a personal concern. The facilitator may warm up a Discussion by beginning with a group exercise. During Pass the Hat, Announcements may include a reminder to inform others about SMART Recovery and an invitation to participate in scientific studies that SMART Recovery is supporting. The Check-Out is often the most interesting part of the meeting, as participants reveal what was most meaningful to them about what occurred. The management of the meeting process requires a confident and trained facilitator.

Because of SMART Recovery's commitment to evolving as scientific findings evolve, the ongoing involvement of professionals (both clinicians and researchers) is essential. At present, about half of the board of directors is professionals, and the other half are participants. Some directors are in both categories. The majority of the organization's approximately 700 volunteers began as participants, but a significant number are volunteer advisors (professionals) who support other volunteers in their localities and in some cases facilitate meetings. The International Advisory Council is listed in Table 2.

EVIDENCE FOR EFFECTIVENESS

Although the SMART Recovery program is based largely on evidence-based CBT techniques and secondarily on motivational enhancement techniques, there has been little research on the effectiveness of SMART Recovery itself. Little is known from an empirical perspective about the potential benefits of attending SMART Recovery meetings or the mechanisms through which involvement in the organization may exert its beneficial effects. Of the existing research, two cross-sectional, survey-based studies have examined characteristics of SMART Recovery members (e.g., religiosity, locus of control) relative to members of other mutual-help organizations, such as Alcoholics Anonymous (AA; Atkins & Hawdon, 2007; Li et al., 2000). One of these studies (Atkins & Hawdon) found a positive relationship between the extent of participation in mutual-help groups, including SMART Recovery, and the duration of continuous abstinence. This relationship did not differ according to the type of mutual-help group in which respondents participated, suggesting that participating in SMART Recovery may be just as helpful as participating in other mutual aid groups.

Another study compared 12-step-based and SMART-based intensive outpatient treatment programs for dually diagnosed patients (Brooks & Penn, 2003). This study found that the SMART Recovery-based treatment was less

TABLE 2 SMART Recovery International Advisory Council

Aaron Beck, M.D. Department of Psychiatry, University of Pennsylvania
Carlo DiClemente, Ph.D. Department of Psychology, University of Maryland at Baltimore
Albert Ellis, Ph.D. (1913–2007) The Albert Ellis Institute
Frederick Glaser, M.D. Greenville, NC
Nick Heather, Ph.D. University of Northumbria at Newcastle Center for Alcohol & Drug Studies
Reid Hester, Ph.D. Behavior Therapy Associates
Harald Klingemann, Ph.D. Institute for Social Planning and Social Management, University of Applied Sciences Berne
Richard Longabaugh, Ed.D. Center for Alcohol and Addiction Studies, Brown University
Alan Marlatt, Ph.D. (1942–2011) Addictive Behaviors Research Center, University of Washington
Barbara McCrady, Ph.D. Center on Alcoholism, Substance Abuse, and Addictions, University of New Mexico
Maxie C. Maultsby, Jr., M.D. Department of Psychiatry, College of Medicine Howard University
Peter Monti, Ph.D. Center for Alcohol and Addiction Studies, Brown University
Stanton Peele, Ph.D. Fellow, The Lindesmith Center
Linda Sobell, Ph.D., ABPP Nova Southeastern University Center for Psychological Studies
Mark Sobell, Ph.D., ABPP Nova Southeastern University Center for Psychological Studies
William L. White, MA Chestnut Health System

effective at reducing alcohol use compared with the 12-step-based treatment, but it was more effective at improving participants' employment status and medical concerns. However, this study also suffered from several methodological problems that limited its internal validity (e.g., high dropout rate, unequal levels of treatment exposure across conditions) and external validity (e.g., intensive outpatient (IOP) treatment context that is not comparable to the context in which SMART Recovery groups typically occur, use of a sample of dually diagnosed individuals who may not be representative of most SMART Recovery members).

A qualitative study conducted in the United Kingdom provides information about the perceived helpfulness of SMART Recovery groups from the perspectives of members (MacGregor & Herring, 2010). This study found that the vast majority of the SMART Recovery attendees who were surveyed found the groups to be very helpful and intended to continue attending within the next 3 months. Most had previously attended other mutual aid groups and reported that SMART Recovery was more useful than these other groups. Some of the benefits mentioned by participants were the emphasis on moving forward, the nonhierarchical nature of groups, and the shared experiences of group members.

RESEARCH OPPORTUNITIES

Because little research on SMART Recovery has been conducted to date, there are numerous research opportunities remaining. One of the most pressing practical issues is how to match participants to groups. For instance, it appears that having an internal locus of control is a predictor of interest in SMART Recovery, but the question has not been asked in a controlled fashion. There is also a small contingent of "atheist" AA meetings, which raises the question of whether participants in these meetings would fare better in SMART Recovery.

Given the comparable degree of success produced by widely divergent approaches to addiction treatment, the question about the effectiveness of a particular mutual aid group seems less important than the matching question. Presumably, all mutual aid groups will be found to be helpful in general, but there may be differences in effectiveness that depend on the goodness of fit between the group and the individual. Knowing more about who is more likely to benefit from SMART Recovery as compared with other mutual aid groups, for example, could save participants time and effort in the search for a suitable group. Given that searching for a suitable group may exhaust a limited supply of motivation, this question appears more pressing than the effectiveness question alone.

A set of questions that may be unique to SMART Recovery concerns facilitators. Numerous anecdotal reports suggest that the facilitator having an authoritative style (vs. laissez-faire or authoritarian style) is generally more important to the success of a SMART Recovery meeting than if the facilitator has knowledge of the SMART Recovery program itself. Unless the meeting is new, participants generally have sufficient knowledge about the program so that the facilitator's knowledge is not essential to the success of the meeting. However, a poorly managed meeting is a poor meeting regardless of the facilitator's program knowledge.

The laissez-faire ("anything goes") leader is unlikely to create a discussion environment in which participants feel safe enough to reveal themselves in any depth. The depth of self-disclosure, in any mutual aid group, is a predictor of the value of the discussion to participants. Typical problems in an "anything goes" meeting include lengthy monologues rather than discussion, arguments, and off-topic discussions. The authoritarian facilitator squelches self-expression with an overemphasis on rules. Although the meeting may appear well organized, the heart of the activity, which is the sharing of personal experiences and perspectives, is lost. The authoritative facilitator balances enforcing a few rules with support for self-disclosure. Related research questions include: How easily can this authoritative style be taught? How can facilitators be selected to minimize training needs?

There are also questions about how to gain greater acceptance for SMART Recovery and other alternative approaches in the United States, where 12-step approaches dominate addiction recovery. Will change need to occur "retirement by retirement" or can overzealous 12-step supporters be persuaded to consider the diversity of recovery rather than insist that all individuals in recovery attend 12-step meetings? How might this persuasion occur? These questions may be as much political as they are scientific.

How should SMART Recovery respond to the numerous individuals who report having negative experiences or even feeling traumatized by their 12-step experiences (often when confronted about wanting an alternative approach)? SMART Recovery has elected to keep its meetings focused on addiction recovery and not focus on trauma experienced in other mutual aid groups. Should these issues be dealt with as part of SMART Recovery, in a separate mutual aid group established for that purpose, or in professional treatment?

Currently, many SMART Recovery participants also attend 12-step meetings. Many report that they attend "SMART Recovery for the tools and 12-step for the fellowship." Will this dual attendance diminish as more SMART Recovery meetings become available? How do dual participants benefit from both approaches?

What remains unknown is whether 12-step groups attract individuals who would have recovered even without a 12-step group, or would have recovered attending other types of groups, or would have recovered by being involved in some aspect of 12-step recovery that may be distant from the basic elements of the 12-step program. For instance, for some participants, the effectiveness of 12-step recovery might arise primarily from being somewhat public about making a commitment to change, or from having a regular activity to attend, or from having a new social network. Another approach to recovery that involved public commitment, regular activity, or a new social network might work as well.

It may be difficult to persuade investigators and funders to study alternative mutual aid groups when their availability is so limited, and 12-step groups are nearly ubiquitous. Nevertheless, a small body of literature on alternatives has emerged, and additional studies are in progress. Of central interest might be the question of efficacy. However, alternatives probably cannot overcome an issue already noted for the conduct of research on

12-step groups: "These studies are necessarily correlational, evaluating the extent to which these two factors—attendance and outcome—covary, without establishing whether one causes the other" (Miller, Forcehimes, & Zweben, 2011, p. 228).

However, efficacy (in controlled scientific trials) may be too high a standard for any mutual aid group, especially given the difficulty of studying them in a controlled fashion. A group could be considered effective (in the real world) if participants elect to attend. By this standard, 12-step groups have been very effective, because so many individual have attended them. However, given that most individuals who are referred to AA do not attend, and most who attend drop out quickly (National Academy of Sciences, 1990), 12-step groups alone are ineffective relative to the size of the population that needs recovery. Although it appears unlikely that any other single mutual aid group would fare better, it is highly plausible that a more diverse array of recovery mutual aid groups would attract a larger portion of the population that needs recovery. Therefore, there would appear to be incentive for studying emerging mutual aid groups and for whom they are a good match, even if for the moment they are not widely available.

FUTURE DIRECTIONS

Future directions for the SMART Recovery program will largely be based on new scientific evidence about what approaches or techniques are effective for helping individuals overcome addiction. Future directions for the organization are largely centered on how to achieve a sufficient size (perhaps 5,000 meetings in the United States) so that participants are not significantly inconvenienced, relative to 12-step meetings, to attend SMART Recovery. To achieve this size, the organization will need to continue to improve its capacity to recruit, train, support, and oversee volunteer nonprofessional facilitators, who are the backbone of the organization.

REFERENCES

Allwood, S., & White, W. (2011). *A chronology of SMART Recovery*. Retrieved from http://www.williamwhitepapers.com/pr/2001%20A%20Chronololgy%20of%20SMART%20Recovery.pdf

Atkins, R. G., & Hawdon, J. E. (2007). Religiosity and participation in mutual-aid support groups for addiction. *Journal of Substance Abuse Treatment*, *33*, 321–331.

Brooks, A. J., & Penn, P. E. (2003). Comparing treatments for dual diagnosis: Twelve-step and self-management and recovery training. *American Journal of Drug and Alcohol Abuse*, *29*(2), 359–383.

Galanter, M., Egelko, S., & Edwards, H. (1993). Rational recovery: Alternative to AA for addiction? *American Journal of Drug and Alcohol Abuse*, *19*(4), 499–510.

Horvath, A. T. (2011). Alternative support groups. In P. Ruiz & E. C. Strain (Eds.), *Substance abuse: A comprehensive text (5th ed.*, pp. 533–542). Philadelphia, PA: Wolters Kluwer.

Horvath, A. T., & Sokoloff, J. (2011). Individuals seeking non-12-step recovery. In G. W. Lawson & A. W. Lawson (Eds.), *Alcoholism and substance abuse in diverse populations* (2nd ed., pp. 75–90). Austin, TX: Pro-ed.

Li, E. C., Feifer, C., & Strohm, M. (2000). A pilot study: Locus of control and spiritual beliefs in Alcoholics Anonymous and SMART Recovery members. *Addictive Behaviors, 25*(4), 633–640.

MacGregor, S., & Herring, R. (2010). *The alcohol concern SMART Recovery pilot project final evaluation report.* London, UK: Middlesex University Drug and Alcohol Research Group.

Manuel, J. K., Hagedorn, H. J., & Finney, J. W. (2011). Implementing evidence-based psychosocial treatment in specialty substance use disorder care. *Psychology of Addictive Behaviors, 25*(2), 225–237.

Miller, W., Forcehimes, A., & Zweben, A. (2011). *Treating addiction: A guide for professionals.* New York, NY: Guilford.

National Academy of Sciences. (1990). *Broadening the base of treatment for alcohol problems.* Washington, DC: Author.

Rational Recovery. (2011). *Mission statement.* Retrieved from http://rational.org/index.php?id=94

SMART Recovery. (2011). *Court cases and mandated 12-step attendance.* Retrieved from http://www.smartrecovery.org/courts/court-mandated-attendance.htm

von Breton, J. (2009). SMART Recovery online news. *SMART Recovery News and Views, 15*(2), 5–6.

Empowering Your Sober Self: The LifeRing Approach to Addiction Recovery

MARTIN NICOLAUS
LifeRing Secular Recovery, Berkeley, California, USA

Addicted persons are torn between the urge to consume addictive substances and the drive to break with the substances and get free of them. The LifeRing approach anchors itself in the addicted person's drive to get free of the substances and works to empower that urge and to enthrone it permanently in the addicted person's character. Positive peer support focusing on small decisions made in everyday life is the primary psychodynamic engine for recovery in the LifeRing context. Working through nine principal domains, each participant constructs a personal recovery program founded on complete abstinence from all drugs of addiction.

ORIGINS AND HISTORICAL DEVELOPMENT

Mutual support groups in the field of addiction recovery have a long history and have come in many flavors. William White's monumental *Slaying the Dragon* (1998) describes a broad panorama of styles and philosophies and suggests that the existence of a diversity of approaches is a positive attribute, given the diversity of personalities, cultures, experiences, and needs among the addicted. One of the new mutual aid groups that have sprung up in this century, adding to the available diversity of approaches, is LifeRing Secular Recovery (LifeRing).

LifeRing held its foundational congress as a national organization in April 2001. Meeting at a retreat center in Florida, two dozen delegates from 15 U.S. states adopted a set of bylaws (LifeRing, 2001) that established a member-run, financially independent, abstinence-based network of peer-led mutual support groups under the name LifeRing Secular Recovery. A number of the organizers had previously participated in Secular Organizations for

Sobriety; some had spent time in 12-step groups. As a broad generalization, the founding members believed that the traditional paradigm was valid in its emphasis on abstinence, its use of peer-based social support, and in many of its organizational/structural features, but that its therapeutic protocol (the 12 steps) was unacceptable due to its reliance on a "higher power" and its emotional negativity, particularly the emphasis on "powerlessness" and all that goes along with it. Members also felt that a recovery organization should encompass all addictive substances instead of segregating people into different groups by "drug of choice."

Early LifeRing group meetings sometimes were little more than sounding boards for members who felt unserved, and in some cases "traumatized," by their 12-step exposure. But within a short time, the group evolved a therapeutically positive meeting format and developed a workbook, *Recovery by Choice* (Nicolaus, 2011),[1] that provides a structured pathway for individuals to build personal recovery programs (PRPs).

LifeRing's leadership at all levels is nonprofessional, as is also the case with the 12-step groups. Meeting facilitators, termed convenors, are "ordinary" persons in recovery and relate to other meeting participants as peers. A convenor's handbook (Nicolaus, 2003) focuses on basic philosophy and on connectivity skills. Treatment professionals occasionally serve as initial convenors to get meetings started, and in a few instances, where client turnover is rapid, they have served as convenors for a longer term. Despite, or perhaps because of its peer-leadership basis, LifeRing's growth owes much to leading addiction treatment professionals who have seen in the organization a useful service for the ever-present portion of their clients who seek an alternative to the 12-step paradigm. The majority of LifeRing meetings convene on the premises of treatment centers, and referrals from treatment professionals formed the leading source of LifeRing membership in the 2005 survey (LifeRing, 2005). A growing number of treatment professionals have opened the door to LifeRing groups because LifeRing groups are abstinence-based and have coexisted peacefully with 12-step groups in the same treatment settings for more than a decade.[2] LifeRing is also an obvious choice in settings involving state coercion over the client; federal court decisions have made it clear that forced referral to 12-step programs violates the Establishment Clause of the Constitution and that secular options must be offered (Nicolaus, 2009a).

MEMBERSHIP

The most recent membership sample survey ($n = 401$) conducted in 2005 yielded the following highlights (LifeRing, 2005):

- The typical member had been clean and sober for an average of 2.74 years.

- Men (58%) outnumbered women. The average age was 47.8 years.
- More than 80% of participants had attended some college, and 44% had an undergraduate degree or higher. Slightly more than half (54%) held professional, technical, or managerial occupations. About 80% were White.
- More than three out of four were raised in a religion. In the past year, nearly 40% (39%) had attended a religious service.
- Participants' "drugs of choice" covered the spectrum, with alcohol, tobacco, marijuana, cocaine powder, prescription drugs, meth derivatives, club drugs, crack cocaine, and heroin each reported by at least 10% of the respondents.
- Nearly half (47%) had participated in some type of professional substance abuse treatment within the past year. Almost that many (45%) had received a diagnosis for a co-occurring mental health disorder, with depression (33%) being the leading item.
- Participants were enthusiastic about LifeRing, with 98% saying they would recommend it to their friends. The parts of the LifeRing experience that gave them the most satisfaction were the absence of religious content and the positive, empowering atmosphere (56%), the encouragement to build a PRP (53%), the encouragement of crosstalk (52%), and the small group setting (51%).
- Close to half used only LifeRing for mutual support; more than one third currently also participated in 12-step groups.
- Asked what improvements they would like to see in LifeRing, participants' leading response by far was "more meetings!"

Initially, the group counted barely a dozen meetings, with most of these in the San Francisco Bay area. Currently (end of 2011), the organization shows more than 140 face-to-face meetings in the United States, Canada, Ireland, and Sweden and continues to grow steadily.

LifeRing has an extensive Internet presence centered on the www.lifering.org Web site. The LifeRing online social network has more than 1,000 members, and there are numerous online meetings in chat rooms. There are also e-mail lists, online forums, and linked LifeRing Web sites, such as www.liferingcanada.org and www.liferingcork.com (Ireland). LifeRing encourages participants to maintain connections outside the meeting hours. Participants exchange phone numbers and e-mail addresses, and social occasions are organized wherever feasible.

LifeRing continues to be financed entirely by member contributions and literature sales. All directors, officers, and meeting convenors are volunteers.

THEORETICAL BASIS

The almost-universal psychological experience of addicted persons is a Jekyll-and-Hyde struggle between the urge to consume the drug heedless of consequences and the drive to get free of the drug and lead a normal life. In the words of William L. White:

> Addicts simultaneously want—more than anything—both to maintain an uninterrupted relationship with their drug of choice and to break free of the drug. Behaviorally, this paradox is evidenced both in the incredible lengths to which the addict will go to sustain a relationship with the drug and in his or her repeated efforts to exert control over the drug and sever his or her relationship with it. (White, 1998 p. 335)

Numerous other students of addiction (cited in Nicolaus, 2009b) have remarked on this fierce tug of war lying at the core of the addiction experience. The addicted person is a person in conflict between two antagonistic drives. It is useful to conceptualize these drives as if they stemmed from two parts of a divided self, or in effect, from two antagonistic selves within the same personality: an Addict Self ("A") and a Sober Self ("S"). To be sure, the picture in any given individual displays numerous complexities and subtleties, many of which are mapped in the 300 pages of the *Recovery by Choice* workbook (Nicolaus, 2011), but the general dichotomy between the "A" and the "S" serves as a useful and easily grasped analytical tool that has numerous reference points in both individual and collective experience.

The LifeRing approach to the addicted person centers strategically on empowerment of the Sober Self. In contradistinction to the 12-step paradigm, LifeRing posits that the psychological map of the addicted person contains not only areas of illness, decay, degeneration, and morbidity in various forms, but also resources of health, vigor, strength, and vitality. The general aim of helping such a person is to facilitate the growth and expansion of these positive assets within the person and to enable their ascension to a stable dominance within the personality structure and behavior. In the loftier idiom of the Rev. Adler Temple, speaking in 1886, the aim of the group toward the addicted is, "by its living spirit of love and fraternity, [to] unlock the wards of their heart and reach the elements of humanness which lay buried there and rehabilitate and re-enthrone them" (quoted in White, 1998, p. 15).

LifeRing's philosophical and therapeutic foundation is abstinence from alcohol and all other medically uncalled-for addictive substances. The organization's hardcore insistence on abstinence is based in part on the personal experience of many members who experimented with moderation and found it a failure. It is based in another part on observation of other groups where moderation led to personal and organizational disaster. This experience suggests that far from enhancing a group's popularity, an effort to bring moderators and abstainers under the same umbrella drives both sides away. Even among recovering persons who reject the 12-step paradigm, abstinence is overwhelmingly the popular choice (Fletcher 2002; Granfield & Cloud, 1999). To be sure, individuals who are undecided on the issue and wish to see whether LifeRing groups are a fit for them are welcome to visit and talk out their concerns, but those who opt for moderation as their recovery goal are firmly invited to seek support elsewhere.

While committed to a comprehensive abstinence, LifeRing maintains a positive attitude toward physician-prescribed pharmaceuticals that address co-occurring disorders. If a participant has been honest with the physician and the physician is knowledgeable in addiction medicine, then the prescription is considered a sobriety tool, and participants are encouraged to take it as prescribed (Nicolaus, 2003, p. 125)

THE RECOVERY PROCESS

In very general terms, the process of empowering the Sober Self has three major components: recognition, activation, and mastery.[3] These elements inspire the LifeRing meeting process and literature.

Recognition

The addicted person not uncommonly suffers from depression and negative self-esteem. These paralyzing states of mind, which emanate from the "A," may become entrenched by repeated exposure to treatment paradigms that teach powerlessness, helplessness, and related attitudes. The first task, then, is to hold up a true mirror and to assist the addicted person to recognize, or rediscover, a spark of inner strength. LifeRing teaches that the mere fact of still being alive is evidence of the addicted person's drive to survive, which is the core of the Sober Self. The act of coming to a meeting is proof positive that the Sober Self is stirring within the person. Your Sober Self brought you here! The LifeRing meeting process, which encourages all participants to speak from Day 1, underlines the message that each person brings something valuable and important to the gathering. Participants frequently come to recognize the Sober Self within themselves by its reflection in the regard of others. The positive atmosphere of the meeting process gradually erodes negative and self-abusive postures and endows individuals with a sense of their own value and power as sober persons.

Activation

Empowerment of inner resources can come about only by their activation. The most common LifeRing meeting format begins, after a very brief opening statement, with the question, "How was your week?" This format, which evolved from the process groups found in many treatment programs, asks each participant to speak about the issues they encountered in their recovery since the last meeting and also to look ahead to the challenges they anticipate in the coming days. Positive cross-talk is encouraged and is a central feature of a successful meeting. Participation by speaking is a form of activating the inner recovery reserves, the Sober Self. As a rule of thumb, speaking engages the speaker in self-discovery and in change more forcefully than listening does. Because the topic is not book-based but life-based, literacy is not required for meeting participation. It is rare for a person to "pass" on this topic, and it is common for people to speak at their first LifeRing meeting. The topic focuses on the here and now and elicits individuals' reporting on the decisions they made in everyday life—the "small" decisions. Participants' explication of their actions both after and before the moment of decision fosters activation of sober emotive-cognitive resources in the decision-making process. Individual participants often say that as they go about their daily life, the awareness that they will report their decisions to the meeting is active in their minds, and it shapes what they do.

Mastery

A comprehensive study of relapse in chemical dependency concluded that the most successful client in resisting relapse is the one who "confidently acts as his or her own therapist" (Dimeff & Marlatt, 1995, p. 177). The largest longitudinal study of alcoholics in the United States concluded, similarly, that "alcoholics recover not because we treat them but because they heal themselves" (Vaillant, 1995, p. 384). It follows that a mutual aid organization for addicted persons needs to have as a strategic goal the empowerment of each of its members to be the "author and arbiter of their own recovery" (Herman, 1997, p. 133). The notion that there exists a universal cure, a silver bullet, a program that works for everyone is a case of magical thinking that has no basis in evidence. Self-treatment, the same as institutional treatment, must be individualized to accommodate the specific needs, personal goals, and cultural perspectives of unique individuals in different stages of change (Substance Abuse and Mental Health Services Administration [SAMHSA], 2006; additional citations in Nicolaus, 2009b, Ch. 4).

PERSONAL RECOVERY PROGRAMS

LifeRing honors these basic findings of modern addiction research by facilitating each participant's development of an abstinence-based PRP.

People develop their PRPs by two principal methods, or a combination thereof: random access and structured progression.

Random Access

At each meeting, and sometimes at encounters outside the meeting context, something happens that holds special significance for the participant and finds a place in long-term memory. This meaningful item is like a mosaic stone. Over time, additional pieces enter and gradually form a picture, which constitutes the person's remade sober identity, their PRP. This method is effective because each of its elements is deeply meaningful to the individual. But the assembly of pieces depends on random events, and the individual has little control over the timing, structure, or coverage of the whole.

Structured Progression

Using the *Recovery by Choice* workbook (Nicolaus, 2011), participants engage, pencil in hand, with a comprehensive and searching series of recovery questions. They may proceed in an organized manner, choosing the whole sequence and content of their recovery planning. Where literacy is an obstacle, persons may choose to partner up with a reader. When done, they have a written product that they can carry, revise, and share. Working the workbook gives them the advantage of permanence, organization, and control—in a word, structure.

NINE DOMAINS

The *Recovery by Choice* workbook (Nicolaus, 2011) organizes the process of building a PRP into nine domains or work areas.

First Domain: The Body

Give yourself a medical checkup. Make a checklist of concerns and plan to see a health care professional as appropriate.

Second Domain: The Immediate Environment

Map the triggers and slippery places in everyday life, create a safe space, and learn daily exercises to solidify your commitment to sobriety.

Third Domain: Time and Activities

Assess how you spend your time and evaluate which activities are safe and which should be avoided for now. Learn how to do an activity clean and sober.

Fourth Domain: People

Some people in your life support your freedom from substances, some do not know that it's an issue for you, and some try to drag you back. Learn to identify these three kinds of people and develop strategies for dealing with them.

Fifth Domain: Feelings

Learn to recapture old sober sources of pleasure and develop new ones that do not involve substance use. Learn to recognize your feelings, cultivate a more vibrant emotional life, and handle emotional crises while staying clean and sober.

Sixth Domain: Lifestyle

Assess the impact of substance use on your work, housing, living situation, social life, housekeeping, personal appearance, sex life, finances, legal situation, and other lifestyle aspects, and make a plan for positive change.

Seventh Domain: History

Review the origins of your substance use, understand the neurobiological dimension of addiction, and let go emotionally of this chapter of life.

Eighth Domain: Culture

Learn to read the messages about drinking and using that come from the culture and decide how you fit into the culture as a sober person.

Ninth Domain: Treatment and Support Groups

Decide what you need in the way of professional help and mutual aid groups to advance your recovery.

The *Recovery by Choice* workbook (Nicolaus, 2011) also contains a big chapter on relapse, but that is not a separate domain; rather, it is a synopsis and review of all the others. A provocative section of the relapse chapter is the "Relapse Planning Worksheet," where participants contemplating relapse can plan it out in all its details—and have a hard look at the probable consequences.

It will be seen that the LifeRing approach arose pragmatically and eclectically out of the experience of recovering persons and is essentially a homespun, rather than an academic, product. However, it draws inspiration from and has affinities with a number of trends in the universities and in the healing professions. It navigates, of course, within the broad stream of cognitive-behavioral science. The LifeRing approach takes many lessons from the client-centered psychology of Carl Rogers (Cain, 2010; Rogers, 1980). It strongly resonates with much of the teaching of Albert Bandura about self-efficacy (Bandura, 1997). It shares many themes with modern strength-based movements in psychology, education, and social work (Maton, Schellenbach, Leadbeater, and Solarz, 2004; Powell, Batsche, Ferro, Fox, and Dunlap, 1997). It is independent of but highly congruent with the motivational interviewing movement in addiction recovery (Miller, 1995) and has much in common with other modern recovery approaches, including William Glasser's choice theory, Ronald Warner's solution-focused therapy, and Marsha Linehan's dialectical behavior theory. It is informed by the most solid findings on addiction and recovery emanating from public and private research institutions.[4] In essence, LifeRing forms an instance of the New Recovery Movement described by William L. White (2000).

EVIDENCE FOR EFFECTIVENESS

The current evidence for LifeRing's effectiveness is of the same nature as the evidence for the traditional paradigm a decade or more after its foundation—anecdotal. Thousands of clean and sober individuals are living evidence that LifeRing participation is associated with long-term, stable abstinence. It remains an open question whether LifeRing contains an active ingredient that causes individuals to recover when they would not have done so otherwise, or whether LifeRing is merely a congenial environment for individuals who bring the active ingredient of their recoveries with them, or whether both are true to some extent, varying with the individual. Basically, LifeRing operates by generating social support for living life free of alcohol and other addictive drugs, and this combination of factors—social support and abstinence—is widely appreciated as the secret of effective recovery approaches.

RESEARCH OPPORTUNITIES

Two senior researchers at the Alcohol Research Group in Emeryville, CA, have applied repeatedly for a federal grant to assess the efficacy of LifeRing as an adjunct to treatment programs, to date without obtaining funding. LifeRing presents a number of facets that may fit within the research interest of qualified professionals; for example:

- What are the pluses and minuses of combining users of different addictive substances in the same recovery group, as distinct from segregating users by "drug of choice"?
- What personality types (or other factors) might be a better fit for an approach where the posited agency of change is internal (the Sober Self) as distinct from external (the higher power)?
- What is the evidence for the efficacy of individualized approaches in related fields (e.g., medicine, occupational training, special education, etc.), as compared with the application of a standardized one-size-fits-all approach?
- What difference is there in outcomes for LifeRing participants who develop their PRPs by the random access method as distinct from the structured approach embodied in the *Recovery by Choice* workbook (Nicolaus, 2011)?
- What features of current chemical dependency treatment programs could be tweaked to encourage clients to recognize, activate, and empower their Sober Self?

Any research effort must, of course, comply with appropriate ethical standards and confidentiality guidelines.

SUMMARY, CONCLUSIONS, AND FUTURE DIRECTIONS

LifeRing is one of the recovery approaches that emerged since the founding of Women for Sobriety in 1975 cracked the hegemony of the 12-step paradigm. Its future depends fundamentally on the continuation of cultural trends that have, since the 1970s, favored a less religiously tinted and a more psychologically positive approach in addiction healing. It depends, secondly, on the continuing good faith of treatment professionals in serving, rather than excluding or punishing, the portion of the clientele that seeks a recovery paradigm other than 12-step. In this regard, although LifeRing has mapped a structured pathway to self-healing with the *Recovery by Choice* workbook (Nicolaus, 2011), LifeRing still faces the challenge of developing a treatment protocol for use by professionals in an institutional setting. LifeRing also needs to solve the problem of developing ever more meeting facilitators to fill the growing demand for new meetings. Finally, although LifeRing has achieved small miracles of growth and publicity with an all-volunteer leadership and a five-figure shoestring budget, a quantum leap to primetime public awareness with a fully staffed back office awaits the involvement of financially capable sustainers.

NOTES

1. The workbook, *Recovery by Choice* (Nicolaus, 2011), was originally published in 2001; it is currently in its fourth edition.

2. Among published professional references are these:

> LifeRing meetings have always been well attended but the Saturday group has been so popular that at times we have had to open a second meeting room to accommodate all the people who wish to attend. I am happy to state that LifeRing has always been able to coexist harmoniously with other support meetings. Patients report being satisfied with the format and some say they attend LifeRing and 12-step support meetings. I am happy to recommend LifeRing to any drug treatment program" (day treatment co-coordinator, Kaiser Permanente Chemical Dependency Recovery Program, Oakland, CA)

> LifeRing has been extremely popular with our clients, and we offer it every Wednesday evening. MPI would recommend LifeRing with enthusiasm and full support to any other drug treatment program (manager, Merritt-Peralta Institute [MPI], Summit Medical Center, Oakland, CA)

Both letters are published in Nicolaus (2003), where facsimiles of the original letters may be found. Additional professional references appear in the advance readers' comments to Nicolaus, 2009b.

3. The reader will recognize here a debt to the Transtheoretical Model of Stages of Change; for a brief introduction, see Prochaska & DiClemente (1992).

4. Nicolaus (2009b) contains extensive citations. Among the findings of note since its publication is the working definition of recovery published in May 2011 by SAMHSA: Recovery "is an individualized process whereby each person's journey of recovery is unique and whereby each person in recovery chooses supports, ranging from clinical treatment to peer services that facilitate recovery" (SAMHSA, 2011). Also noteworthy is one of the first neurological explorations of innate recovery resources, "Discovery of Brain's Natural Resistance to Drugs May Offer Clues to Treating Addiction" (National Association of Alcoholism and Drug Abuse Counselors, 2012). Neurological research has concentrated almost exclusively on the addictive pathways, practically ignoring the vital mechanisms of recovery.

REFERENCES

Bandura, A. (1997). *Self-efficacy: The exercise of control.* New York, NY: W.H. Freeman.

Cain, D. J. (2010). *Person-centered psychotherapies.* Washington, DC: American Psychological Association.

Dimeff, L., & Marlatt, A. (1995). Relapse prevention. In R. K. Hester & W. R. Miller (Eds.), *Handbook of alcoholism treatment approaches* (2nd ed.). pp. 176–194. Boston, MA: Allyn & Bacon.

Fletcher, A. (2002). *Sober for good: New solutions for drinking problems—advice from those who have succeeded.* Boston, MA: Houghton Mifflin.

Granfield, R., & Cloud, R. (1999). *Coming clean: Overcoming addiction without treatment.* New York, NY: New York University Press.

Herman, J. (1997). *Trauma and recovery: The aftermath of violence—from domestic abuse to political terror.* New York: Basic Books.

LifeRing Secular Recovery. (2001). *Bylaws.* Oakland, California: LifeRing Press.

LifeRing Secular Recovery. (2005). *2005 LifeRing participant survey: Results.* Retrieved from http://lifering.org/wp-content/uploads/Survey_Final.pdf

Maton, K. I., Schellenbach, C. J., Leadbetter, B. J., and Solarz, A. L. (2004). *Investing in children, youth, families and communities: Strengths-based research and policy.* Washington, DC: American Psychological Association.

Miller, W. (1995). Increasing motivation for change. In R. K. Hester & R. Miller (Eds.), *Handbook of alcoholism treatment approaches: Effective alternatives* (2nd ed., pp. 89–104). Boston, MA: Allyn & Bacon.

National Association of Drug Abuse Counselors, The Association for Addiction Professionals. (2012, March 13). Discovery of brain's natural resistance to drugs may offer clues to treating addiction. *NAADAC News Brief.*

Nicolaus, M. (2003). *How was your week? Bringing people together in recovery the LifeRing way: A handbook.* Oakland, California: LifeRing Press.

Nicolaus, M. (2009a). Choice of support groups: It's the law. *Counselor, 10*(5), 40–46.

Nicolaus, M. (2009b). *Empowering your sober self: The LifeRing approach to addiction recovery.* New York, NY: Jossey-Bass.

Nicolaus, M. (2011). *Recovery by choice: Living and enjoying life free of alcohol and other drugs, a workbook* (4th ed.). Oakland, California: LifeRing Press.

Powell, D. S., Batsche, C. J., Ferro, J., Fox, L., and Dunlap, G. (1997). A strength-based approach in support of multi-risk families. *Topics in Early Childhood Special Education, 17*(1), 1–26.

Prochaska, J., & DiClemente, C. (1992). In search of how people change: Applications to addictive behaviors. *American Psychologist, 47*(9), 1102.

Rogers, Carl. (1980). *A way of being.* New York, NY: Houghton-Mifflin.

Substance Abuse and Mental Health Services Administration. (2006). *Overarching principles to address the needs of persons with co-occurring disorders.* Washington, D.C.

Substance Abuse and Mental Health Services Administration. (2011). *Recovery defined—a unified working definition and set of principles.* Retrieved from http://blog.samhsa.gov/2011/05/20/recovery-defined-a-unified-working-definition-and-set-of-principles/#comments%20

Vaillant, G. (1995). *The natural history of alcoholism revisited.* Cambridge, MA: Harvard University Press.

White, W. L. (1998). *Slaying the dragon: The history of addiction treatment and recovery in America.* Chicago, IL: Chestnut Health Systems/Lighthouse Institute.

White, W. L. (2000). Toward a new recovery movement: Historical reflections on recovery, treatment and advocacy. Retrieved from www.williamwhitepapers.com/pr/2000TowardANewRecoveryMovement.pdf

Moderation Management: A Mutual-Help Organization for Problem Drinkers Who Are Not Alcohol-Dependent

ANNA LEMBKE

Department of Psychiatry and Behavioral Sciences, Stanford University, Stanford, California, USA

KEITH HUMPHREYS

Department of Psychiatry and Behavioral Sciences, Stanford University, Stanford, California, USA, and Veterans Affairs Health Care System, Palo Alto, California, USA

Moderation Management (MM) is a mutual-help organization for problem drinkers who are not alcohol-dependent. MM members pursue a goal of moderate drinking as defined by specific guidelines for frequency and quantity of alcohol consumption. MM's program for change is based primarily on cognitive restructuring and behavioral self-control enhancement and has no inherent spiritual component. MM's definition of the "nondependent" problem drinker is based on the individual's ability to adhere to MM guidelines, which include an initial 30-day abstinence period followed by limits on daily consumption. MM's members, on average, are less alcohol-dependent and have higher social capital than individuals who participate in Alcoholics Anonymous or seek inpatient alcohol treatment. Although no longitudinal studies to date have examined the efficacy of MM, there are positive outcome data for similar cognitive and brief behavioral interventions delivered by health care professionals. Critics of MM claim the organization feeds denial among dependent drinkers and thereby delays abstinence-oriented treatment, but its defenders point out that MM may prevent some problem drinkers from progressing to a more deteriorated state such that abstinence would be necessary. Randomized trials examining whether MM is more effective than no treatment, or if it is

Dr. Humphreys was supported by a Senior Research Career Scientist Award for the Department of Veterans Affairs Health Services Research and Development Service.

comparable to existing evidence-based ambulatory treatments, are needed to resolve this debate. That many MM members have never sought help before suggests the organization has some public health value by widening the range of attractive options available to people with alcohol use disorders.

INTRODUCTION

Moderation Management (MM) is the only alcohol-related mutual-help organization (MHO) with the stated goal of moderate drinking rather than abstinence only. It is designed for problem drinkers who are not alcohol-dependent. Audrey Kishline founded MM in 1994 as an alternative to Alcoholics Anonymous (AA). Kishline was inspired to start MM out of her frustration with her own participation in AA and 12-step-oriented residential alcoholism treatment. She believed that her drinking problem was less severe than that of most other AA members and did not feel that the AA philosophy and program for change suited her needs. She started MM with the intention of helping others like herself who acknowledged a problem with alcohol but did not consider it a disease, did not embrace abstinence, and believed that with the right kind of fellowship, drinking in moderation without negative consequences could be a reasonable option. Ironically, Kishline herself ultimately was unable to maintain moderate drinking, leading her to quit her own organization and join AA. Her subsequent relapse, during which she killed two people in a car accident, has helped make MM a continuing subject of significant controversy, even though Kishline was no longer a member of MM at the time of the accident (Humphreys, 2004).

The organization Kishline created continued to grow after her departure. Although it remains small in terms of absolute number of members, MM's central text, *Moderate Drinking: The Moderation Management Guide for People Who Want to Reduce Their Drinking* (Kishline, 1994), has sold more than 50,000 copies (Humphreys, 2004). Active membership was about 500 in 2000 (Humphreys & Klaw, 2001) and is probably several thousand today, due to a large number of meetings occurring online. Indeed, MM has the unique distinction of being the first alcohol self-help organization to be accessed as much or more online as in person (Humphreys & Klaw; Kosok, 2006).

This manuscript reviews the available literature to answer four important questions regarding MM: (1) What is MM's program for change? (2) How is MM's target population of "nondependent problem drinkers" defined? (3) Does MM actually attract nondependent problem drinkers? And (4) does MM work? In conclusion, this manuscript comments on whether MM provides a useful public health service for the population of people with alcohol use disorders.

WHAT IS MODERATION MANAGEMENT'S PROGRAM FOR CHANGE?

MM has the universal features of all MHOs (Humphreys, 2004), such as being free of charge, operated by peers rather than helping professionals, consisting of members who share a common problem, valuing experiential knowledge and reciprocal helping (i.e., that individuals with similar problems can come together to help each other overcome that problem), and including personal-change goals. Like many MHOs, it outlines specific goals for personal change in a written document (as described earlier) and has a structured program of behavior change (the nine steps) that members are recommended to follow.

The Nine Steps (Kishline, 1994)

1. Attend meetings or online groups and learn about the program of MM.
2. Abstain from alcoholic beverages for 30 days and complete Steps 3 through 6 during this time.
3. Examine how drinking has affected your life.
4. Write down your life priorities.
5. Take a look at how much, how often, and under what circumstances you had been drinking.
6. Learn the MM guidelines and limits for moderate drinking.
7. Set moderate drinking limits and start weekly "small steps" toward balance and moderation in other areas of your life.
8. Review your progress and update your goals.
9. Continue to make positive lifestyle changes and attend meetings whenever you need ongoing support or would like to help newcomers.

Unlike all other alcohol-related MHOs, the prototype being AA, MM's primary goal is moderate drinking (abstinence is allowed as a goal, but at most, 1% of MM members choose it; Humphreys & Klaw, 2001). MM maintains that there are certain types of problem drinkers who can reduce drinking to a controlled, healthy level, without having to give up alcohol altogether. MM rejects the idea that loss of control is a core aspect of all problem drinking, while at the same time accepts that there are some alcohol-dependent individuals for whom this is true. MM furthermore rejects the notion that all alcohol misuse represents a disease, arguing instead that its members' alcohol misuse is a behavioral problem that can be remedied with behavior-modification techniques, such as setting a goal, identifying barriers to achieving that goal, and taking action to meet the goal (Kishline, 1994). Note, however, that MM does not deny the existence of uncontrolled alcohol addiction, any more than the founders of AA denied that some problem drinkers could return to moderate drinking (Humphreys, 2003). MM accepts that "alcoholism" (i.e., alcohol dependence) is a real condition but asserts that there is also a separate population of drinkers who are not well served by resources that were designed for severely dependent drinkers.

MM also differs from AA by having no explicit spiritual component. Whereas the notion of a "higher power" is central to AA's program for change, MM's nine steps present a rationalistic approach with no spiritual content. The locus of control is presumed to reside within the self, whereas AA asks the individual to admit the futility of self-control and "surrender to a higher power." For some individuals, the absence of spirituality and the emphasis on self-efficacy, as much as the goal of moderate drinking, draws them to MM and away from AA. As one prospective MM member phrased it, "I believe there is power in the mind, attitude, practice, and discipline that I have been careless about. Assuming responsibility is important. I have two options—practice responsibility or choose abstinence" (p. 387) (Klaw, Luft, & Humphreys, 2003).

Another fundamental difference between AA and MM is that MM is not open to all problem drinkers, only to those who are not alcohol-dependent. MM defines "nondependent problem drinkers" as those who can meet MM's specific criteria for membership, namely a 30-day abstinence period, preferably prior to or just after joining, and the ability to maintain the drinking limits set by the organization. For women, the drinking limits are no more than 9 standard (i.e., 12 ounces of beer, 5 ounces of wine, 1.5 ounces of hard liquor) drinks per week, with a maximum of 3 drinks on any 1 day. The corresponding limits for men are no more than 14 standard drinks per week with a maximum of 4 on any given day. Both men and women are to have 3 to 4 nondrinking days per week (Sanchez-Craig, Wilkinson, & Davila, 1995).

HOW IS A 'NONDEPENDENT PROBLEM DRINKER' DEFINED?

MM defines appropriate prospective members (i.e., nondependent problem drinkers) as anyone with an alcohol use problem who demonstrates the ability to complete an initial 30-day abstinence trial and then subsequently adhere to MM's guidelines on quantity and frequency. Such criteria for eligibility are harder for a prospective member to judge than are AA's (anyone with a sincere desire to stop drinking can join), because they depend on particular behavioral achievements that the person may not yet have attempted. Some critics of MM are uncomfortable with the fact that problem drinkers themselves make the judgment of whether MM is appropriate for them. But this reflects the fact that MM (just like AA) is a peer-led MHO rather than a professionally led organization with a gatekeeper who certifies people as potential members.

The issue of whether problem drinkers can decide for themselves if they are alcohol-dependent is a nontrivial one and a source of intense debate in the addiction field. Proponents of MM argue that the fact that Kishline recognized that she had become alcohol-dependent and left MM to join AA prior to the accident is evidence that MM's selection process is well-founded. Opponents of MM argue that alcoholic individuals will never appropriately self-select, because they invariably consider their drinking to be under better control than it is (Humphreys, 2004).

From a population public health perspective, the world is not divided conceptually into "alcoholics" and those who have no drinking problem. Rather, alcohol use disorders are conceptualized as a spectrum ranging from "risky use,"—the least problematic—to "problem drinking," to "harmful use" (abuse), to "alcohol dependence." "Risky use" is defined as a pattern of alcohol use exceeding a certain quantity and frequency of consumption (i.e., more than 7 standard drinks per week or more than 3 drinks per occasion for women; more than 14 standard drinks per week or more than 4 per occasion for men), but excluding those with dependence (although one third in this "risky use" group are at risk for dependence; Saitz, 2005). The quantities of alcohol consumption defined as "risky use" by the medical community are similar but not identical to those put forth by MM and are based on an ever-growing body of evidence linking quantity and frequency of alcohol consumption to overall morbidity and mortality, demonstrating that those who drink above a certain level are at increased risk for numerous poor health outcomes, including gastrointestinal problems (Lembke, Bradley, Henderson, Moos, & Harris, 2011), trauma (Harris, Bryson, Sun, Blough, & Bradley, 2009), and all-cause mortality (Harris, Bradley, Bowe, Henderson, & Moos, 2010).

"Problematic drinking" and "harmful use," by contrast, are defined as alcohol-related consequences, independent of quantity of consumption, in individuals who do not meet threshold criteria for "dependence." Likewise, the definition of "alcohol dependence" is not based on quantities of alcohol consumption but is rather defined by the *Diagnostic and Statistical Manual of Mental Disorders* (DSM) as "significant impairment and distress" due to alcohol-related compulsion, loss of control, and consequences, often accompanied by physical symptoms of tolerance and withdrawal but not necessarily requiring tolerance or withdrawal to meet diagnostic criteria (American Psychiatric Association, 2000). The DSM definition of alcohol dependence does not specify how much alcohol is too much but rather emphasizes the physical, psychological, and psychosocial impact of alcohol addiction.

MM's target population of nondependent problem drinkers theoretically encompasses risky use, problematic drinking, and harmful use (abuse), but not alcohol dependence. In relying on quantity and frequency and a 30-day abstinence trial, MM sidesteps the complex interpretation of consequences of use, which are harder to measure, are subject to interpretation, and are usually reliant on health care professionals for determination. As an interesting side note, the United Kingdom once had a moderate drinking organization (Drinkwatchers), which could only be accessed by individuals certified as appropriate by a professional. It struggled for members, as many potential members did not want professional involvement and some of the professionals involved were extremely wary of approving anyone for participation (Humphreys, 2004).

In sum, MM's target population of nondependent drinkers is defined on the one hand as individuals who are able to abstain for 30 days and then maintain moderate drinking below a certain threshold; and on the other hand, this population is defined as individuals who are not alcohol-dependent as defined by the DSM (i.e., compulsive, out-of-control use with adverse consequences, with or without physiological dependence). The question of whether MM succeeds in capturing its target population of nondependent problem drinkers is best answered by examining the drinking patterns, histories, and trajectories of those who join MM.

DOES MM ATTRACT NONDEPENDENT PROBLEM DRINKERS?

Three cross-sectional studies have examined the drinking patterns of MM members in the 6 months prior to MM participation.

The first study, by Humphreys and Klaw (2001), found that among 177 surveyed MM participants, the majority reported drinking 4 or more days per week, with five or more drinks per drinking day prior to joining MM. For reported frequency of drinking days, 8% reported drinking 2 to 4 days per month, 5% reported drinking 2 to 3 days per week, and 85% reported drinking 4 or more days per week. Fifty-four percent reported five or more drinks per drinking day. Those who were participating online reported drinking more on average compared with those who were participating in person, in the 6 months prior to joining MM. The second survey, by Kosok (2006), showed that of 272 MM members surveyed, the majority were regular, heavy drinkers in the 6 months prior to joining MM. Sixty-one percent of members drank daily and consumed on average six drinks per drinking day. Again, members participating in online groups drank more compared with those attending groups in person. A survey by Klaw et al. (2003) examined characteristics of 445 problem drinkers who telephoned MM's national information referral line and found 1% reported drinking monthly or less, 9% reported drinking 2 to 4 days per month, 24% reported drinking 2 to 3 days per week, and 55% reported drinking 4 or more days per week. On typical drinking days, 44% consumed five or more drinks per drinking day, and 14% consumed seven or more drinks per drinking day.

None of the surveys evaluated "alcohol dependence" as defined by the DSM or any other major diagnostic manual. However, each survey employed scales that assessed physical and psychological markers of dependence, as well as drinking- and health-related consequences. Humphreys and Klaw (2001) used the Alcohol Dependence Scale (Skinner & Allen, 1982) and the Health and Daily Living Form (Moos, Cronkite, & Finney, 1992) and found that MM members' scores for the whole sample were one standard deviation lower than AA members' scores completing the same three instruments (Timko, Finney, Moos, Moos, & Steinbaum, 1993). Respondents reported 4 alcohol-dependence symptoms, 5 alcohol-related problems, and 7 to 8 intoxicated days per month; this was compared with AA members in the study by Timko et al. using the same measures, who reported 11 alcohol-dependence symptoms, 10 alcohol-related problems, and 13 intoxicated days per month. Kosok's (2006) survey used the Short-Form Alcohol Dependence Data (SADD) Questionnaire (Raistrick, Dunbar, & Davidson, 1983). (The SADD was developed to be sensitive to drinkers who are moderately alcohol-dependent, and in addition to being validated in three studies [Davidson & Raistrick, 1986], it is also used by MM members to track their own progress [Kishline, 1994; Miller & Wilbourne, 2002].) Kosok found that the mean of summed scores for all subjects was 11, which ranks in the medium dependency range. The breakdown of the entire sample was as follows: 28% low dependency range, 62% medium dependency range, and 10% high dependency range.

The survey by Klaw et al. (2003), using the same measures as the Humphreys et al. survey (Humphreys & Klaw, 2001), the Alcohol Dependence Scale (Skinner & Allen, 1982) and the Health and Daily Living Form (Moos et al., 1992), found that average scores on measures of dependency and alcohol-related problems were even lower. Respondents reported one alcohol-dependence symptom, two alcohol-related problems, and 5 intoxicated days per month. In asking about specific markers of physiologic dependence, Klaw et al. (2003) found that 48% experienced amnesic periods due to drinking ("blackouts") in the 6 months prior, 38% had become physically ill through drinking in the 6 months prior, and 22% had physiologic symptoms of withdrawal in the 6 months prior ("shakes").

In answer to the primary question, does MM primarily attract nondependent problem drinkers, the answer appears to be a tentative "yes." The majority of prospective MM members meet the medical definition for "at-risk" drinking based on quantity and frequency. That is to say, they are drinking in the hazardous range and could be classified as problem drinkers. Furthermore, prospective MM members on average represent a less severely dependent population than those seeking help from AA. It is likely that some people who try MM meet medical criteria for alcohol dependence, but the data imply that a minority meet criteria for severe alcohol dependence (i.e., close to 10%).

DOES MM WORK?

To our knowledge, there are no prospective, longitudinal studies of MM face-to-face group participation, much less a randomized clinical trial. Given the limited evidence base, any conclusion about MM's effectiveness must remain tentative, but four lines of evidence should be noted.

First, there are ample data demonstrating that problem drinkers can return to moderate drinking (Cunningham, Lin, Ross, & Walsh, 2000; Sobell, Cunningham & Sobell, 1996). There is a growing literature on the positive impact of brief office-based interventions by health care providers for problem drinkers with mild-to-moderate alcohol use, who have been shown to reduce their drinking and improve health outcomes in response to advice about healthy drinking (Babor et al., 2007). MM may function in a similar way, mediated by consumers rather than professionals.

Second, there is a growing evidence base demonstrating that Web-based interventions to reduce drinking- and alcohol-related problems have similar efficacy as brief interventions delivered by practitioners (Witkiewitz & Marlatt, 2006). MM, with its relatively strong online presence, with some members accessing participation online only, certainly counts among these. In a randomized clinical trial, Hester, Delaney, and Campbell (2011) compared efficacy of MM online participation among nondependent problem drinkers, with MM online participation plus a Web-based program for moderate drinking. This moderate-drinking Web-based program is grounded in principles of self-control training, much like MM, but in addition gives users feedback on their progress based on computerized inputs of self-monitored drinking and mood data (Hester, Delaney, Campbell, & Handmaker, 2009). Hester et al. found that both groups reduced their drinking significantly from baseline, as measured by percentage of abstinent days and number of drinks per drinking day, with a medium-to-large effect size (Hester et al., 2009) (0.70). The absence of an assessment-only control group precludes saying anything definitive about the effectiveness of MM online participation alone, but the data do imply that those in this sample who participated in MM online showed reduced drinking at 3-, 6-, and 12-month follow-up.

Third, MM is based fairly closely on principles of cognitive-behavioral psychotherapies and also is to some extent informed by motivational enhancement interventions. These types of professionally developed therapies have been exhaustively researched and are judged as effective treatments by researchers and evidence-synthesizing bodies (Miller & Wilbourne, 2002). For example, cognitive-behavioral therapy (CBT) encourages the individual to examine his or her automatic negative thoughts and then reflect on how these thoughts affect mood and behavior. Likewise, MM's nine steps encourage members to "examine how drinking has affected your life" and "take a look at how much, how often, and under what circumstances you had been drinking" (Kishline, 1994), which in turn leads them to make connections between their drinking and their behavior, much the way CBT encourages making connections between automatic negative thoughts and mood and behavior. Behavioral activation is another important aspect of CBT, in which individuals are urged to take "baby steps" to accomplish their goals (i.e., to break down the challenge into manageable and discrete units). So too do MM's nine steps advocate that the individual "set moderate drinking limits and start weekly 'small steps' toward balance and moderation in other areas of your life" (Kishline, 1994).

Fourth, ample evidence demonstrates that lower-dependence, higher-social-capital drinkers are more likely to achieve moderate drinking (Marshall, Humphreys, & Ball, 2010). For example, a study by Humphreys, Moos, and Finney (1995) empirically demonstrates that there is a pathway for more severe drinkers that involves AA and results in abstinence, and a different pathway that leads to moderate drinking for people who have less severe drinking problems and more social capital to begin. This resonates with the finding that MM attracts less-dependent drinkers (Humphreys & Klaw, 2001; Kosok, 2006), the majority of whom are college-educated, employed, and have good social support.

Some critics may argue that people with more severe problems drop out of the organization quickly, giving the illusion of effectiveness through selective attrition. Careful research has debunked this explanation, however. Individuals who call MM's national helpline but then never go on to attend a meeting have less severe alcohol problems than those who attend a meeting. And those who attend for an extended period have even more serious alcohol problems prior to joining than do the other two groups (Klaw, Horst, & Humphreys, 2006). Selection into MM is thus prognostically adverse rather than being a case of "creaming" (i.e., only the easy cases stay). These observations do not prove that MM works, only that any successful moderate drinking with MM typically reflects change in someone who had a genuine drinking problem, rather than selective attrition making current members a sample of the "worried well."

CONCLUSION

In summary, MM provides an alternative to abstinence-oriented MHOs by offering a goal of moderate drinking. MM limits membership to nondependent problem drinkers, defined by MM as those who can adhere to a 30-day abstinence trial and specified drinking guidelines. MM attracts problem drinkers who are less severely dependent than those who seek to join AA and have high social capital. MM's philosophy is in concert with current trends in public health conceptualizing alcohol use disorders as representing a continuum, with different treatment goals for individuals at different places on that continuum. There is ongoing controversy around whether individuals with alcohol use disorders can determine for themselves their place on that continuum, and in turn the best goal for their type of drinking problem. There is also controversy as to whether, as some claim, allowing problem drinkers to choose MM delays the abstinence-only treatment, which they really need.

For alcohol-dependent individuals, the evidence shows that AA is clearly helpful (Humphreys, 2004). The question is whether there is a positive role for an organization like MM for those with less severe alcohol use problems. Epidemiologic studies show that individuals with mild-to-moderate drinking problems outnumber those with severe alcohol problems 4 to 1 (Committee on Treatment of Alcohol Problems, 1990). Approximately 75% of individuals who recover from a diagnosed alcohol problem for a year or more do so without treatment, and between 30% and 60% of them return to moderate drinking rather than abstinence (Sobell et al., 1996). Those who return to moderate drinking without treatment tend to be people who initially had less severe drinking problems (Cunningham et al., 2000). Among problem drinkers who seek help, the majority (53%–83%) report using AA (Sobell et al.).

MM widens the range of attractive options available to people with alcohol use disorders, particularly for problem drinkers who wish to return to moderate drinking rather than abstinence but who have heretofore spurned AA and other abstinence-oriented treatment options in favor of "going it alone." By its own description, MM is "a good place to begin" and may "shorten the discovery process" by providing guidelines for healthy drinking (Miller & Wilbourne, 2002). MM may well provide a useful and necessary public health service for problem drinkers who are unlikely to participate initially in abstinence-oriented programs but who would benefit from some basic guidelines about healthy drinking. MM may serve primarily to point individuals in the right direction in terms of deciding what kind of treatment they need. It is worth mentioning that a portion of individuals who seek treatment for a moderate drinking goal come over time to pursue abstinence as they learn that moderate drinking is not attainable.

What is needed going forward are studies of MM's efficacy based on where on the use–disorder continuum the individual resides, examining whether MM participation reduces drinking from hazardous to moderate use and in what population. These data should include comparisons of MM online participation to MM face-to-face participation. The evidence suggests that those who participate online are heavier drinkers than those who attend face-to-face meetings and thus may represent a slightly different population of problem drinkers. Future research should also explore prior treatment utilization of individuals who seek MM to investigate the claim that MM delays treatment.

It is the belief of these authors that MM provides a useful public health service by offering guidelines about healthy drinking in the context of a fellowship of individuals with similar problems. It remains for a well-designed outcome study to determine definitively whether the MM organization itself is the primary mechanism that drives such behavior change, or whether it is more a signpost for healthier goals for individuals seeking to improve their well-being.

REFERENCES

American Psychiatric Association. (2000). *Diagnostic and statistical manual of mental disorders* (4th ed., text rev.). Washington, DC: Author.

Babor, T. F., McRee, B. G., Kassebaum, P. A., Grimaldi, P. L., Ahmed, K., & Bray, J. (2007). Screening, Brief Intervention, and Referral to Treatment (SBIRT). *Substance Abuse, 28*(3), 7–30.

Committee on Treatment of Alcohol Problems, I. o. M. (1990). *Broadening the Base of Treatment for Alcohol Problems: Report of a Study by a Committee of the Institute of Medicine*. Washington, D.C.: Division of Mental Health and Behavioral Medicine.

Cunningham, J. A., Lin, E., Ross, H. E., & Walsh, G. W. (2000). Factors associated with untreated remissions from alcohol abuse or dependence. *Addictive Behaviors, 25*(2), 317–321.

Davidson, R., & Raistrick, D. (1986). The validity of the Short Alcohol Dependence Data (SADD) Questionnaire: A short self-report questionnaire for the assessment of alcohol dependence. *British Journal of Addiction, 81*, 217–222.

Harris, A., Bradley, K. A., Bowe, T., Henderson, P., & Moos, R. (2010). Associations Between AUDIT-C and Mortality Vary by Age and Sex. *Population Health Management, 13*(5), 263–268.

Harris, A. H. S., Bryson, C. L., Sun, H., Blough, D., & Bradley, K. A. (2009). Alcohol Screening Scores Predict Risk of Subsequent Fractures. *Substance Use & Misuse, 44*(8), 1055–1069.

Hester, R. K., Delaney, H. D., Campbell, W., & Handmaker, K. (2009). A web application for moderation training: Initial results of a randomized clinical trial. *Journal of Substance Abuse Treatment, 37*, 266–276.

Hester, R. K., Delaney, H. D., & Campbell, W. (2011). ModerateDrinking.com and Moderation Management: Outcomes of a randomized clinical trial with non-dependent problem drinkers. *Journal of Consulting and Clinical Psychology, 79*, 215–224.

Humphreys, K. (2003). Alcohol & drug abuse: A research-based analysis of the Moderation Management controversy. *Psychiatric Services, 54*(5), 621–622.

Humphreys, K. (2004). Circles of recovery: Self-help organizations for addictions. In G. Edwards (Ed.), *International research monographs in the addictions*. Cambridge, UK: Cambridge University Press.

Humphreys, K., & Klaw, E. (2001). Can targeting nondependent problem drinkers and providing Internet-based services expand access to assistance for alcohol problems? A study of the Moderation Management self-help/mutual aid organization. *Journal of Studies on Alcohol, 62*, 528–532.

Humphreys, K., Moos, R. H., & Finney, J. W. (1995). Two pathways out of drinking problems without professional treatment. *Addictive Behaviors, 20*, 427–441.

Kishline, A. (1994). *Moderate drinking: The Moderation Management guide for people who want to reduce their drinking*. New York, NY: Crown.

Klaw, E., Horst, D., & Humphreys, K. (2006). Inquirers, triers, and buyers of an alcohol harm reduction self-help organization. *Addiction Research & Theory, 14*(5), 527–535.

Klaw, E., Luft, S., & Humphreys, K. (2003). Characteristics and motives of problem drinkers seeking help from Moderation Management self-help groups. *Cognitive and Behavioral Practice, 10*, 385–390.

Kosok, A. (2006). The Moderation Management programme in 2004: What type of drinker seeks controlled drinking? *International Journal of Drug Policy, 17*(4), 295–303.

Lembke, A., Bradley, K., Henderson, P., Moos, R., & Harris, A. (2011). Alcohol Screening Scores and the Risk of New-Onset Gastrointestinal Illness or Related Hospitalization. *Journal of General Internal Medicine, 26*(7), 777–782.

Marshall, J., Humphreys, K., & Ball, D. (2010). *The treatment of drinking problems* (5th ed.). Cambridge, UK: Cambridge University Press.

Miller, W. R., & Wilbourne, P. L. (2002). Mesa Grande: A methodological analysis of clinical trials of treatments for alcohol use disorders. *Addiction, 97*(3), 265–277.

Moos, R. H., Cronkite, R. C., & Finney, J. W. (1992). *Health and daily living form manual*. Palo Alto, CA: Consulting Psychologists Press.

Raistrick, D., Dunbar, G., & Davidson, R. (1983). Development of a questionnaire to measure alcohol dependence. *British Journal of Addiction, 78*, 89–93.

Saitz, R. (2005). Unhealthy alcohol use. *New England Journal of Medicine, 352*(6), 596–607.

Sanchez-Craig, M., Wilkinson, D. A., & Davila, R. (1995). Empirically based guidelines for moderate drinking: 1-year results from three studies with problem drinkers. *American Journal of Public Health, 85*(6), 823–828.

Skinner, H. A., & Allen, B. A. (1982). Alcohol dependence syndrome: Measurement and validation. *Journal of Abnormal Psychology, 91*, 199–209.

Sobell, L. C., Cunningham, J. A., & Sobell, M. B. (1996). Recovery from alcohol problems with and without treatment: Prevalence in two population surveys. *American Journal of Public Health, 86*(7), 966–972.

Timko, C., Finney, J. W., Moos, R. H., Moos, B. S., & Steinbaum, D. P. (1993). The process of treatment selection among previously untreated help-seeking problem drinkers. *J Subst Abuse 5*, 203–220.

Witkiewitz, K., & Marlatt, G. A. (2006). Overview of harm reduction treatments for alcohol problems. *International Journal of Drug Policy, 17*, 285–294.

Women for Sobriety: 35 Years of Challenges, Changes, and Continuity

REBECCA M. FENNER and MARY H. GIFFORD
Women for Sobriety Inc., Quakertown, Pennsylvania, USA

This article examines Women for Sobriety (WFS), an abstinence-based, secular recovery organization for women created as an alternative recovery strategy in contrast to the well-known 12-step approach. This comprehensive overview is intended to familiarize treatment professionals with WFS for its potential application in their treatment programs and referrals. Also considered in this article are how the WFS organization has fared during the past 20 years and where the organization is today, through comparison of results from two previously conducted WFS surveys in 1991 and 2011. Survey results suggest that the organization has evolved through the years by facing challenges and embracing change yet preserving necessary continuities.

Until the late 1970s, little research had been done specifically on women alcoholics and their treatment; consequently, all referrals were generally made to an Alcoholics Anonymous (AA) group using the 12-step program. This program was designed by male alcoholics for other men and treated all alcoholics, men and women, the same. There were no alternatives (Kaskutas, 1994, p. 185). Shortly thereafter, with the rise of the women's movement,

The Women for Sobriety (WFS) organization is greatly indebted to Lee Ann Kaskutas, Ph.D., of the Alcohol Research Group in Berkeley, CA. Her research, analysis, and professional attention during the past two decades has been invaluable, from her initial contact with WFS founder Dr. Jean Kirkpatrick through WFS today. Without her insightful contributions to our understanding of ourselves, especially in her seminal work on the first survey of WFS in 1991, this article would not have been possible. We thank Dr. Kaskutas for her ongoing support as an interested friend of the organization.

and consistent with the thinking of sociologist Dr. Jean Kirkpatrick, women's needs in recovery and their treatment began to be viewed differently. Kirkpatrick's position was that a woman's experience as an alcoholic is a distinct phenomenon—as is her recovery from her drinking—and she requires a separate approach as well as separate meetings (Kaskutas, 1994, p. 186). Likewise, as researcher, Dr. Lee Kaskutas surmised, "The AA philosophy and its approach to sobriety are not for everyone, irrespective of gender" (Kaskutas 1992b, p. 632). Fortunately, in 2012, there is greater acknowledgment that women pursuing recovery need to be treated separately and differently from men; therefore, different but equally effective treatment approaches are needed as alternatives. Women for Sobriety (WFS) is considered one of these unique solutions.

This article examines WFS, an abstinence-based, secular recovery organization for women, founded in 1975. WFS and its program were created as an alternative recovery strategy in contrast to the well-known 12-step approach.[1] As a nonprofessional, self- and mutual-help organization, WFS has no physical treatment facilities; it offers the WFS "New Life" Program, group meetings, and other support materials to help women pursue a positive recovery. Also considered in this article is how the WFS organization has fared during the past 20 years and where the organization is today, based on the results of two surveys of the WFS organization conducted 20 years apart, in 1991 and 2011. The comparisons indicate that the organization has evolved through the years by facing challenges and embracing change yet preserving necessary continuities.

WFS HISTORY

In 1973, Jean Kirkpatrick was 50 years old with a doctorate in sociology and dwindling job prospects; she was also an alcoholic with a 29-year history of problem drinking and only a collective 3 years sober, until she was able to achieve lasting sobriety on her own, using her own methods. In her search for a new profession and meaningful work, she realized that in addition to her education and experience in teaching and research, she had considerable expertise as an alcoholic, more specifically a *woman* alcoholic, who overcame alcoholism using a means other than the traditional AA 12-step program in widespread use at that time. Also, she had worked with and sponsored women alcoholics in her previous years in AA, and she was planning work with Marty Mann, the founder of the National Council on Alcoholism. Above all, though, she viewed herself as an expert on female alcoholics, based on her extensive firsthand experience with her own addiction.

She had found a cause and, at last, what became her life's work. "No woman need die from the disease of alcoholism" became her battle cry, and she fought that battle with every weapon she could think of, with very little money and, at times, very little help, as she worked to effect positive change. A prolific writer, she began to organize her thoughts, notes, and perspectives on alcoholism, women, and recovery, based on her research and her personal experience. Eventually, her original trial-and-error methods gelled into a new program designed by a woman alcoholic specifically for women alcoholics. Her approach to sobriety was influenced by the writings of American transcendental author and thinker Ralph Waldo Emerson and the Unity Movement of New Thought, another product of the late 19th century; her exploration and practice of meditation; the emerging women's movement; her experience with AA and her own battle with alcohol; and her studies of sociology. These intellectual, introspective, and experiential pursuits combined to result in a cognitive-based program that would address what she believed to be the fundamental problem of women alcoholics: low self-esteem (Kaskutas, 1996c, p. 274).

Further, Kirkpatrick concluded that the concept of "one size fits all" should no longer apply to recovery efforts and that women's needs not only vary by individual but also differ greatly from men's recovery needs. Therefore, she reasoned, there are many women for whom a 12-step approach is simply not the right fit, for various reasons, and these women may be more successful using a different, women-only strategy for their personal recovery.

By 1974, she was ready to inaugurate her new program. The WFS organization, with its "New Life" Program and "13 Statements of Acceptance," was incorporated as a nonprofit charitable organization in 1975. Following a United Press International feature, which appeared in 50 newspapers nationwide, within a week, WFS received letters from more than 500 women alcoholics seeking information and requests about starting groups in 50 major cities. As an additional resource for WFS members, Kirkpatrick began a monthly newsletter, *Sobering Thoughts,* which she envisioned as a way to provide expanded information about the WFS program and other issues affecting women alcoholics. She suggested using the newsletter's topics as subjects for discussion at group meetings, as a way to help "lead each [group] member to some kind of self-examination" (Kirkpatrick, 1976, p. 4). In addition, Kirkpatrick developed a pen-pal service as a way to connect new WFS members with other women who had more experience with the program and sobriety yet shared the common bond of dealing with their drinking and wanting a new life.

Recognizing the applicability of the WFS approach to other addictions, Kirkpatrick expanded the scope of the "New Life" Program to include women dealing not only with alcohol but also with other chemical substance abuse issues, including street drugs and prescription drugs. In addition, Kirkpatrick discovered interest among some men in recovery who responded well to the "New Life" Program's positive approach. As a result, in 1983, she created a companion version of the program to meet that need, which she called Men for Sobriety. Eventually, Kirkpatrick customized a version of her program called the "New You Program," this time for women struggling with food addictions.

The organization's greatest accomplishment during the 1990s was its early recognition of the Internet as the future of communication and, more importantly, of the Internet's potential role in the future of WFS. Through development of internal systems and recognition of ongoing technological opportunities, WFS became well positioned to meet the needs of members and of its own survival.

Through the generosity and talent of a member, WFS created its first Web site and went online in December 1995. The site provided information about the organization and a basic overview of the "New Life" Program, which women were able to access and use free of charge. A bookstore function was also part of the site so that women could purchase recovery materials. To deliver communications in an immediate and more effective way, WFS began development of an online forum, which went live in the spring of 1998. America Online hosted the first WFS chat meeting, in which 25 women participated. The immediate success of the online forum meant the inevitable demise of the pen-pal service, as WFS chose to focus on less dated and more productive support activities.

On June 19, 2000, Kirkpatrick passed away at the age of 77. Throughout her life, Kirkpatrick remained adamant about preserving the purpose of her original program and the makeup of her meetings, so that the "New Life" Program focused exclusively on women's recovery from alcohol and drug addiction. In her final years, her wish was that after her passing, WFS would continue on as her legacy, so that no woman would have to take the journey to recovery alone. Through the efforts of the WFS Board of Directors, headquarters staff, and the women who have benefited from her program, her wish is being accomplished, and WFS continues into the 21st century.

THE WFS 'NEW LIFE' PROGRAM

Any woman with a sincere desire to achieve lasting recovery and who is willing to try using the WFS program is welcome. There is no membership fee to join.

The program is designed especially for women who are addicted to or who abuse alcohol and/or drugs. It is cognitive-behaviorally based and emphasizes that women can draw on their inner strength to change their thinking and use the power of their minds to likewise change their habits and their lives. The vehicle Kirkpatrick uses for accomplishing change is the power of positive thinking. This approach teaches women how to put into practice a positive, active growth process of self-discovery; during this process, women acquire coping skills and tools to deal with life and its underlying issues, past and present, without resorting to the mind crutch of addiction.

The WFS program emphasizes empowerment: assuming responsibility for one's choices, one's actions, and one's life. Another fundamental component of the program is that negative thoughts are at the root of women's drinking and drugging. WFS holds that women start drinking in reaction to "faulty thinking," which underlies destructive behavior. WFS teaches that women have the power to change their way of thinking—that their own mental images, either negative or positive, shape their actions accordingly. Thus, recovery is predicated on a change in outlook at the most basic level, the inner self (Kaskutas, 1989, p. 179).

Central to the WFS program are 13 affirmations, called the Statements of Acceptance. These statements emphasize positive thinking, personal responsibility, and personal growth; they are the tools with which women can learn to establish a secure, self-confident base from which to move forward in their recovery.

WFS Statements of Acceptance

1. I have a life-threatening problem that once had me.
   I now take charge of my life and my disease. I accept the responsibility.
2. Negative thoughts destroy only myself.
   My first conscious sober act must be to remove negativity from my life.
3. Happiness is a habit I will develop.
   Happiness is created, not waited for.
4. Problems bother me only to the degree I permit them to.
   I now better understand my problems and do not permit problems to overwhelm me.
5. I am what I think.
   I am a capable, competent, caring, compassionate woman.
6. Life can be ordinary or it can be great.
   Greatness is mine by a conscious effort.
7. Love can change the course of my world.
   Caring becomes all important.
8. The fundamental object of life is emotional and spiritual growth.
   Daily I put my life into a proper order, knowing which are the priorities.
9. The past is gone forever.
   No longer will I be victimized by the past. I am a new person.
10. All love given returns.
    I will learn to know that others love me.
11. Enthusiasm is my daily exercise.
    I treasure all moments of my new life.
12. I am a competent woman and have much to give life.
    This is what I am and I shall know it always.

13. I am responsible for myself and for my actions.
    I am in charge of my mind, my thoughts, and my life.
    Copyright 2012 WFS Inc.

The statements are not steps. Therefore, after the starting point of the program, acceptance of Statement #1, the affirmations can be used in any order or combination that a woman chooses. This flexibility permits each woman to customize these program components to meet her specific needs in pursuit of her recovery. In addition, Kirkpatrick developed a sample arrangement of the affirmations for women who might prefer a ready-made recovery plan that is proven effective for others. Based on her own recovery efforts, Kirkpatrick grouped the statements into a blueprint for recovery, which she describes as a "stepwise progression toward liberation and happiness" (quoted in Kaskutas, 1996a, p. 83). She suggests arranging the affirmations into the following six levels of personal progress:

1. *Acceptance.* Accepting that alcoholism and drug addiction are a physical disorder. Statement #1.
2. *Cleaning House.* Getting rid of negative thoughts, putting guilt behind us, and practicing a new way of viewing problems. Statements #2, 4, and 9.
3. *New Thinking.* Creating and practicing a new view of self. Statements #5 and 12.
4. *New Attitudes.* Using new attitudes to enforce new behavior patterns. Statements #3, 6, and 11.
5. *Relationships.* Working on relationships as a result of our new feelings about self. Statements #7 and 10.
6. *A New Self.* Recognizing life's priorities: emotional and spiritual growth, plus self-responsibility. Statements #8 and 13.

Copyright 2012 WFS Inc.

As part of their ongoing recovery efforts, women are directed to practice the affirmation statements daily, preferably just after awakening, in a period of personal meditation and introspection, and to actively apply the statements to the situations they encounter in the course of everyday living. Then, through diligence, determination, repetition, and practical application of the program's affirmations, and by using the power of her own mind, a woman can break the hold of her addiction, herself.

Although both organizations have the same objectives (i.e., abstinence and the achievement of lasting recovery), WFS clarifies that it is not affiliated with 12-step programs because of the significant difference in the two approaches to accomplish those objectives. However, WFS does not discourage participation in AA. In keeping with its belief that each woman's personal preference should decide her choice of recovery alternatives, WFS encourages women to choose and pursue whatever recovery approach (or combination of approaches) best suits their needs.

WFS MEETINGS

Consistent with the WFS program and its affirmations, group meetings reflect the concepts of cognitive behavior modification, as group members literally learn to change their thoughts from negative to positive. Further, participants discover how to eliminate their negative habits associated with drinking and to introduce new habits through which they think, behave, and respond to life in new, healthier, more positive ways.

Face-to-Face Groups

WFS offers face-to-face groups so that women can meet together in person for mutual encouragement while using the program. However, Kirkpatrick emphasized that the program is self-help (i.e., she designed the program with that specific flexibility in mind), so that women can be successful using its positive approach without attending a group. As a result, while face-to-face groups are a valuable additional resource, attending them does not preclude a woman's ability to use the WFS program successfully on her own.

WFS face-to-face meetings are held weekly; they are closed meetings, not open to the public, and only women pursuing recovery may attend. Group size is routinely small, ranging from 3 to 4 women in some groups and up to 11 or 12 in others. Occasionally, groups may reach as many as 24 members, but this overcrowding is addressed by splitting the group into smaller units.

The meeting process begins with brief introductions, during which participants identify themselves by saying, "My name is Mary and I am a competent woman." Then the affirmation statements are read, either by individual members or the group. Thereafter, each woman may share a positive action (how they have handled a situation differently) or a feeling (how they were able to identify and respond differently) and relate their experience to one of the affirmation statements. All participants are offered this opportunity to speak, but no one is compelled to do so.

Next, the discussion topic for the meeting is introduced. Moderators prepare a topic for each week, but if the need arises, a different, more immediate topic can be substituted. Again, women speak out as they feel inclined. At this point, the meeting format is rather like a focused conversation; questions, feedback, and discussion are encouraged without the artifice of taking turns. At some point during the meeting, a voluntary donation earmarked for the WFS organization is requested; however, this contribution is entirely free will, and no one is turned away from meetings because she cannot afford a donation.

There are no slogans or sponsors in WFS. Introspection, insight, and problem solving are encouraged, and honest, nonjudgmental conversation is the atmosphere this format creates. Compassionate give-and-take affords opportunities for individualized mutual support. Members do not repeatedly share their drinking history; rather, they reflect on it and use it to learn different approaches to handling specific situations, challenges, and people. This approach is consistent with WFS philosophy, which views the recapitulation of drinking histories as a negative, an action that emphasizes guilt and shame and hinders emotional and spiritual growth, especially among women. At the end of each meeting, the group repeats the program motto together: "We are capable and competent, caring and compassionate, always willing to help another, bonded together in overcoming our addictions."

Sponsors, as provided in 12-step programs, are not a part of the WFS program or its meetings. WFS believes that utilizing sponsors is inconsistent with its philosophy of self-respect and empowerment and can promote dependency instead of responsibility for one's own choices and behaviors. Most groups offer a list of group members who can be contacted between meetings for help, but these women do not act as sponsors. Rather, encouragement and support are engendered through the sisterhood of the groups, and self-help is effected through organization membership. Further, additional support is readily accessible at any time between face-to-face meetings through the online forum.

Online Meetings

The WFS online forum puts women in touch with many other caring and compassionate women who share a common bond, use the WFS program in their recovery, and are willing to help one another. Currently, the forum is the most popular of all WFS support resources, one that is used by thousands of members on a daily basis. Especially helpful in areas where no face-to-face groups are available, forum participation is likewise very effective between regular group meetings. So, for example, when cravings strike, women can choose to reach for their keyboard instead of a drink and talk to someone online who understands. Rapid access is readily at hand, 24/7 for support, when help is needed quickly. The forum offers multiple message boards as well as 14 formal chat meetings per week across many time zones. The forum is a private site, so women must register before permission is given to log on for the first time. However, there are no membership fees involved; voluntary donations are used to support this site.

Phone-Support Alternatives

In areas where no face-to-face groups are available, WFS offers phone support provided by volunteers—women who are experienced using the WFS program and who have consistent, strong sobriety. Phone-support volunteers talk with women in need about the WFS program, answer questions, offer encouragement and support, and provide practical tips to help newcomers learn to use the program. As it does for its group moderators, WFS approves phone-support volunteers through an official application process.

Moderator Certification

To ensure that the WFS program and its meetings are presented according to the organization's guidelines, the volunteers who facilitate WFS groups must be certified to do so by the WFS organization. Likewise, the women who volunteer to be chat leaders for the online forum are certified based on the same competencies that WFS requires for its face-to-face group moderators.

The process of certification is competency-based. Each volunteer moderator is a woman in recovery with consistent, sound sobriety for a minimum of at least 1 year, in-depth understanding of the WFS organization and its philosophy, and considerable experience in the practical application of the WFS program in her daily recovery efforts. Required reading of some of Kirkpatrick's literature is also necessary before minimum application requirements can be met to apply for certification. Individual competency is determined through a combination of written questionnaires, interviews, recommendations (from other moderators or treatment professionals), and board review. Moderators are expected not only to follow the guidelines and facilitate the group but also to take care of administrative details associated with running the group, such as handling meeting materials, collecting and forwarding donations to the main office, maintaining support/contact lists, planning discussion topics for meetings, and providing local publicity about meetings and the WFS organization.

CHALLENGES, CHANGES, AND CONTINUITIES

Society, technology, and humanity have come a long way in the 37 years since the founding of WFS. Nevertheless, the organization and its philosophy have demonstrated enduring vitality despite mind-boggling changes in how we communicate, work, live, and view addiction and its treatment. This ability to evolve and adapt as conditions and circumstances change is the essence of survival, not only for individuals but also for organizations, and recovery organizations are no different. Fortunately, WFS has been able to recognize and plan for new opportunities to remain viable into the 21st century.

In particular, with the explosion of communication alternatives made available by the Internet, getting in touch and keeping in touch have never been easier or more instantaneous. The WFS organization is now able to offer its philosophy and program in many different delivery forms, increasing access to its program and providing more choices for women hoping to avail themselves of the help that WFS offers. Depending upon their circumstances, women can choose to contact WFS by Internet, phone, or postal mail; learn about WFS from its Web site; utilize print, audio, and digital materials obtained through the online catalog/bookstore; attend face-to-face or online meetings for support; use the program "on their own" as independent self-help; or utilize any combination of these resources that works for them. The following are some quick comparisons of how the organization has grown and changed.

Methods of Contact

Any woman contacting WFS—by e-mail, phone, or postal mail—receives information free of charge; further, responsiveness to inquiries from women seeking help is the organization's first priority. Originally, Kirkpatrick answered every letter, until the volume became such that office assistance was necessary. Her tradition of individual attention to each woman seeking help has continued and is now expedited by Internet communications. The organization's current database is more than 100,000 strong and growing, with the overwhelming majority of contacts made almost exclusively by e-mail now, roughly 90% of the time.

WFS Web Site

The program's first Web site in 1997 averaged 1,000 page views per month; in comparison, consistent with the Internet explosion during the next 20 years, the newly revised and updated Web site in 2012 currently averages 30,000 views per month. The site, http://www.womenforsobriety.org, is now a worldwide information resource for not only women with addictions and their families and friends, but also for treatment professionals and their clients. A brief description of the program and suggestions for using it, as well as a list of informative pamphlets, brochures, and articles, can be downloaded and printed out from the site free of charge.

Online Bookstore/Catalog

For more than 25 years, the only way to distribute the WFS catalog was via postal mail. Today, linked on the WFS homepage, the catalog site is online and easy to use, with a variety of shipping options including foreign orders. Ninety-nine percent of WFS orders come through the online bookstore.

The Online Forum

Since its inception with one chat meeting and 25 participants, the WFS online community has continued to grow, showing in 2011 a 31% increase in forum membership and participation compared with the previous year. Additional statistics for 2011 reveal a total of 291,529 posts on the message boards and 49,000 private messages among the members.

Face-to-Face Groups

WFS has roughly 100 active face-to-face groups nationwide and is fairly well represented in Canada, with groups in the provinces of Ontario, Alberta, British Columbia, and Nova Scotia. There are also a number of groups across Australia, Finland, and Iceland, with a few groups scattered in other foreign countries. The current total represents a decline from the 125 face-to-face groups active at the time of the Kaskutas survey in 1991 (Kaskutas, 1992a, p. 2).

WFS believes that going forward, the trend may be to have a fairly static number of face-to-face groups, but not because of a decline in popularity of the WFS program. Rather, WFS attributes the major reason for the decline to changes in communication preferences, as demonstrated by the popularity of Internet communications. Today's women are much more skilled and comfortable using the Internet for their conversations, work, recreation, purchasing, and research; further, for many, choosing the Internet for help with recovery is more private, more convenient, more immediate, more comfortable, and less risky (in the sense of being seen at a group) than is attending a face-to-face group meeting.

A lesser reason for the decline in face-to-face groups is the ongoing challenge WFS faces in attracting women volunteers who are willing to pursue moderator certification to start and maintain a group. Many women seek to attend a WFS group meeting, but few of them are willing to assume the responsibility for facilitating a weekly meeting, and even fewer of those who express interest in starting a group actually complete the required certification process to do so.

E-mail Updates Service

The E-mail Updates Service came online for WFS early in 2011 as another way to communicate and to keep women connected with WFS. Even more important, by converting to another Internet-based communication, the organization was able to rectify three financial-related concerns: declining subscriptions for the still paper-based newsletter, escalating subscription costs, plus increasing costs in production and distribution of printed materials. The electronic-mail only communication service is designed to keep members and friends of WFS informed about news, projects, new groups forming, and the new e-newsletter. Subscribers can choose to receive only the information that interests them by requesting special interest selections. Designed by WFS headquarters staff, the E-mail Updates Service is private, secure, and free.

Reaching out to an even greater audience, WFS created a Facebook page in 2011 so that women have another way to keep in touch with the organization. A member of the WFS Board of Directors posts a weekly recovery statement about which women may make comments.

Sobering Thoughts Newsletter

The 35 years during which the WFS newsletter, *Sobering Thoughts,* was published monthly represent thousands of pages of positive messages, practical tips, and insights into the recovery process, written by WFS women for other women in recovery. At first, Kirkpatrick authored and edited newsletter contents and continued this practice until her passing; however, early on, she expanded the newsletter so that each issue also offers opportunities for members to submit personal comments and articles on various recovery topics.

In 2011, subscriptions reached women using the WFS program in not only the United States and Canada, but also in Australia, Bermuda, China, England, Finland, France, Germany, Iceland, Ireland, Israel, New Zealand, Northern Ireland, Scotland, South Africa, Sweden, and Switzerland. Recognizing the signs that the traditional newsletter publication method was becoming outdated, WFS transformed *Sobering Thoughts* into an e-newsletter format, so that it is currently available electronically, free of charge. Although it has been less than a year since the change, e-subscriptions have already reached 3 times the former paper subscription rate.

Sources of Funds

WFS remains unfunded by any outside agencies or grants; consequently, fundraising remains an ongoing challenge. Fortunately, the ability to provide most WFS resources and services free of charge is made possible in large part because of the generosity of members. For example, the costs of the WFS Web site and software, the online bookstore and shopping cart, and the online forum and its ongoing management were all created and continue to be supported by donations from several creative and generous individual members. Overall, WFS continues to derive its operating income from three main sources: donations from individuals and WFS groups, including an automatic monthly deduction feature; sales of program materials and other recovery-support materials; and profits from the annual conference and fundraising auction held each June.

DEMOGRAPHICS: WHO USES WFS?

How is success measured? Can success be measured? In self-help organizations, measures of success are hard to determine, because evaluation depends not only on the quality of a given program but also on the determination of individuals using it. Consequently, few research studies have been conducted on self-help recovery programs because of the difficulty in developing scientifically valid testing instruments (Kaskutas, 1996a, p. 78). Nevertheless, WFS points to a number of statistics that help support its claims of continuing relevance, based on comparative information compiled from two surveys conducted 20 years apart, in 1991 and 2011.

In 1991, Dr. Lee Kaskutas worked with Kirkpatrick to develop the first formal survey conducted on the WFS membership. At that time, the entire membership of the organization was surveyed. Participation was anonymous and voluntary. Moderators of the 125 WFS groups in the United States and Canada distributed survey questionnaires at their groups' weekly meetings. WFS members were permitted to take their surveys home to complete, and they were also provided with a stamped, preaddressed envelope in which to mail their responses back. This approach generated 600 usable responses. Twenty years later in 2011, the WFS organization conducted its own internal survey of its membership. Again, participation was anonymous and voluntary, and members were invited to complete the survey electronically online. A total of 671 usable responses were obtained by this method. Please note that in some cases, percentages given in the survey data equal more than 100%, because survey participants were given the opportunity to select more than one reason or preference for their responses.

Comparison of the demographic information from the two surveys provides some insight on the typical 4C women[2] who use the WFS program and also shows how aspects of their profiles, motivations, preferences, and recovery resources have both changed and also, in some important ways, remained consistent over time. Results also reveal how the WFS organization has fared over time in terms of maintaining its essential identity and message.

Age

In Kaskutas's survey, respondents were on average 46 years of age (ranging from ages 23 to 78 years), and 53% were aged 45 years and older (Kaskutas, 1996a, p. 86). In 2011, only 13% of respondents are younger than age 40; the largest single age group is 51 to 60 years old and represents 41% of the survey replies. Consequently, with 75% of respondents older than age 40, it appears that the WFS program continues to find its greatest appeal among women of early middle age. In addition, both surveys show that the majority of WFS members are Caucasian.

Marital Status

Half of the members in the 1991 survey were married (53%) and many had children, while 29% were divorced, separated, or single (Kaskutas, 1996a, p. 87). A greater percentage of WFS women are married today—a total of 61%—and 63% indicated that they have children. Showing a slight increase, 32% of those in last year's survey are single, separated, or divorced. While marital status remains fairly consistent in both surveys and across 20 years, there is a slight increase in the most recent survey in both married and divorced/single numbers.

Work Status

In 1991, 47% of the survey participants were employed full-time; 19% were part-time employees; and 9% were self-employed. In total, then, 75% of the women surveyed were employed in a formal job situation (Kaskutas, 1996a, p. 87). Kirkpatrick commented at the time that this percentage of employed women indicated definite progress regarding women's changing roles and their access to employment outside the home. In the 2011 WFS survey, full-time employment showed a decline from 1991, with only 42% of participants working full-time. Part-time employment accounted for 12%; and self-employed represented another 14%. In total, then, at 68% of participants, employment in 2011 showed a 7% decline after 20 years. One immediate explanation that comes to mind as a cause is the recent economic downturn and concomitant loss of jobs, which resulted in 6% of survey respondents indicating that they are currently unemployed. Less visible were some of the unpaid positions given by the participants, including student (2%), retired (12%), homemaker (10%), and on disability (3%).

Family Alcoholism

Not surprisingly, the incidence of alcoholism in survey participants' families was high in the Kaskutas survey (Kirkpatrick, 1992, p. 4) and was similarly high 20 years later in the WFS survey; however, during the span of two decades, there were concerning increases—roughly 10%—in the number of participants with alcoholic mothers and fathers. A majority (48% in 1991 and 58% in 2011) had alcoholic fathers; fewer reported alcoholic mothers (22% in 1991 and 30% in 2011); and the number with alcoholic siblings remained almost the same (50% in 1991 and 48% in 2011).

Other Addictions

Some women alcoholics in the 1991 survey reported that they were also dealing with other addictions (Kirkpatrick, 1992, p. 7). Twenty-six percent were also addicted to drugs, and 47% smoked cigarettes. In comparison, the WFS survey respondents 20 years later indicated that 20% are addicted to street and/or prescription drugs, and 33% smoke cigarettes. Perhaps the noticeable decrease in smoking would indicate that smoking cessation efforts and ongoing media attention to the health risks have had an impact on smokers.

Education Level

In the Kaskutas study, 22% of participants attended or finished high school (Kaskutas, 1996a, p. 87). Although 20 years later the high school level shows a drop in survey participants (11%), the number of women attending or finishing college in the WFS group (54%) remains very close to the number in the original survey (52%). Also, interestingly, the number of women who chose to continue their education by attending or completing graduate school is slightly higher, increasing from 26% in the original study to 35% in the 2011 study.

Overall

Summarizing the demographic makeup of her survey respondents, Kaskutas observed that the WFS approach to recovery is especially attractive to mostly middle-aged, well-educated, White women (Kaskutas, 1996a, p. 87). Interestingly, her description applies equally well to the women participating in last year's survey, a result indicative of the consistent, ongoing appeal of the program's philosophy and message to women in that particular demographic profile during a 20-year time span. Some have labeled the WFS program as a "thinking woman's program"; and to an extent, this description fits when one considers that it is a woman's thoughts, focused intently on making positive changes, that are responsible for her willingness to follow through and attain her goal. Similarly, willingness to think in new ways is necessary considering the program's emphasis on introspection, analysis, and problem resolution. WFS believes any woman can apply the power of her mind to effect positive change, provided that she is determined and actually wants to change.

MOTIVATIONS, TURNING POINTS, AND PREFERENCES

Why Women Drink: Reasons They Turn to Alcohol/Drugs

A fundamental part of the WFS philosophy is that women have different needs in recovery compared with their male counterparts, because they drink for different reasons, gender-based reasons, and therefore require different treatment strategies. Kaskutas did not include a specific question on her 1991 survey regarding why participants drank. However, in an article during the same time period based on other research, Kaskutas assembled a number of reasons why women drink, which, like Kirkpatrick, she felt were "associated with sexuality and gender roles" (Kaskutas, 1994, p. 186). The WFS 2011 survey did include the "why" question, so some meaningful comparison across the two decades is possible.

The role of alcohol as a social lubricant has not changed; Kaskutas mentioned reasons in this vein, which included: to get along socially, on dates, to feel more womanly. Comparably, in the 2011 survey, roughly 60% of respondents said they drank to get high or have fun, or to be sociable. Also continuing large on the list is drinking to fill emotional needs, which 59% mentioned on the 2011 survey. Feelings of inadequacy and worthlessness, both as an individual and as a woman, were also key reasons for drinking in Kaskutas's investigations (Kaskutas, 1996c, p. 274); similarly, 50% of women in the 2011 survey said they drank to counter feelings of worthlessness, guilt, and shame and to booster their self-confidence.

Kaskutas also included response to family problems/relationships as a reason women drank—a reason that still ranks high with the 2011 WFS members, at 50%. Another reason for drinking mentioned in Kaskutas's list is in response to sexual or physical abuse; unfortunately, the same reason exists in 2011, although it was mentioned by only 20% of the survey respondents. Interestingly, although it would certainly be a corollary lurking behind all her previous reasons, Kaskutas did not specifically mention that women drink because of stress (Kaskutas, 1994, p. 185). However, 60% of respondents in the 2011 survey mentioned that they began drinking to reduce stress, help them relax, and help them sleep.

Notice that all of these reasons, and their similarity past and present, suggest an underlying feeling of inadequacy; that is, the lack of self-esteem that Kirkpatrick posited was at the heart of women's relationships with alcohol. Because of low self-esteem, women start drinking and the result becomes a downward spiral of alcoholism, even more negative feelings, and consequences.

Why/When Did They Seek Help?

Participants in both surveys were asked what prompted them to seek help with their addictions. A number of reasons were indicated, but in both cases, the outstanding reason mentioned by survey participants was loss of control over their drinking/drugging, as well as the feeling that they and their lives were likewise out of control (Kaskutas, 1996b, p. 266). This situation as a primary reason was mentioned by just 20% of WFS members in 1991, but it has risen to a whopping 80% among women in the 2011 survey. Physical signs and health issues were also important motivators in both surveys, with women listing several specifics (blackouts, cirrhosis, withdrawal, and feeling sick) in the 1991 survey (which collectively amount to about a 30% cumulative response). The later survey showed a similar concern (40%) with health issues (which were not itemized). Emotional issues (53%) were more significant reasons for seeking help in the 2011 survey, compared with only 29% who mentioned this category as causative in 1991.

Less significant motivational factors appeared to be fairly constant in both surveys. For example, 20% of both survey groups felt that family/life problems caused them to seek help; further, legal issues, such as citations for driving under the influence, remained as a change agent, but at only 8% in both survey groups. Similarly, exposure to others with the same problem motivated about 6% of women in both surveys.

Two other reasons for seeking help showed mirror-opposite changes among survey participants, possibly because of societal changes during the two intervening decades. Work issues as a catalyst for change moved only 6% of survey respondents in 1991, but today's women expressed greater concern about their jobs, with 15% of respondents mentioning this factor as a reason for change. With the opposite result, only 6% of women in the 2011 survey cited intervention as a motivating tactic for them to seek help, while intervention seemed to be more frequently attempted in 1991, based on mention by 15% of the respondents.

Early in her work with women using the WFS program, Kirkpatrick mentioned the average age for this "awakening" to the need for help as being 55 years old (Kirkpatrick, 1984, p. 2). The survey results in 1991 showed a slightly earlier average age, at 46 years old (Kaskutas, 1996b, p. 265). And the WFS survey in 2011 showed the change occurred in a similar but somewhat younger age group, the 41- to 50-year-olds.

How Did They Find WFS?

In addition to questioning survey participants about what caused them to recognize their need to change, women in both surveys were also asked about their main resource in choosing WFS, among several potential communications pathways. Although two decades apart, the majority of the women tested said that they found WFS and decided to try it based on self-referral, a personal decision; they found WFS on their own. Before the growth of the Internet, women in the 1991 survey relied on what they had found through media sources (24%), such as newspapers, magazines, books, television, radio—possibly because of Kirkpatrick's frequent exposure in these media, as well as the growing interest at that time in women's alcoholism as a topic for debate (Kaskutas, 1996b, p. 271). The 2011 results revealed that the overwhelming majority of women still find WFS on their own, now primarily through an Internet search (52%), with the other media currently representing only 16% of their information resources.

In addition, 23% of the women in the Kaskutas survey (1992a) cited WFS literature as their main resource; however, reflecting profound changes in communication preferences, now only 5% located WFS through its literature. Information gained through concerned family members and friends was the source for more than one quarter of the women in the first survey, compared with apparently much smaller direct communication efforts by family and friends in 2011, a path which represented only 6% of those surveyed as a route for finding WFS (Kaskutas, 1996c, p. 271).

In the Kaskutas study (1992a), 34% found WFS through professional resources, such as counselors, treatment facilities, and personal physicians. Significantly, however, professional referrals are the least frequently cited source for finding WFS in 2011, representing only 17% of participants. Among professional referrals overall, women's personal physicians finished last in both surveys, at 5% of physicians in 1991 and only 2% in 2011. What appears to be a decline in professional referrals in the more recent survey may be a function of the rise of the Internet as a "first response" when women are seeking help on their own; today's women most frequently investigate resources to meet their needs by going online, quite possibly even before they seek professional help (Kaskutas, 1996b, pp. 272–273).

Length of Sober Time Versus Length of Time in WFS

The chart in Table 1 compares the length of sober time for each survey's participants 20 years apart and compares the length of sober time with the participants' respective length of time as WFS members (Kaskutas, 1992a, p. 4). Notice the percentages for both sobriety time and time as a member, especially when the length of time measured is less than a year. The similarity seems to indicate that the majority of newcomers to the WFS program are also newcomers to sobriety; in addition, these very similar percentages seem

TABLE 1

	Length of Sobriety Time			
	Less than 1 year	1 year to 1 year and 11 months	2 years to 4 years	5 years or more
In 1991	35%	14%	25%	26%
In 2011	48%	20%	13%	24%
	Length of Time as WFS Member			
	Less than 1 year	1 year to 1 year and 11 months	2 years to 4 years	5 years or more
In 1991	45%	15%	24%	17%
In 2011	47%	20%	11%	20%

to confirm that for these newcomers, their most recent continuous sobriety time came as a result of their time in the WFS program.

Although similar percentages continue through the years, the 5-year mark in both sobriety and membership is apparently some form of watershed point for these women, because thereafter, although both sober time and membership time percentages remain similar in both surveys, the numbers do indicate a decrease after 5 years. Looking at the percentages another way, with 74% of respondents in 1991 and 91% in 2011 having less than 5 years of sobriety time, the discrepancy after the 5-year point becomes more apparent. Similarly, if one looks at the combined amount of WFS membership less than 5 years—84% in 1991 and 78% in 2011—a similar discrepancy also occurs.

Notice also that even though surveyed two decades apart, many women come to WFS having already achieved some sobriety, a result that indicates that they have probably tried other avenues of recovery beforehand; in addition, the result may also suggest that women are drawn to the WFS tenets with their emphasis on the need for positive thinking, the importance of self-esteem, and the notion of taking responsibility for their addictions—whether they are looking for a different recovery approach, something for additional "sobriety insurance," or simply seeking something different that will help them continue to move forward in their journey. Some WFS members who have previously used a 12-step program express this phenomenon when they say that AA got them sober, but WFS keeps them sober (Kaskutas, 1992a, p. 13).

Relapses

Reflecting the WFS belief that views recovery as a process that takes time, determination, and practice, the organization's reaction to relapses encourages women to see such backsliding incidents as unfortunate, but primarily as a learning opportunity; that is, relapse can help them uncover situations or triggers that result in their automatic drinking response. Further, these discoveries also provide an opportunity to make plans for handling the situation or trigger when it reoccurs and to be prepared to implement a planned defense. Likewise, rather than chastising themselves or feeling organizational or fellow-member disapproval, women are advised to mentally pick themselves up, start over, and move forward, until sobriety eventually sticks. In other words, relapse is not failure; failure is when one ceases to try.

Also, the WFS approach to relapse may reflect Kirkpatrick's own personal trial-and-error experience before creating her program. Furthermore, the WFS position allows for more tolerance of relapse because of its cognitive-behavioral basis, which views addiction as a habit, an automatic situational response; therefore, replacing this coping mechanism with new habits of sobriety is expected to require considerable repetition and practice, as well as focus and determination, before a new, more desirable behavior becomes equally habitual.

Statistically, in the Kaskutas study (1996b, p. 275–276), about 33% of participants experienced a relapse after joining WFS; in comparison, a surprising 50% of women in the 2011 survey have experienced a relapse after becoming a WFS member. To offset that concerning comparative statistic, however, notice that a much larger number of the 2011 respondents (80%) had experienced relapse(s) before they found WFS, a fact that indicates that 30% did not have any relapses after joining. As anticipated in both surveys, relapse occurred more frequently among the "pure" newcomers—that is, those women who are both newcomers to sobriety and newcomers to the WFS approach. In addition, about equal numbers in both surveys reported that they either had taken or were still currently taking medication, including Antabuse, to assist them in their recovery (e.g., for cravings or withdrawal symptoms). These numbers, however, represented only a small percentage in each survey, 10% in 1991 and 7% in 2011 (Kaskutas, 1996b, p. 274).

Treatment Resources Found Most Beneficial in Getting Sober

In both surveys, WFS is the most desirable resource for getting sober; further, the preference and the percentage have increased during the 20-year time period, a result that tends to indicate the WFS program's continuing appeal. For example, based on their personal experience in pursuing recovery, in 1991, 45% of women surveyed felt that WFS was most beneficial in helping them achieve sobriety (Kirkpatrick, 1992, p. 1); in 2011, almost double that number, 89%, came to the same conclusion.

Other methods attempted were felt to be less beneficial in achieving sobriety. Women in the original survey placed AA considerably further behind, at 11%; this ranking fell below their preference for inpatient treatment (17%) but above their preference for outpatient treatment (8%) as helpful resources. Based on their pursuit of recovery, women in the 2011 survey moved 12-step programs ahead a bit to 14% preference, still much below the WFS mark, but were much less satisfied with inpatient treatment (at 7%) and slightly more satisfied with outpatient treatment (10%).

Another question that both surveys asked involves what the survey participants found most beneficial from attending WFS; or asked another way: *What do women get out of attending WFS?* Kaskutas asked this as an open-ended question, which generated many different individual responses; she grouped the five most-frequently mentioned reasons as follows (Kaskutas, 1994, p. 191): At the top of the list (54%), most women felt that WFS gave them support and nurturance. Another 42% appreciated the ability to share women's issues with other women; further, 39% found the focus on self-esteem and self-reliance most beneficial, and 38% appreciated the program's positive emphasis. A bit further behind, 26% of participants found it beneficial to be in a safe environment where they could speak freely.

Looking at what women in the 2011 survey found most beneficial about WFS, the percentages that indicated the ongoing appeal of WFS are even greater in the more recent survey. Note, however, that in this more recent survey, the topic was not open-ended, so a limited number of selections were offered, although participants could select as many as applied. This approach tends to concentrate the choices rather than diffusing the possible answers as in the 1991 survey. Nevertheless, survey participants were still consistent about the WFS appeal, with an overwhelming 88% who stated its benefit is because the program encourages positive thinking and letting go of the past; an additional 87% said it was the program's emphasis on self-empowerment; 77% cited its women-only approach; and 75% pointed to its promotion of emotional and spiritual growth. Reason 5 on the 2011 survey, interestingly, did not make the top five in the Kaskutas survey (1992a); in 2011, 74% of respondents said that they found WFS most beneficial because the program can be applied to life in general, not just to recovery.

As a counterpoint to get at the previous question in a different way (i.e., what women get out of attending WFS), Kaskutas also asked a related question in her survey, phrased as, *Why did the participants choose not to attend AA?* This was another open-ended question that prompted at least 25 different reasons. Some of the most frequently cited reasons were: not comfortable, didn't fit in at AA (20%); AA was too negative (18%); didn't like the religious/God part (15%); and AA was too male-oriented, geared toward men's needs (15%). A final 15% said that WFS offers more support, understanding, and growth opportunities. Although all of these answers are posed in the negative (i.e., what they did *not* get or did *not* find beneficial from AA), by surmising the opposite of each of these responses, one comes back to most of the same positive reasons why women chose WFS, an interesting approach to a double check (Kaskutas, 1994, p. 191–192). However, the 2011 survey did not ask a comparable question of its participants.

The 2011 survey did ask a further refinement of the question, *What did you find most beneficial about WFS?*, by asking respondents which of the resources that WFS offers have proved most beneficial to them on a daily/weekly basis. As anticipated, by far, the most useful resource cited is the online forum, at 86%, because logging into the online forum offers opportunities to read, post, reach out for support, encourage other members, and/or participate in an online chat. Another useful practice mentioned, at 59%, is actively applying the acceptance statements throughout the day; and not too far behind is the 37% who find morning meditations and journaling with the acceptance statements useful. Other beneficial aspects of the WFS program are daily reading of the WFS Program Booklet or other WFS literature; and although the actual number of face-to-face groups nationwide is comparatively small, attending face-to-face meetings is mentioned by 30% as beneficial on a weekly basis. No similar question refining specific WFS resources was asked in the Kaskutas survey (1992a).

WFS and Religion

Another topic Kaskutas chose to explore among WFS members was their spiritual beliefs and practices as they related to WFS and sources of sobriety. Her preliminary expectation was twofold: Because many survey participants said they joined WFS because they disliked AA's emphasis on God in the recovery equation, then the lack of emphasis on God must be part of the WFS program's appeal. Therefore, women attracted to WFS should be a more agnostic or atheistic, less spiritually oriented group than were women in recovery who pursued other approaches to sobriety, especially those women who had participated in AA (Kaskutas, 1992a, p. 11).

However, Kaskutas's initial assumption proved *not* to be the case. In her survey, participants represent many religious affiliations, including 63% Christian, 16% Other (Jewish, Eastern, other), with only 20% indicating no religion/agnostic. Further, of those who worshipped, 63% said they did so at least annually; and 37% said they worshipped as often as weekly or several times per month (Kirkpatrick, 1992, p. 7). Like the previous survey, 2011 survey results support that the majority of WFS members are religious or believe in God. Again, Christian members were the largest category of survey participants, at 47%. The "Other" category shows an increase, at 35%, perhaps reflecting a trend for women seeking spiritual growth to explore other than traditional religious approaches. And finally, those women who identified themselves as atheist/agnostic declined to 17%. Kirkpatrick has explained why WFS members' religious dimensions prove the exception to what might be reasonably expected. She said:

> It's not that the women in WFS are any less believers in [G]od—they are not. You aren't going to find that fewer of our members believe in [G]od, or that fewer of our members have religious or spiritual commitment. What is important is that unlike AA, WFS members do not base their sobriety on [G]od or on religious beliefs. Spirituality does not equate to sobriety in WFS. Belief in [G]od does not equate to sobriety in WFS. But our members do care about spirituality, and they do believe in [G]od. At least, many of them do. The difference is that their sobriety is not based upon that belief and that belief alone. (Kaskutas, 1992a, p. 11)

Professionals and Referrals

A number of women in both surveys turned to professionals for help, both before and after trying other avenues of recovery on their own. Exclusive of mutual help, these professional services include one-on-one therapy, group therapy led by a professional, inpatient treatment, and outpatient treatment. Further, it is often through professional treatment providers that clients are given referrals to mutual-help programs as part of their ongoing recovery plans. In the 1991 survey, only 13% of the participants were referred to WFS by a treatment facility, possibly because of less recognition of and little experience with the newer program (Kaskutas, 1996a, p. 86). Proportionately, more than twice that percentage of respondents (27%) in a 1992 triennial AA survey (Kaskutas, 1996b, p. 266) indicated that they were referred to AA by a treatment facility. Similarly, in the WFS (2011) survey, 40% of the women who had gone to a counselor were referred to WFS, again compared with twice that percentage (80%) referred by individual counselors to AA.

In the 1991 survey (Kaskutas, 1996b, p. 271), the four most frequently cited sources for finding WFS were self-referral (40%); media, at that time newspaper, radio, or television (31%); family, friends, or neighbors (25%); and counselor or treatment facility (29%). However, in this 1991 survey, participants were limited to only two choices among the referral sources provided. Comparing again AA's 1992 survey, the major ways individuals found AA were through treatment or counseling (36%), another AA member (34%), self-referral (29%), and family (21%) (Kaskutas, 1996b, p. 271). Results show that professional referrals (36%) were most frequently responsible for individuals coming to AA, compared with professional referrals as the impetus in the Kaskutas survey (1992b); (29%). Interesting also is that in the AA survey, self-referral (29%) occurred less frequently than did professional referrals; however, in the Kaskutas survey, the percentage of self-referral was much higher (40%; Kaskutas, 1996b, pp. 272–273).

In 2011, however, the main way to locate self- and mutual-help resources, according to the WFS women in the survey, is through their own efforts, primarily directed at the Internet (52%) and to a lesser extent through other media (16%). As a result then, 68% of the survey respondents reflect the preference for using information technology personally to find referrals, rather than depending on other sources. Counselors and treatment facilities fell far behind with only 15% of survey participants citing them as a referral source, about the same frequency as referrals from friends and family.

Currently, the WFS organization's contact with professionals or facilities seeking information is almost exclusively via e-mail, with a small number who still call for direct conversation. These professionals are given general instructions about obtaining group-meeting information and other information for themselves and their women clients. WFS does not give specific meeting information on the Internet because of confidentiality concerns, out of consideration for group participants and for the group moderators. Instead, WFS prefers that women in need contact the organization directly for group and other information, rather than through an intermediary source, given the importance for women seeking help to assume responsibility for pursuing their recovery. Further, the contact procedure helps ensure that women will receive the most current local meeting information; for example, once a woman has gathered the courage to try attending a group, how unfortunate if she should go to a location and find an empty room because the meeting has been temporarily relocated or rescheduled.

Similarly, because lists can become quickly outdated, professionals are discouraged from compiling such resources for local WFS information unless they have specific permission to do so from the women involved. Rather, professionals are advised to direct their women clients to the WFS Web site, where clients can complete and submit an e-mail "request for information" form to receive local group-meeting and other information. For immediate information, a phone call remains the fastest way, either from the client's home or from the professional's office. Also emphasized with professionals is that women can be successful using the WFS positive self-help approach without attending formal group meetings, given that Kirkpatrick designed the program with that specific flexibility in mind. Professionals are also referred to the WFS Web site for more detailed and free downloadable information.

WFS communications with professionals also ask if there is any interest in starting a WFS group for the benefit of their women clients. Many counseling professionals believe—erroneously—that they must be in recovery themselves to start a WFS group. That requirement is true for individual women in recovery seeking certification, but not so for addictions counseling professionals. Obviously, WFS expects professionals to conduct WFS meetings according to its guidelines; however, the requirements and process for starting groups are more streamlined for professionals and treatment facilities. The intention is to allow faster startup for these groups. Professionals who lead a WFS group do not need to be in recovery themselves, nor are they required to use the WFS program personally. Very important, however, they do need to be *women* to lead a WFS group. To have other than same-sex facilitators is contrary to the WFS philosophy that the needs and issues of women and men vary greatly in recovery. Most importantly, before professionals start a group, WFS requires that they read Kirkpatrick's book *Turnabout* (Kirkpatrick, 1997), which describes her personal struggle with alcohol and how she came to create WFS, as well as her philosophy and objectives regarding the "New Life" Program and its use.

For groups in treatment facilities, WFS applies a "blanket" approach, in which the facility purchases a professional group starter kit for staff professionals to use and the facility retains the certification to conduct WFS meetings. This blanket accommodation provides the flexibility for any counselor in the facility who understands the WFS program to facilitate the WFS meetings. In some cases, professionals eventually turn over leadership of a group to one of the women in the group, provided she meets the WFS minimum certification requirements for individuals in recovery and is recommended by the counselor. This approach works well for professionals who have neither the time nor the desire to make a long-term commitment to leading a WFS meeting but are willing to help get one started in areas where face-to-face resources are lacking. Once necessary materials are purchased and a group is ready to start, WFS is willing to send an experienced group moderator to visit the facility and demonstrate how WFS groups are conducted, provided a moderator is available within a reasonable traveling distance. WFS offers a group starter kit designed for use by professionals in treatment facilities. Packets are likewise available and provide basic materials to help clients learn to use the "New Life" Program while attending a WFS group.

In the new century—and perhaps coincidentally as more women have chosen to enter the addictions treatment and counseling professions—WFS has experienced a steady increase in professionals and facilities seeking to refer clients to WFS groups and exploring the WFS approach as a potential treatment solution for women clients who do not like or do not respond well to the 12-step method. Also, in the increasing number of states that require court-mandated attendance in treatment and/or support groups, the WFS program is recognized as a secular treatment alternative to religious-based programs. These promising trends may reflect recognition of the need for and value of multiple treatment solutions and choices for effective recovery. In addition, the Internet has become a powerful tool for referrals and education, both for women who are self-referring and interested counselors, facilities, or researchers (Kaskutas, 1996b, p. 277).

CONCLUSIONS

WFS continues to flourish in the dozen years since the founder's passing, and the program has remained faithful to Kirkpatrick's original vision and goals. In 2011, with the goal of continuing relevance, the WFS Board of Directors unanimously approved a revision of Kirkpatrick's "Statement of Purpose," a document which, except for minor adjustments, had remained essentially unchanged since she created it in 1975. The resulting "WFS Mission Statement" repeats the organization's original core purpose and focus in an updated version for the new century.

WFS MISSION STATEMENT

'A Mission Statement for the New Century'

Women for Sobriety (WFS) is an organization whose purpose is to help all women find their individual path to recovery through discovery of self, gained by sharing experiences, hopes and encouragement with other women in similar circumstances. We are an abstinence-based self-help program for women facing issues of alcohol or drug addiction. Our 'New Life' Program acknowledges the very special needs women have in recovery—the need to nurture feelings of self-value and self-worth and the desire to discard feelings of guilt, shame, and humiliation.

WFS is unique in that it is an organization of women for women. We are not affiliated with any other recovery organization and stand on our own principles and philosophies. We recognize each woman's necessity for self-discovery. WFS offers a variety of recovery tools to guide a woman in developing coping skills which focus on emotional growth, spiritual growth, self-esteem, and a healthy lifestyle. Our vision is to encourage all women in developing personal growth and continued abstinence through the 'New Life' Program.

WFS believes that addiction began to overcome stress, loneliness, frustration or emotional deprivation in daily life—dependence often resulted. Physical, mental, and emotional addiction are overcome with abstinence and the knowledge of self gained through the principles and philosophies of WFS. Membership in WFS requires a sincere desire for an abstinent 'New Life.' WFS members live by the philosophy: 'Release the past—plan for tomorrow—live for today.'

Revised: June 10, 2011

WFS Board of Directors

The success of WFS and its "New Life" Program is vetted by the organization's ability to survive and remain meaningful, as indicated by its almost 40 years in existence and by survey data spanning 20 years, as well as success stories and positive feedback from women using the program through the years. Its longevity has occurred without agency funding or grants, accomplished largely through consistent support from its members, in spite of economic downturns and the incredible speed of change. And yet, a misconception still seems to persist that because the organization is smaller and does not have as much "name recognition" in the public eye, it must be somehow less valuable. The reality is that WFS has maintained its relevance and continues to succeed as an *important alternative recovery choice for women*, despite its modest, low-key—but determined—profile.

Consider, for example, that WFS by its stated mission limits its own appeal; because it is an organization and program developed by a woman for other women—and it remains the only self-help organization designed specifically for women—logically it can appeal to only half the total population. Further, of the potential women-only audience, WFS seems to be found most appealing by a specific demographic segment. Similarly, the

WFS philosophy also requires what amounts to a complete redesign of these women's perspectives about themselves and their lives, an effort that may not be appealing or acceptable to all women. However, rather than designing the program as a way to ensure lifelong dependence on the organization, in keeping with its belief in choices, WFS encourages women to find and use an approach that works best for them. Consequently, in terms of sheer bulk, WFS can never realistically match the size of 12-step organizations. However, it is erroneous to conclude based on its size that WFS is a "less popular" alternative.

The continuing stigmatization of addiction, and of women addicts in particular, contributes to the low-key profile of WFS. Although progress has been made during the past 40 years, this stigma still exists in society, and it is felt even more keenly in the guilt- and shame-ridden minds of the women addicts themselves. As a consequence, anonymity often remains a woman's choice, and the women who choose WFS may be reluctant to reveal their addiction. In other words, women may be more willing to seek help than are men, but they may also be less willing to talk about their efforts publicly and prefer to shun the spotlight. Also, limited resources restrict WFS access to the wide exposure afforded by advertising in major media markets; likewise, free publicity through feature-type media interest is limited, without a professional publicist to pursue these venues. And finally, WFS tends to receive less attention and exposure from the national-level recovery organizations, which have been more familiar with and more invested over time in the 12-step approach, because it aims at both men and women and thus offers wider appeal.

In reality, the WFS approach to recovery has increased in popularity because it fills the now-recognized need for customized recovery alternatives. Likewise, WFS is immensely popular through its Internet resources, and this popularity will continue as a major way to spread the word about the organization's approach to women in recovery. Remember, as well, that Kirkpatrick always viewed WFS—and the organization still views itself—as "offering a self-help choice in the community—in competition neither with AA nor with other treatment options" (Kaskutas, 1994, p. 193). This consistent attitude of coexistence, not competition, has revealed itself as a wise business decision, as well as a key reason for the program's longevity. In the face of an older, larger organization with a much wider appeal, Kirkpatrick and WFS management since her time have successfully positioned WFS as a niche organization, providing a valuable service as a treatment alternative for certain women: those who may be more successful using a different, for-women-only strategy for their recovery; those women who find a 12-step approach is not the right fit; and those women who are looking for a different way to enrich and enhance their ongoing recovery efforts.

When Jean Kirkpatrick's writings were first penned in the 1970s and 1980s, the feminist movement and concern with women's issues were just beginning to gain serious attention, and the instant information revolution was just starting to gain momentum. As a result, some of her earliest work may sound a bit dated today, because she describes certain societal perspectives about the roles of men and women that may seem somewhat outdated; after all, societal mores as well as communication technologies have moved forward since that time. Some societal "carryover" issues do remain, though (e.g., the continuing stigma attached to women addicts); but women today face additional challenges that are unique to the new century and a new generation, women raised with different values, expectations, and pressures.

With its focus on taking personal responsibility, empowerment, and positive thinking, WFS and its message resonate even more consistently and meaningfully with the needs and beliefs of many women who are struggling with addiction today. With their gifts of empowerment, self-respect, and spiritual and emotional growth, the 13 affirmation statements are just as relevant for women today as they were when created in 1975, and they will continue to be relevant for women seeking recovery in the future. Jean Kirkpatrick's message remains timeless, and the WFS program is evergreen, a guide for life and for living beyond its proven effectiveness for women in recovery.

NOTES

1. Throughout the article, the descriptions of and discussion of the WFS organization, its program, philosophy, and other WFS-specific content reflect the views and writings of WFS founder Dr. Jean Kirkpatrick and the organization today; further, unless it is specifically noted otherwise in the text, information comes in most part from the body of written materials produced and copyrighted by WFS since its inception.

2. The term "4C" refers to the four qualities emphasized in the WFS motto: capable, competent, caring, compassionate. To be a 4C woman is to be part of the sisterhood of WFS.

REFERENCES

Kaskutas, L.A. (1989). Women for Sobriety: A qualitative analysis. *Contemporary Drug Problems, 16*, 177–200.

Kaskutas, L.A. (1992a). Results from a survey of Women for Sobriety, 1991 (unpublished summary produced for WFS). From *An Analysis of Women for Sobriety,* doctoral dissertation, University of California, Berkeley.

Kaskutas, L.A. (1992b). Beliefs on the source of sobriety: Interactions of membership in Women for Sobriety and AA. *Contemporary Drug Problems, 19*, 631–648.

Kaskutas, L.A. (1994). What do women get out of self help? Their reasons for attending Women for Sobriety and AA. *Journal of Substance Abuse Treatment, 11* (3), 185–195.

Kaskutas, L. A. (1996a). A road less traveled: Choosing the Women for Sobriety program. *Journal of Drug Issues, 26*, (1), 77–94.

Kaskutas, L. A. (1996b). Pathways to self-help among Women for Sobriety. *American Journal of Drug and Alcohol Abuse, 22* (2), 259–280.

Kaskutas, L.A. (1996c). Predictors of self esteem among members of Women for Sobriety. *Addiction Research*, *4* (3), 273–281.

Kirkpatrick, J. (1976). Program note. *Sobering Thoughts*, *1*, 4.

Kirkpatrick, J. (1977). *Turnabout: New Help for the Woman Alcoholic*. New York: Bantam.

Kirkpatrick, J. (1984). Some answers about us. *Sobering Thoughts*, *6*, 1–2.

Kirkpatrick, J. (1992). A Report on the First-Ever Survey of the WFS Membership (Unpublished conference presentation). WFS Annual Conference; Cedar Crest College, Allentown PA, June 1992.

Part II: Mutual Support Groups for Addiction for Specific Populations

Ethnic-Specific Support Systems as a Method for Sustaining Long-Term Addiction Recovery

ARTHUR C. EVANS, JR and IJEOMA ACHARA-ABRAHAMS
Philadelphia Department of Behavioral Health & Intellectual Disability Services, Philadelphia, Pennsylvania, USA

ROLAND LAMB
Office of Addiction Services, Philadelphia Department of Behavioral Health & Intellectual Disability Services, Philadelphia, Pennsylvania, USA

WILLIAM L. WHITE
Lighthouse Institute, Chestnut Health Systems, Punta Gorda, Florida, USA

Although addiction-recovery mutual-aid support groups have grown dramatically and now span secular, spiritual, and religious frameworks of recovery, most of what is known from the standpoint of science about these groups is based on the early participation of treated populations in Alcoholics Anonymous. Many questions remain about the effects of participation in other mutual-aid groups and different pathways and styles of recovery within and across diverse ethnic groups. This article reviews existing data on ethnic group participation in recovery mutual-aid groups, summarizes the history of culturally indigenous recovery movements within Native American and African American communities in the United States, and describes strategies aimed at increasing recovery prevalence and the quality of life in recovery for persons of color in Philadelphia, PA.

INTRODUCTION

The prevalence of alcohol and other drug (AOD) use and related problems and access to and participation in treatment and recovery support resources are not equally distributed across racial/ethnic groups in the United States (Caetano, Baruah, & Chartier, 2011; Chartier & Caetano, 2011; Mulia, Ye, Greenfield, & Zemore, 2009; Wallace, 1999). Although non-Whites experience remission from substance use disorders at rates comparable to Whites (Arndt, Vélez, Segre, & Clayton, 2010), AOD problems within communities of color have been historically portrayed in the mainstream media through a lens of pathology rather than through the perspectives of resilience, resistance, and recovery (White & Sanders, 2008). Pejorative racial stereotypes long embedded within antidrug campaigns in the United States have misrepresented the source, scope, and solutions to AOD-related problems within communities of color (Helmer, 1975; Leland, 1976; Musto, 1973; Neuspiel, 1996). If there is a yet-untold addictions-related story at public and professional levels, it is the rich tradition through which communities of color have actively resisted the infusion of alcohol and drugs into their cultures, adapted mainstream recovery support resources for cultural fit, and mounted indigenous responses to the rise of AOD-related problems (Coyhis & White, 2006; James & Johnson, 1996; White & Sanders, 2002; White, Sanders, & Sanders, 2006).

This article: (1) reviews the diffusion and adaptation of recovery mutual-aid resources within communities of color; (2) outlines the history of abstinence-based religious and cultural revitalization movements as frameworks of addiction recovery within Native American and African American communities; and (3) describes culturally indigenous recovery support resources (CIRSR) that are being utilized as adjuncts and alternatives to mainstream recovery mutual-aid and addiction treatment organizations in the City of Philadelphia. An introductory caution is in order. U.S. *communities of color*—as a collective concept and in reference to particular ethnic groups—are characterized by substantial intragroup and intergroup differences. The resulting limitations in drawing broad conclusions will require readers to test the viability of suggested principles and strategies within their respective local communities.

ETHNIC PARTICIPATION IN CONTEMPORARY ADDICTION-RECOVERY MUTUAL-AID ORGANIZATIONS

Addiction-recovery mutual-aid organizations are assemblies of individuals who have joined together for the sole purpose of rendering each other peer-based, nonprofessional support for the resolution of AOD problems. Such groups have risen around the world within highly diverse cultural contexts, including the Swedish Links, Vie Libre (Free Life Movement), the Polish Abstainers Club, the Danshukai movement in Japan, and the Pui Hong Self-Help Association in China, to name just a few (White, 2004a). Alcoholics Anonymous (AA) and other 12-step groups have dominated addiction-recovery mutual aid in the United States even as the spectrum of secular and explicitly religious alternatives to 12-step programs has grown in recent decades. This dominance elicited early criticisms that the 12-step program was based on the experience of White men and therefore was inappropriate for historically disenfranchised minorities (for review, see White, 1998).

This particular criticism has not withstood historical and scientific analysis. First, AA and other 12-step programs exist and continue to grow throughout much of the world, including Latin America, the Middle East, Africa, and Asia, and representation of people of color in 12-step programs has progressively increased in the United States since their founding (White, 1998, 2004a). Second, scientific studies of ethnicity and AA have concluded that:

1. AA's view of alcoholism and its solution are widely accepted within communities of color (Caetano, 1993; Goebert & Nishimura, 2011).
2. Non-Whites affiliate with AA at similar or higher rates than Whites following professional treatment (Humphreys, Mavis, & Stöfflemayr, 1991, 1994).
3. African Americans have lower dropout rates in AA than do Whites (Kelly & Moos, 2003).
4. Twelve-step program emphasis on mutual support with a community of shared experience and its elevation of the role of spirituality in healing personal wounds are themes quite congruent with the cultures of many communities of color (Humphreys et al., 1994; White & Sanders, 2008).

Such conclusions may challenge the experience of many clinicians who have witnessed low engagement rates of clients of color within predominantly White communities and mutual-aid groups. It is the authors' experience that the engagement of people of color in predominantly White mutual-aid groups remains difficult until a certain critical mass of participation is reached, after which ethnic representation can grow quite dramatically.

There has been very little research on ethnic group participation across the spectrum of addiction-recovery mutual-aid organizations, but a glimmer of such participation can be gleaned from survey data published by key recovery mutual-aid organizations. Table 1 summarizes the latest available survey data reported by White (2009b) for AA, Narcotics Anonymous (NA), Cocaine Anonymous (CA), Secular Organization for Sobriety (SOS), Women for Sobriety (WFS), LifeRing Secular Recovery (LSR), and Moderation Management (MM).

Table 1 suggests substantial participation of non-Whites in 12-step programs but low rates of such participation in most secular mutual-aid groups, although comparison of these groups is difficult because of varying survey methodologies and different years in which available data were collected. Membership profile data are not available for faith-based addiction-recovery support groups such as Celebrate Recovery.

TABLE 1 Demographic Characteristics of Recovery Mutual-Aid Societies (Excerpted from White, 2009a, with permission)

Membership Ethnicity	AA (2007)	NA (2007)	CA	SOS (1992)	WFS (1992a, 1992b)	LSR (2005)	MM (2004)
Caucasian	85.1%	70%	68%	99.4%	98%	77%	98%
African American	5.7%	11%	19%	*	1%	5%	
Hispanic	4.8%	11%	6%	*	0%	4%	
Asian American	2.8%	—	1%	*	0%	1%	
Native American	1.6%	—	5%	*	0%	1%	
Other (or no answer)	—	8%	1%	0.6%	0%	12%	2%

Most of the critical research questions raised by Caetano in 1993 about ethnic group participation in AA and other recovery mutual-aid groups remain unanswered nearly 20 years later, but some conclusions can be drawn. First, there is clear evidence of efforts by 12-step groups to reach out to people of color (e.g., specialized literature; AA, 2001). Second, AA and NA now have an established presence within most urban ethnic communities in the United States. Third, although these groups were birthed within a particular historical and cultural context, they have been nuanced for cultural fit as they spread across ethnic boundaries (Caetano; Hoffman, 1994; Womak, 1996).

ABSTINENCE-BASED RELIGIOUS AND CULTURAL REVITALIZATION MOVEMENTS WITHIN COMMUNITIES OF COLOR

CIRSR are recovery mutual-aid efforts organized by and on behalf of members of particular ethnic cultures. CIRSR mobilize distinctive cultural features (e.g., history, language, values, symbols, rituals, art, music, humor) to buttress successful recovery from addiction. To illustrate the role of indigenous recovery-focused cultural and religious revitalization movements as a framework of long-term addiction recovery, we will briefly describe the evolution of such movements within Native American and African American communities.

Organized mutual support for addiction recovery first occurred within Native American tribes experiencing a rise in alcohol problems in tandem with efforts to revive their cultural traditions in the face of physical and cultural assaults on their communities. These blended religious/cultural revitalization and personal healing movements date to the Delaware Prophets of the 1730s and extend historically through the Handsome Lake Movement, the Shawnee Prophet Movement, the Kickapoo Prophet Movement, Indian Christian evangelism, Indian temperance societies, the Indian Shaker Church, Peyote Societies, the American Indian Church, the ghost dance movements and the more recent "Indianization of AA," the Red Road, and the contemporary Wellbriety Movement (Coyhis & White, 2002; Womak, 1996). These movements were birthed by charismatic "wounded healers" who escaped addiction through a transformational change experience that was sudden, unplanned, positive, and permanent—similar to that of AA cofounder Bill Wilson in late 1934 (White, 2004b).

Early milestones in the rise of indigenous addiction-recovery movements among African Americans include the use of early mainstream temperance societies as a framework for recovery initiation (Sigorney & Smith, 1833) and Frederick Douglass's 1845 personal commitment to sobriety and his call for sobriety as a preparatory step toward full citizenship (White et al., 2006). Douglass played a key leadership role in the "colored temperance movement" and the growth of local African American temperance societies (e.g., the Black Templars; Cheagle, 1969; Herd, 1985).

This tradition extended into the mid-20th century through creation of AA groups specifically for African Americans (beginning in Washington, DC, in 1945), the subsequent racial integration of AA and NA, the growing use of the Black Church as a place of healing and recovery, Malcolm X's conversion to the Nation of Islam (NOI), and NOI outreach efforts to addicted African Americans (C., Glen, 2005; White, 1998; White et al., 2006). Addiction ministries of the 1950s and 1960s rose in response to rising heroin addiction among African Americans—with drugs framed as tools of genocide by the Black Panthers and other Black Nationalist organizations (Tabor, 1970). The past two decades have witnessed the rise of indigenous faith-based recovery movements within predominantly African American communities and the birth of recovery advocacy and peer-support organizations serving predominantly African American communities (Whiters, Santibanez, Dennison, & Clark, 2010; Williams & Laird, 1992). Collectively, these religious and cultural revitalization movements have provided diverse Africentric pathways of addiction-recovery initiation and maintenance. Clergy now constitute a major recovery support resource within African American communities (Bohnert et al., 2010; Sexton, Carlson, Siegal, Leukefeld, & Booth, 2006). Faith-based organizations may be particularly well suited to provide nonclinical addiction-recovery support services (DeKrall, Bulling, Shank, & Tomkins, 2011).

CIRSR exist alongside the growth of AA and NA within Native American and African American communities, with individuals picking which resources best met their needs, participating in both simultaneously, or using one program to initiate recovery (e.g., AA/NA) only to then migrate to another to maintain that recovery (the Black Church/Celebrate Recovery)—the latter having been reported among a population of African American women in recovery in the urban centers of Illinois (White, Woll, & Webber, 2003). Whether individuals within communities of color respond best to mainstream groups, culturally specific recovery mutual-aid resources or combinations of such resources may be linked to different degrees of cultural affiliation (Bell, 2002).

DISTINCTIVE FEATURES OF CULTURALLY INDIGENOUS RECOVERY SUPPORT RESOURCES

CIRSR share many features with the mainstream spiritual, religious, and secular recovery support groups described elsewhere in this special issue of *Journal of Groups in Addiction & Recovery*. Nearly all are founded and led by people in recovery. Most share an abstinence-based approach to problem resolution. All involve a reconstruction of personal identity, daily lifestyle, and interpersonal relationships, although to different degrees of intensity. All but MM contain the elements of problem admission, commitment to abstinence, service to others, and sober fellowship. That said, there are distinctive differences between mainstream recovery mutual-aid groups and CIRSR.

Etiology of Addiction

CIRSR share a broader understanding of the etiological roots of addiction. Addiction is often viewed within communities of color as an outgrowth of historical/intergenerational trauma, the targeted promotion of drugs to communities of color (a tool of economic and political exploitation), and as a personal response to present social, economic, and political marginalization (Brave Heart, 2003). Sharing of cultural pain within CIRSR as a dimension of personal recovery may include discussions of slavery, the loss of land, extermination campaigns, epidemic diseases, the purposeful breakup of families and tribes, the loss of families and culture via immigration or deportation, forced internment as prisoners of war, other forms of physical sequestration, immigration distress, acculturation pressure, racism, and discrimination. Within CIRSR, the sharing of such experiences is viewed as a valuable step in consciousness raising, identity reconstruction, and embracing recovery as an act of personal/cultural healing rather than as strategies of denial, diversion, or rationalization as they are sometimes cast in mainstream mutual-aid and addiction treatment contexts (Green, 1995; White & Sanders, 2008).

Ecology of Recovery

Within CIRSR, personal recovery is nested in broader concerns for the survival and healing of families, neighborhoods, and communities—recovery as *a people*. Recovery is often framed as a political as well as a personal act—a means of cultural survival and revitalization. Recovery of the person, family, and community are viewed as inseparable, suggesting that one part of the recovery ecosystem cannot be treated or healed without treating and healing the whole. This is reflected in the Wellbriety Movement's concept of the *Healing Forest* (Coyhis, 1999) and the concept of *community recovery* that is gaining salience in predominately African American communities

(White, Evans, & Lamb, 2010). This simultaneous focus on person, family, and community can be evidenced in Reverend Cecil Williams's personal recovery/community revitalization work in the Tenderloin district of San Francisco (Williams & Laird, 1992) and in the historic recovery and renewal of the Alkali Lake community following decades of pervasive alcoholism (Chelsea & Chelsea, 1985; Taylor, 1987).

Culture as an Agent of Healing

One of the underlying premises of many CIRSR is that AOD problems rose in tandem with the loss of cultural traditions and that the renewal of those traditions and their adaptation to contemporary needs can provide a framework for recovery of the person, family, and community (Bowser & Bilal, 2001; Sanders, 2002; for studies of the association of recovery with increased cultural identification, see Flores, 1985, and Westermeyer & Neider, 1984).

Continuity of Support

Within CIRSR, what is traditionally called "relapse" is not viewed as a moral failure deeming someone unworthy of further support. The individual who has resumed AOD after seeking recovery is viewed as a fallen warrior in the struggle for personal/cultural survival. The corollary to that belief is that no warrior should be left on the battlefield—that the community has a responsibility to care for its wounded warriors—a concept exemplified in White Bison's Warrior Down relapse prevention and intervention initiative for Native Americans (White Bison, 2012).

Multiplicity Versus Singularity of Purpose

Where 12-step and many secular recovery mutual-aid groups adhere to a singularity of purpose and avoid getting involved in what are perceived as "outside issues," CIRSR tend to see AOD problems nested in multiple contexts that deserve attention. Organizations promoting CIRSR have much more boundary fluidity (e.g., involvement in mutual aid, professional treatment, and policy advocacy as well as simultaneous involvement in such issues as addiction, mental illness, domestic violence, child neglect and abuse, homelessness, HIV/AIDS, health care disparities, cultural revitalization, and economic development).

Mutual Support and Political Advocacy

The greater link between recovery support and personal and political advocacy seen in CIRSR may stem from awareness that recovery of persons within communities of color involves finding ways to survive and thrive in the face of multiple sources of stigma and discrimination—first described by Bell and Evans (1981) as *double consciousness*.

Respect for Transformational Change Experiences

CIRSR share a deep respect for life-transforming conversions, epiphanies, defining moments, peak experiences, and the personal "calling" to service that often emanates from such experiences. Service to others in this context is less a task to be completed to support one's own recovery and more a manifestation of the newly reborn person. The affirmation of the transformational power of spiritual experience that permeates CIRSR draws on deep traditions within communities of color and unapologetic respect for the multiple therapeutic functions served by culturally indigenous religious institutions (Thompson & McRae, 2001; Whitley, 2012; Wright, 2003).

Hope Versus Pain

CIRSR rise from communities in which the members have lived a literal and metaphorical "bottom." In this context, hope is a greater motivator for addiction recovery than new increments of physical or psychological pain. CIRSR serve communities, families, and individuals with unfathomable capacities for prolonged physical and psychological pain. Pain in this context is not viewed as a motivator for recovery in the absence of hope. Hope is viewed as the key catalytic ingredient in recovery initiation.

Catalytic Metaphors

Hope is conveyed within CIRSR through *catalytic metaphors* that are culturally vibrant ("hot"). Such metaphors encompass words, ideas, and stories that, by creating dramatic breakthroughs in perception of self and the world, spark and anchor processes of personal transformation. These catalytic metaphors are linked to recovery and are integrated as prominent themes in an overarching culture of recovery. In a very real sense, culture and its stories and metaphors become the "treatment" (Spicer, 2001).

Witnessing

Within the CIRSR context, one is expected to give, as well as receive, hope. That is achieved by becoming a recovery carrier—one who makes recovery contagious through the act of personal witnessing in the community. Such assertive and public recovery evangelism, in contrast to the anonymity practiced by most mainstream recovery support groups, is a way of offering hope (living proof) of the transformative power of recovery and the fruits it can bear through community service and cultural awakening.

Indigenous Healers and Institutions

CIRSR within communities of color emanate from or subsequently engage culturally indigenous healers and institutions. Such healing roles include the medicine man/woman, cacique (Indian healer), curandero (Mexican folk healer), Espiritista (Puerto Rican spirit healer), minister, priest, shaman, monk, and herbalist (Abbott, 1998; Brave Heart & DeBruyn, 1998; Jilek, 1974, 1978; Singer & Borrero, 1984; White & Sanders, 2008).

Community Credentialing

Credibility of recovery carriers inside communities of color is based on *experiential knowledge* (lived knowledge of the problem and its solution) and *experiential expertise* (the ability to translate personal knowledge into skills in helping others within the community—living proof of one's power as a healer; Borkman, 1976). This vetting is guided by community elders and is conveyed through community storytelling. It constitutes a credential that no university, professional association, or governmental body can bestow (White & Sanders, 2008).

THE PHILADELPHIA STORY

Community recovery capital is the quantity and quality of extrapersonal/extrafamilial assets available to individuals to initiate and maintain addiction recovery and enhance the quality of personal/family life in long-term recovery (White & Cloud, 2008). There have been recent calls to develop and mobilize community recovery resources beyond professionally directed addiction treatment and recovery mutual-aid organizations (White, 2009a; White, Kelly, & Roth, this issue)—particularly within communities of color (Coyhis, 1999; White & Sanders, 2008). The goals of these efforts include increasing the ethnic diversity and level of representation within mainstream recovery mutual-aid groups, increasing the presence and capacity of CIRSR within ethnic communities, and building bridges of collaboration between these natural resources and mainstream addiction treatment and allied health and human service organizations.

The authors have been involved for 7 years in efforts to achieve these goals within a larger recovery-focused transformation of the City of Philadelphia's behavioral health care system facilitated by the Philadelphia Department of Behavioral Health and Intellectual DisAbility Services (DBH/IDS; see Achara-Abrahams, Evans, & King, 2011; Evans, 2007). The importance of achieving these goals is indicated in part by Philadelphia's growing racial diversity: 43.4% Black; 41% White; 0.5% American Indian or Alaskan Native; 12.3% persons of Hispanic or Latino origin; 6.3% Asian persons; and 2.8% persons reporting two or more races (U.S. Census Bureau, 2010). Table 2 outlines those strategies consistently reported through service recipient and provider focus groups and town meetings as well as through internal DBH/IDS evaluations that have been identified as most important in increasing recovery capital within communities of color in the City of Philadelphia. The strategies are organized within six core functions: (1) mapping recovery resources, (2) celebrating recovery at a community level, (3) mobilizing culturally diverse peers, (4) assuring representation, (5) assertive community outreach, education, and collaboration, and (6) targeted funding.

DBH/IDS used a mix of funding mechanisms to support the strategies outlined. These included reinvesting savings from Community Behavioral Health, Philadelphia's own nonprofit, managed behavioral health organization for Medicaid recipients, as well as assertive efforts to increase federal support for behavioral health services. In addition, consistent with the larger recovery-focused transformation that is underway in Philadelphia, many DBH/IDS staff roles and responsibilities have been realigned to support the transformation effort. As a result, many of the strategies employed to expand CIRSR were cost-neutral. For example, existing staff conducted focus groups to explore people's experiences with accessing services, led storytelling trainings, and identified and mobilized people in recovery who volunteered their time to conduct street outreach and provide community education. This realignment of staff roles has been critical to the sustainability of these efforts, as many of these efforts are now embedded in the culture of the organization.

The specific strategies outlined in Table 2 were developed in response to Philadelphia's local culture, needs, and resources. Most importantly, they were developed in partnership with diverse stakeholders in the community, including people receiving services, treatment providers, recovery advocacy organizations, and faith-based organizations. We have found that CIRSR can be strategically increased within a community through efforts by federal, state, and local planning and funding authorities. Although the specific strategies might change across communities, many of the outlined core functions of CIRSR can serve as a framework for developing and organizing efforts to promote more community recovery capital for diverse ethnic groups.

A warning caveat is pertinent for systems seeking to facilitate the development of CIRSR. There is a long tradition of harm in the name of help in the relationship between culturally dominant institutions and poor communities of color. For generations, politicians, philanthropists, researchers, educators, and armies of professional helpers and social control agents have tried to rally local ethnic communities with promises of outside help. All too often, these efforts were ill-informed, ill-timed, inadequately resourced, too

TABLE 2 Strategies to Increase Community Recovery Capital for Diverse Ethnic Groups

Strategy	Reported Effects
Core Function: Mapping Recovery Resource	
Health disparities and recovery resource mapping: analysis of service utilization across ethnic communities; identification of all treatment providers, recovery support meetings, recovery homes, recovery ministries, etc., by zip code.	1) Increased ability to assure recovery resources as close as possible to areas with the highest density of AOD problems. 2) Increased choices and improved matching of individuals to treatment and recovery support resources. 3) Increase in targeted Request for Proposals for recovery support in underserved areas. 4) Creation of "learning community" to generate lessons for whole service system.
Biannual recovery prevalence survey: included within a larger public health survey.	Increased capacity to measure: (1) recovery prevalence by ethnic groups; (2) health status of people in recovery across ethnic groups; (3) perceptions of quality of addiction treatment by areas of the community and by ethnic groups; and (4) changes in recovery prevalence over time in areas of focused recovery support initiatives.
Focus groups and town meetings: exploring issues related to accessing services and supports in communities of color.	1) Increased understanding of the barriers related to service access and retention. 2) Increased dialogue and collaboration between people in recovery, CIRSR, and treatment providers.
Core Function: Celebrating Recovery at a Community Level	
Support for public *recovery celebration events* and visible *celebration of multiple pathways of recovery* across diverse ethnic communities.	People from diverse and previously closed recovery groups beginning to see themselves as part of a larger entity: *People in Recovery*. Persons from diverse backgrounds seeking recovery see "people like me."
Core Function: Mobilizing Culturally Diverse Peers	
Work with treatment providers to develop *consumer councils/alumni associations* and *assertive linkage procedures* to mutual-aid and other recovery support entities.	1) Transition from treatment culture to a recovery culture within provider agencies. 2) Recovery leadership development within all geographical areas of the City of Philadelphia.
Youth Leadership Initiative: developed Philadelphia Youth MOVE (Motivating Others Through Voices of Experience). Focused on increasing peer supports for children and adolescents, promoting advocacy for and by youth of color, addressing stigma through education and sharing of personal recovery stories, and providing youth of color with leadership training.	1) Inclusion of child/adolescent/family recovery support needs within all strategic planning efforts. 2) Increase in adolescent peer recovery support groups.
Assertive outreach to recovering people of color to promote their participation in storytelling trainings.	1) Increased sharing of hope-based recovery stories by people of color. 2) Increased representation of recovering people of color during community events. 3) Development of informal peer-based recovery network in communities of color.

(Continued on next page)

TABLE 2 Strategies to Increase Community Recovery Capital for Diverse Ethnic Groups *(Continued)*

Strategy	Reported Effects
Peer-based community outreach through the Taking It to the Streets Initiative: focus on peer outreach to underserved populations in the community at venues such as homeless shelters and safe havens.	1) Increased awareness of recovery support services among people of color. 2) Assertive linkages of persons in treatment to CIRSR.
Core Function: Assuring Representation	
Assuring ethnic diversity and recovery representation in DBH/IDS staff and all DBH/IDS policy and advisory councils.	Improved constituency representation in DBH/IDS leadership initiatives across ethnic communities and diverse pathways of recovery.
Expectation of cultural competence within practice guidelines governing treatment and recovery support services.	Increased recruitment, retention, and long-term recovery support for underserved populations. Concept of cultural competence now extended to encompass diverse communities of recovery.
Core Function: Assertive Community Outreach, Education, and Collaboration	
Cross-systems collaborations to bring increased recovery orientation to systems with high representation of persons of color (e.g., drug, mental health, and juvenile courts; recovery homes for prison reentry; assertive linkage to communities of recovery within child welfare projects).	Increased access of historically underserved populations to addiction treatment and recovery support services.
Faith & Spiritual Affairs Initiative: aimed at mobilizing recovery support within faith communities, including a special initiative aimed at enhancing service access and recovery support within the African American Muslim community.	1) Increased acceptance of and support for people of recovery within Philadelphia's religious institutions. 2) Religious leaders embracing role of their organizations as CIRSR. 3) Growth of 12-step support group adaptations for the Muslim community.
Use of Community Coalitions Initiative and mini grants: embed recovery support services within nontraditional service providers and forge education, outreach, and recovery support coalitions of treatment providers, community service providers, recovery community organizations, and faith organizations.	1) Increased recovery orientation of treatment providers. 2) Enhanced community capacity for delivery of peer-based recovery support services. 3) Increased utilization of treatment and recovery support services via their integration into nonstigmatized service sites.
Creation of culture-specific community task forces: identify and respond to education and recovery support needs within various communities of color.	1) Recovery-focused education and support embedded within indigenous culture-specific service organizations. 2) Mobilization of indigenous community leaders to serve as recovery advocates and promote the sustained development of community recovery capital. 3) Ensured that strategies and solutions were community-driven.

TABLE 2 Strategies to Increase Community Recovery Capital for Diverse Ethnic Groups *(Continued)*

Strategy	Reported Effects
Committee-led efforts to *address stigma of medication-assisted recovery* and increasing the recovery orientation of medication-assisted treatment.	Increased advocacy related to stigma attached to medication-assisted treatment and recovery within ethnic communities.
Published and posted articles, interviews, and video clips that increase *visibility of CIRSR*.	Heightening the visibility, resistance, resilience, and recovery within ethnic communities.
Core Function: Targeted Funding	
Financial and volunteer support for *recovery mural arts projects*.	Increased public visibility and celebration of recovery within ethnic neighborhoods.
Funding support for Pennsylvania Recovery Organization-Achieving Community Together (PRO-ACT) (recovery advocacy organization) to operate *recovery community centers* accessible to people of color.	1) Heightened visibility of PRO-ACT as a recovery advocacy organization. 2) Recovery community centers serve as a central meeting place for diverse recovery support organizations and a peer-based service hub.

narrowly focused, and too short in their vision and execution. In retrospect, most such projects drew more resources out of the community than they put into it.

What poor communities of color do not need is another outside organization or charismatic rescuer conveying the message, "You have the problem, I/we have the solution" (Humphreys & Hamilton, 1995). A long history of colonization in the name of empowerment (and the inevitable aftermath of the experience of betrayal and mistrust) dictate efforts to build recovery support structures that assure sustained continuity of commitment and contact and a sustained partnership with indigenous community leaders—both community elders and vetted recovery carriers within ethnic communities (White & Sanders, 2008). Strategies to promote CIRSR must be designed to ensure that solutions come from within and remain in the control of these communities and their CIRSR (Humphreys & Hamilton).

SUMMARY

There has been a progressive increase in the participation of persons of color within 12-step mutual-aid groups in the United States, and research to date suggests that affiliation, retention, and recovery rates of ethnic minority members within these groups is comparable to such rates for Whites. Rates of participation of persons of color within most secular recovery mutual-aid societies remain quite low, while such rates of affiliation are currently unknown for explicitly religious recovery mutual-aid societies. Significant progress is being made in understanding diverse secular, spiritual, and religious frameworks of recovery. The next frontier will be the greater understanding of how pathways and styles of addiction recovery differ across cultural contexts. There is some evidence that as minority representation increases within recovery mutual-aid societies, culturally nuanced adaptations of core ideas and meeting rituals occur that enhance affiliation rates and benefits of participation.

There is an equally rich history of CIRSR within communities of color, particularly within Native American and African American communities. CIRSR share many characteristics with culturally dominant recovery mutual-aid organizations, but they differ in such areas as their conceptualization of the etiology of addiction, a whole personal/family/community recovery perspective, an openness to transformational change as a primary medium of recovery initiation, and the inclusion of culturally salient catalytic metaphors and healing practices. Coparticipation in CIRSR, mainstream recovery mutual-aid groups, and professionally directed addiction treatment is common and warrants study to determine what particular service combinations and sequences create recovery outcomes for persons of color superior to those experienced with any of these elements in isolation. CIRSR have historically risen spontaneously within communities of color, but CIRSR may also be increased strategically through carefully crafted social policies and programs. Such resources have increased within the City of Philadelphia as part of the city's recovery-focused transformation of its behavioral health care system. Several strategies were suggested for possible replication in other communities, but a caution was added on the critical importance of nesting these strategies within a long-term commitment to and partnership with local communities of color. Supporting the development and mobilization of CIRSR that are nonhierarchical, reciprocal, noncommercialized, and neighborhood- and family-based may be particularly important within communities in which historical experiences have engendered distrust of offers of help from culturally dominant social institutions.

REFERENCES

Abbott, P. J. (1998). Traditional and Western healing practices for alcoholism in American Indians and Alaska Natives. *Substance Use and Misuse*, *33*, 2605–2646.

Achara-Abrahams, I., Evans, A. C., & King, J. K. (2011). Recovery-focused behavioral health systems transformation: A framework for change and lessons learned from Philadelphia. In J. F. Kelly & W. L. White (Eds.), *Addiction recovery management: Theory, science and practice* (pp. 187–208). New York, NY: Springer Science.

Alcoholics Anonymous. (2001). *Can AA help me too? Black/African Americans share their stories*. New York, NY: Alcoholics Anonymous World Services.

Arndt, S., Vélez, M. B., Segre, L., & Clayton, R. (2010). Remission from substance dependence in U.S. Whites, African Americans, and Latinos. *Journal of Ethnicity in Substance Abuse*, *9*, 237–248. doi:10.1080/15332640.2010.522889

Bell, P. (2002). *Chemical dependency and the African American*. Center City, MN: Hazelden.

Bell, P., & Evans, J. (1981). *Counseling the Black client: Alcohol use and abuse in Black America*. Minneapolis, MN: Hazelden.

Bohnert, A. S. B., Perron, B. E., Jarman, C. N., Vaughn, M. G., Chatters, L. M., & Taylor, R. J. (2010). Use of clergy services among individuals seeking treatment for alcohol use problems. *American Journal on Addictions*, *19*(4), 345–351. doi:10.1111/j.1521-0391.2010.00050.x

Borkman, T. (1976). Experiential knowledge: A new concept for the analysis of self-help groups. *Social Service Review*, *50*, 445–456.

Bowser, B. P., & Bilal, R. (2001). Drug treatment effectiveness: African American culture in recovery. *Journal of Psychoactive Drugs*, *33*(4), 391–402. doi:10.1080/02791072.2001.10399924

Brave Heart, M. Y. (2003). The historical trauma response among natives and its relationship with substance abuse: A Lakota illustration. *Journal of Psychoactive Drugs*, *35*(1), 7–13. doi:10.1080/02791072.2003.10399988

Brave Heart, M. Y., & DeBruyn, L. M. (1998). The American Indian Holocaust: Healing historical unresolved grief. *American Indian and Alaska Native Mental Health Research Journal*, *8*(2), 60–82.

Glen, C. (2005). *Early Black A.A.* Retrieved from http://hindsfoot.org/m/black1.html

Caetano, R. (1993). *Ethnic minority groups and Alcoholics Anonymous: A review*. In B. McCrady & W. Miller (Eds.), *Research on Alcoholics Anonymous: Opportunities and alternatives* (pp. 209–231). New Brunswick, NJ: Rutgers Center of Alcohol Studies.

Caetano, R., Baruah, J., & Chartier, K. G. (2011). Ten-year trends (1992–2002) in sociodemographic predictors and indicators of alcohol abuse and dependence among Whites, Blacks, and Hispanics in the United States. *Alcoholism: Clinical and Experimental Research*, *35*(8), 1458–1466. doi:10.1111/j.1530-0277.2011.01482.x

Chartier, K. G., & Caetano, R. (2011). Trends in alcohol services utilization from 1991–1992 to 2001–2002: Ethnic group differences in the U.S. population. *Alcoholism: Clinical and Experimental Research*, *35*(8), 1485–1497. doi:10.1111/j.1530-0277.2011.01485.x

Cheagle, R. (1969). *The colored temperance movement* (Unpublished master's thesis). Howard University, Washington, DC.

Chelsea, P., & Chelsea, A. (1985). *Honour of all: The people of Alkali Lake* [Video]. BC, Canada: The Alkali Lake Tribal Council, Alkili Lake, British Columbia.

Coyhis, D. (1999). *The Wellbriety journey: Nine talks by Don Coyhis*. Colorado Springs, CO: White Bison.

Coyhis, D., & White, W. L. (2002). Alcohol problems in Native America: Changing paradigms and clinical practices. *Alcoholism Treatment Quarterly*, *20*(3/4), 157–165. doi:10.1300/J020v20n03_10

Coyhis, D., & White, W. L. (2006). *Alcohol problems in Native America: The untold story of resistance, resilience and recovery*. Colorado Springs, CO: White Bison.

DeKrall, M. B., Bulling, D. J., Shank, N. C., & Tomkins, A. J. (2011). Faith-based organizations in a system of behavioral health care. *Journal of Psychology and Theology, 39*(3), 255–267.

Evans, A. C. (2007). The recovery-focused transformation of an urban behavioral health care system: An interview with Arthur Evans, PhD. In W. White (Ed.), *Perspectives on systems transformation: How visionary leaders are shifting addiction treatment toward a recovery-oriented system of care* (pp. 39–58). Chicago, IL: Great Lakes Addiction Technology Transfer Center.

Flores, P. J. (1985). Alcoholism treatment and the relationship of Native American cultural values to recovery. *International Journal of the Addictions, 20*(11/12), 1707–1726. doi:10.3109/10826088509047258

Goebert, D., & Nishimura, S. (2011). Comparison of substance abuse treatment utilization among Native Hawaiians, Asian Americans and Euro Americans. *Journal of Substance Use, 16*(2), 161–170. doi:10.3109/14659891.2011.554594

Green, W. (1995). *Dysfunctional by design: The rebirth of cultural survivors.* Evanston, IL: Chicago Spectrum.

Helmer, J. (1975). *Drugs and minority oppression.* New York, NY: Seabury.

Herd, D. (1985). We cannot stagger to freedom: A history of Blacks and alcohol in American politics. In L. Brill & C. Winick (Eds.), *The yearbook of substance use and abuse: Vol. III* (pp. 1–82). New York, NY: Human Sciences Press.

Hoffman, F. (1994). Cultural adaptations of Alcoholics Anonymous to serve Hispanic populations. *International Journal of the Addictions, 29*(4), 445–460.

Humphreys, K., & Hamilton, E. G. (1995, Winter). Alternating themes: Advocacy and self reliance. *Social Policy*, 24–32.

Humphreys, K., Mavis, B., & Stöfflemayr, B. (1991). Factors predicting attendance at self-help groups after substance abuse treatment: Preliminary findings. *Journal of Consulting and Clinical Psychology, 59*(4), 591–593. doi:10.1037/0022-006X.59.4.591

Humphreys, K., Mavis, B. E., & Stöfflemayr, B. E. (1994). Are twelve-step programs appropriate for disenfranchised groups? Evidence from a study of posttreatment mutual help group involvement. *Prevention in Human Services, 11*, 165–180.

James, W., & Johnson, S. (1996). *Doin' drugs: Patterns of African American addiction.* Austin, TX: University of Texas Press.

Jilek, W. G. (1974). Indian healing power: Indigenous therapeutic practices in the Pacific Northwest. *Psychiatric Annals, 4*(11), 13–21.

Jilek, W. G. (1978). Native renaissance: The survival and revival of indigenous therapeutic ceremonials among North American Indians. *Transcultural Psychiatry, 15*, 117–147. doi:10.1177/136346157801500201

Kelly, J. F., & Moos, R. (2003). Dropout from 12-step self-help groups: Prevalence, predictors, and counteracting treatment influences. *Journal of Substance Abuse Treatment, 24*, 241–250. doi:10.1016/S0740-5472(03)00021-7

Leland, J. (1976). *Firewater myths: North American Indian drinking and alcohol addiction* (Monographs of the Rutgers Center of Alcohol Studies, No. 11). New Brunswick, NJ: Rutgers Center of Alcohol Studies.

Mulia, N., Ye, Y., Greenfield, T. K., & Zemore, S. E. (2009). Disparities in alcohol-related problems among White, Black and Hispanic Americans.

Alcoholism: Clinical & Experimental Research, 33(4), 654–662. doi:10.1111/j.1530-0277.2008.00880.x

Musto, D. (1973). *The American disease: Origins of narcotic control.* New Haven, CT: Yale University Press.

Neuspiel, D. R. (1996). Racism and perinatal addiction. *Ethnicity and Disease, 6*, 47–55.

Sanders, M. (2002). The response of African American communities to alcohol and other drug problems: An opportunity for treatment providers. *Alcoholism Treatment Quarterly, 20*(3/4), 167–174. doi:10.1300/J020v20n03_11

Sexton, R. L., Carlson, R. G., Siegal, H. A., Leukefeld, C. G., & Booth, B. M. (*2006*). The role of African-American clergy in providing informal services to drug users in the rural South: Preliminary ethnographic findings. *Ethnicity in Substance Abuse, 5*(1), 1–21. doi:10.1300/J233v05n01_01

Sigorney, L., & Smith, G. (1833). *The intemperate and the reformed.* Boston, MA: Seth Bliss.

Singer, M., & Borrero, M. G. (1984). Indigenous treatment for alcoholism: The case of Puerto Rican spiritualism. *Medical Anthropology: Cross-Cultural Studies in Health and Illness, 8*, 246–273. doi:10.1080/01459740.1984.9965908

Spicer, P. (2001). Culture and the restoration of self among former American Indian drinkers. *Social Science & Medicine, 53*(2), 227–240. doi:10.1016/S0277-9536(00)00333-6

Tabor, M. (1970). *Capitalism plus dope equals genocide.* Black Panther Party, U.S.A.

Taylor, V. (1987). The triumph of the Alkali Lake Indian band. *Alcohol Health and Research World, 12*(1), 57.

Thompson, D. A., & McRae, M. B. (2001). The need to belong: A theory of the therapeutic function of the Black church tradition. *Counseling and Values, 46*, 40–53.

U.S. Census Bureau. (2010). *US Census Bureau quick facts: City of Philadelphia.* Retrieved from http://quickfacts.census.gov/qfd/states/42/4260000.html

Wallace, J. M. (1999). The social ecology of addiction: Race, risk and resilience. *Pediatrics, 103*(Suppl. 2), 1122–1127.

Westermeyer, J., & Neider, J. (1984). Predicting treatment outcome after ten years among American Indian alcoholics. *Alcoholism: Clinical and Experimental Research, 8*(2), 179–184. doi:10.1111/j.1530-0277.1984.tb05833.x

White, W. L. (1998). *Slaying the dragon: The history of addiction treatment and recovery in America.* Bloomington, IL: Chestnut Health Systems.

White, W. L. (2004a). Addiction recovery mutual aid groups: An enduring international phenomenon. *Addiction, 99*, 532–538. doi:10.1111/j.1360-0443.2004.00684.x

White, W. L. (2004b). Transformational change: A historical review. *Journal of Clinical Psychology, 60*(5), 461–470. doi:10.1002/jclp.20001

White, W. L. (2009a). The mobilization of community resources to support long-term addiction recovery. *Journal of Substance Abuse Treatment, 36*, 146–158. doi:10.1016/j.jsat.2008.10.006

White, W. L. (2009b). *Peer-based addiction recovery support: History, theory, practice, and scientific evaluation.* Chicago, IL: Great Lakes Addiction Technology Transfer Center and Philadelphia Department of Behavioral Health and Mental Retardation Services.

White, W. L., & Cloud, W. (2008). Recovery capital: A primer for addictions professionals. *Counselor, 9*(5), 22–27.

White, W. L., Evans, A. C., & Lamb, R. (2010). *Community recovery.* Retrieved from http://www.facesandvoicesofrecovery.org

White, W. L., & Sanders, M. (2002). Addiction and recovery among African Americans before 1900. *Counselor, 3*(6), 64–66.

White, W. L., & Sanders, M. (2008). Recovery management and people of color: Redesigning addiction treatment for historically disempowered communities. *Alcoholism Treatment Quarterly, 26*(3), 365–395. doi:10.1080/07347320802072198

White, W. L., Sanders, M., & Sanders, T. (*2006*). Addiction in the African American community: The recovery legacies of Frederick Douglass and Malcolm X. *Counselor, 7*(5), *53–58.*

White, W. L., Woll, P., & Webber, R. (2003). *Project SAFE: Best practices resource manual.* Chicago, IL: Illinois Department of Human Service, Office of Alcoholism and Substance Abuse.

White Bison. (2012). *Warrior down.* Retrieved from http://www.whitebison.org/prisons/Warrior%20Down.pdf

Whiters, D., Santibanez, S., Dennison, D., & Clark, H. W. (2010). A case study in collaborating with Atlanta-based African-American churches: A promising means for reaching inner-city substance users with rapid HIV testing. *Journal of Evidence-Based Social Work, 7*(1/2), 103–114. doi:10.1080/15433710903175981

Whitley, R. (2012). 'Thanks you God': Religion and recovery from dual diagnosis among low-income African Americans. *Transcultural Psychiatry, 49*(1), 87–104. doi:10.1177/1363461511425099

Williams, C., & Laird, R. (1992). *No hiding place: Empowerment and recovery for troubled communities.* New York, NY: Harper San Francisco.

Womak, M. L. (1996). *The Indianization of Alcoholics Anonymous: An examination of Native American recovery movements* (Unpublished master's thesis). Tuscon, AZ: University of Arizona, Native American Research and Training Center.

Wright, E. M. (2003). Substance abuse in African American communities. In D. J. Gilbert & E. M. Wright (Eds.), *African American women and HIV/AIDS: Critical responses* (pp. 31–51). Westport, CT: Praeger.

Methadone Anonymous and Mutual Support for Medication-Assisted Recovery

WALTER GINTER

Medication-Assisted Recovery Support (MARS) Project, Port Morris Wellness Center, Bronx, New York, USA

Patients in medication-assisted treatment for opioid addiction have been historically excluded or marginalized within mainstream recovery mutual-aid societies. The resulting isolation has sparked the rise of indigenous support structures organized by and for people in medication-assisted recovery. This article reviews the obstacles methadone maintenance patients experience in seeking to participate in mainstream 12-step groups and describes how Methadone Anonymous and other alternatives are providing recovery support for current and former methadone maintenance patients.

INTRODUCTION

Methadone maintenance (MM) patients have historically encountered many obstacles in their transition from active addiction to recovery, including barriers to participation in such recovery support groups as Narcotics Anonymous (NA) and Alcoholics Anonymous (AA; Ginter, 2009; Obuchowsky & Zweben, 1987; White, 2011; White & Torres, 2010). These obstacles stem in great part from the myths, misconceptions, and professional and social stigma attached to methadone maintenance treatment (MMT) since its inception (Murphy & Irwin, 1992; Vigilant, 2005; Zweben & Sorensen, 1988). This article will discuss the challenges MM patients face in participating in mainstream recovery mutual-aid groups, review the history and program of Methadone

The author would like to thank the following individuals for their assistance with this article: Bruce Casey, Fredrick Christie, Anthony Scro, William White, and Joycelyn Woods.

Anonymous (MA), and discuss other recovery supports currently available to MM patients.

Brief accounts of MA have been previously published in the professional literature (Gilman, Galanter, & Dermatis, 2001; Glickman, Galanter, Dermatis, & Dingle, 2006; McGonagle, 1994). This review is based primarily on interviews with key individuals who have been close participants in or observers of efforts to develop recovery support groups for MM patients.

CHALLENGES FACED BY INDIVIDUALS IN MEDICATION-ASSISTED TREATMENT

In the early years following the introduction of MM treatment in the United States, MM patients were limited to whatever supports were or were not provided at the methadone clinic at which all patients received their medication. Tony Scro (personal communication, December 12, 2011), an early and very influential proponent of what would later become MA, notes that MMT was not held in high regard by either the addiction treatment community or the general public. In the early 1970s, there were major philosophical differences between the proponents of drug-free therapeutic communities (TCs) and the medical models of treatment (outpatient methadone centers). TCs supported a non-medically supervised, abstinence-based approach that sought to reconstitute the client's basic personality and promote positive changes in behavior in an intensive long-term (18 to 24 months) residential setting. These programs viewed MMT as ineffective and MM patients as active users. Early TCs that offered community-based support did so through linkage of clients to NA or AA. MM patients, according to Scro, were not readily accepted either by NA or AA. It was not uncommon during these and subsequent years for MM patients attending NA meetings to be denied the right to speak during a meeting if that individual disclosed participation in methadone—a practice that continues today in some NA groups (White, 2011).

In 1991, at the height of the HIV/AIDS epidemic, MA came into being due in great part to the discrimination that MM patients experienced within AA and NA. The benefits imparted by the 12-step organizations were well known to MM patients, but because they were considered a "different breed of cat" by these mainstream recovery support groups, key ingredients of AA and NA were not available to them—full acceptance as members, ability to share at meetings, ability to participate in service work, and inclusion in fellowship-related social activities. By the early 1990s, there was growing realization within the MM patient community that the true usefulness and effectiveness of these groups were not being realized by MM patients—whether they disclosed their status as patients or concealed such status.

Scro (personal communication, December 12, 2011) attended his first MA meeting in the early 1990s in his professional role with the New York

State Office of Alcoholism and Substance Abuse Services (OASAS). In that same role, he was assigned to provide technical assistance to a methadone program that had been set up at New York City's St. Clare's Hospital. A counselor in that program named Fred Christie was an advocate and proponent of the 12-step approach to recovery and organized an on-site MA group for HIV-infected patients. The success Christie had with that group led to the development and foundation of a group called "Advocates for the Integration of Recovery and Methadone" (AFIRM).

AFIRM believed that MMT providers working together with traditional 12-step support afforded patients the best opportunity to achieve long-term recovery from opiate addiction. The primary difference between mainstream AA and NA meetings and the newly organized MA was that MA groups were initiated in the methadone clinics where the drug was dispensed, and these MA groups were cofacilitated by a staff person and a patient/member. The long-term goal, still unachieved in 2012, was to spin MA out of the clinic to be freestanding in the community like AA, NA, and other recovery mutual-aid groups.

The leaders of OASAS supported the mission of AFIRM and the establishment of MA groups in each methadone clinic. AFIRM also partnered with the other treatment modalities to help bridge the traditional gap between drug-free and medication-based treatment approaches. As a result of AFIRM's efforts, MA spread to other cities, states, and countries. Since the mid- to late 1990s, due in great part to the efforts of groups like AFIRM and the National Alliance of Medication-Assisted (NAMA) Recovery, MM patients have become much more visible and vocal in asserting their rights as patients and in demanding respect. As the scientific credibility of MM treatment was increasingly affirmed in the 1990s, patients began to feel better about their choice of this approach to treatment and began demanding greater access to other recovery support systems. In 1997, the National Institute of Health Consensus Development Panel (1997) concluded that MM in conjunction with other psycho/social interventions was the "gold standard" of effective opiate addiction treatment. MM programs providing only medication were no longer considered as providing effective treatment, opening a huge door for a program-sited support like MA. More importantly, the word "recovery" no longer was the exclusive property of NA and AA. Stabilized MM patients as a group began to assert that they were in recovery.

NARCOTICS ANONYMOUS—PAST AND CURRENT PROBLEMS FACED BY MM PATIENTS

To fully understand the value of MA, what it does, and how it does it, it is very important to review findings related to other alternative peer-support groups, particularly NA, in more detail. This will facilitate a more accurate understanding of the problems faced by MM patients in NA and allow us to contrast their experiences with patients recovering from opiate addiction through affiliation with MA. White, in his 2011 monograph on NA and medication-assisted treatment, collected reports of MM patients on their experiences in NA. He reports four overlapping responses: (1) respect and appreciation for NA as a recovery support institution; (2) confusion and shame related to what they perceive as their demeaned status within NA; (3) hurt, anger, and increased defiance related to limitations on their degree of NA participation due to their medication status; and (4) avoidance or abandonment of NA and exploration of other recovery mutual-aid alternatives.

The key underlying and repetitive theme reported in White's (2011) monograph and heard across MM patient advocacy circles is that MM patients in NA are not treated as equals. Even the most stable and highest-functioning MM patients are viewed in most NA groups as active users who have not achieved the status of recovery. The view of MM treatment encountered in NA is in stark contrast to the near-universal endorsement of MM by the scientific and professional community. White noted in his summary a hope for the future expressed by MM patients: "[I]f there is a final theme emerging from the comments of patients collected by the author, it was hope that attitudes toward medication-assisted treatment might one day change in NA" (White, p. 29).

The work done by White (2011) in gathering the data for his paper confirms that many patients in medication-assisted treatment are greatly benefiting from NA and that there are NA members who were able to taper successfully from medications with the support of NA. White raises the need for the continued study and comparison of clients who get either full participation or restricted participation opportunities from recovery groups like NA:

> ... the collected comments raise the question of potential harm that might occur to patients from the attitudes they encounter towards medications within NA—either the consequences of precipitously terminating their medication use or through being denied the key ingredients of the NA program ... No studies are available detailing the influence of NA on tapering decisions or comparing the recovery outcomes of patients in medication-assisted treatment and non-restrictive NA groups to the recovery outcomes of medication-assisted patients whose degree of participation in NA is restricted. However, there are studies suggesting the possible effects of restricted participation. First is a collection of studies, small in number compared to studies of AA, that reveal that NA attracts and retains a portion of opioid-dependent persons and a broader set of studies concluding that participation in NA elevates recovery outcomes for adults and for adolescents. These studies underscore the assertions

> that access to NA and full participation in NA are important issues for the long-term recovery of patients in medication-assisted treatment. (White, p. 30, reprinted with permission)

White goes on to report:

> A second class of studies links these positive effects to several 'active ingredients' of 12-step programs. ... there are four such ingredients that relate specifically to the restricted levels of NA participation often faced by patients in medication-assisted treatment. The first is the critical role of identity transformation within addiction recovery—a transformation that occurs in great part through the acts of story-reconstruction and storytelling. Members achieve this through the normal experience of sharing in NA meetings and in being invited to share their stories in a more expansive manner (e.g., at a speaker's meeting or in other NA venues). The second critical ingredient is the use of NA to replace an addiction-supportive social network with a recovery-supportive social network. The third ingredient is participation in rewarding, recovery-focused social activities. The fourth ingredient involves the therapeutic effects of helping. Serving as a sponsor to others elevates the recovery stability of the sponsor, and such helping activity is often subsequently extended to broader patterns of fellowship service and community service.
>
> The therapeutic potency of these four ingredients has been confirmed in the far more extensive studies on Alcoholics Anonymous, particularly in studies focusing on the importance of social network reconstruction and the therapeutic effects of helping. The effect of these key ingredients on recovery outcomes is further underscored by the finding that they are influenced by the frequency and intensity of participation in these activities. In a 33-year follow-up study of recovery from heroin addiction, Yih-Ing Hser (2007) found recovery associated with greater self-confidence in the hope of achieving permanent recovery, stronger coping skills, and a non-drug-using social network—all aspects of recovery that are targets of influence within NA.
>
> It could be argued based on such studies that a warm welcome and full NA membership participation by patients in medication-assisted treatment enhances recovery outcomes via such mechanisms as sustained and strengthened commitment to the recovery process, enhanced self-efficacy, improved coping, recovery-based social supports, and the therapeutic effects of helping others. It could further be argued that a combination of cool welcome and restricted NA participation reduces NA attraction and engagement, denies patients access to recovery-based relationships, and pushes them towards continued enmeshment in the drug culture. NA members in medication-assisted treatment have limited

> access to several critical ingredients of the NA program to the extent that they are denied the right to speak in NA, socially ostracized by at least a portion of NA members, and denied access to the therapeutic benefits of helping others. Given these possible outcomes, addiction treatment programs utilizing pharmacological adjuncts within the treatment process will need to assess recovery support options for their patients carefully. (White, pp. 29–32, reprinted with permission)

White (2011) concludes by noting increased efforts by opioid treatment programs (OTPs) to develop or link patients to community-based recovery mutual-aid societies, suggesting strategies for how such participation can be enhanced and noting that such efforts are warranted based on the following three conclusions that can be drawn from available scientific studies:

1. Participation in peer-based recovery support structures elevates recovery initiation and stabilization, facilitates the transition to recovery maintenance, and enhances the quality of personal and family life in long-term recovery.
2. Combining participation in recovery mutual aid societies and professionally directed medication-assisted treatment creates recovery outcomes greater than those of either intervention in isolation.
3. The highest rates of patient engagement in recovery mutual aid societies during and following addiction treatment are associated with assertive linkage procedures and sustained recovery coaching. (White, pp. 32–33, reprinted with permission)

White's findings and subsequent recommendations offer excellent guidelines for addiction professionals wishing to increase recovery supports for MM patients.

In conclusion, MM patients continue to face prejudice within NA and other recovery mutual-aid groups because of their participation in treatment for which the efficacy and effectiveness have been repeatedly validated through scientific studies and clinical experience. All too often, MM patients are told they can attend the meeting of a recovery fellowship but not speak, claim "clean time," sponsor others, or hold a service position. The message at an experiential level is that the MM patient is actively diseased and may infect, contaminate, or corrupt the meeting/group by anything other than his or her silenced presence. While some NA and other 12-step groups have become more liberal in their attitudes toward medication, addiction professionals are advised to closely monitor the local attitudes of these groups before referring MM patients. If MM patients are not able to receive important ingredients of local NA or other mainstream recovery support meetings, other referral options, such as MA, are warranted.

METHADONE ANONYMOUS AS A RECOVERY SUPPORT ALTERNATIVE

The History of Methadone Anonymous Addiction Treatment

In 1991, Gary Sweeny, the education director at Man Alive, a large MMT center in Baltimore, MD, was attending an NA meeting to watch a client receive an "Anniversary Chip" (an award for sobriety time). When the woman stood to speak, she included reference to the important role MMT played in her recovery. In response, she was directed to return the chip because the group viewed methadone as just another illicit drug and cited her as a "nonclean" user. The woman fled the spotlight and the meeting in tears, having been victimized by the very tool that she thought was in place to provide support. In a sense, she had been bitten by the hand that had fed her (McGonagle, 1994).

Sweeny was outraged at what happened and decided to create a place where patients like this woman would be realistically helped and supported with full support for their medical assistance rather than being rejected because of it. Sweeny created MA in the image of AA's 12-step approach specifically for MM patients. Sweeny made one primary change in MA's 12 steps and inserted "illicit drugs including alcohol" in lieu of "alcohol" in AA's 1st step. Sweeny was promptly joined by Duncan McGonagle, RN (Beth Israel), and by Fred Christie, the founder of AFIRM (Long Beach Medical Center). Together, they spread the word of a new recovery fellowship and have subsequently been responsible for the startup of hundreds of MA groups not only in the United States but all over Europe and now Asia ("Program update," 2001, p. 7).

The MA Program

From their inception through the present, most MA meetings are hosted by MM clinics, now known as OTPs. Sweeny emphasized that the clinic's primary role was to provide meeting space that could be rented by MA groups in the same manner many AA and NA groups meet in local churches or community centers. In Sweeny's view, the OTP should not exert control over any aspect of MA meetings. The intention was to replicate AA traditions in requiring that each group be independent and fully self-supporting through its own contributions. A collection basket is usually passed at the meetings, and the normal contribution is $1 or $2, if the attendee is able to afford it.

MA group leaders are not professionals but are "trusted servants"; they do not make decisions for the group or act as therapists. Discussion of controversial issues is not permitted; MA meetings are not meant to be platforms for debating treatment concerns or politics. MA is not an advocacy organization;

it neither endorses nor opposes any causes relating to addiction treatment or other matters. Each group's primary purpose is to help members abstain from illicit drugs and alcohol and to help others achieve such sobriety.

Coparticipation

Because there are relatively few MA meetings in most locations, MA members are advised and encouraged to attend AA meetings on a regular basis. Some patients may choose to attend NA or Cocaine Anonymous meetings in settings where they are fully welcomed. Christie ("Program update," 2001, p. 7) explains that "there are usually many different AA groups in any metropolitan area and MMT patients should search out in which they feel most welcomed and comfortable."

In most AA groups today, the medications taken by a participant are a nonissue and a personal matter. Discussions of medical treatments are discouraged because there is an unwritten tradition that "[n]o AA member should play doctor" (Ginter, 2009). Regarding methadone, a patient openly commenting on his/her MMT program would be an irrelevant distraction from full participation in AA, or in an MA group for that matter. Sweeny also made frequent reminders that there was need at these outside meetings for patients to discuss their medications, including methadone or other prescribed drugs. McGonagle agrees, adding, "Abstinence from all mood altering chemicals not prescribed by a physician, is the primary goal of all chemical-addiction-oriented 12-step programs. Methadone should not be an issue even at MA meetings—it is just another medication, period" ("Program update," 2001, p. 7).

Spirituality

As with AA and similar 12-step programs, MA relies on underlying principles of spirituality. Although this is not the same as religion, it is often a source of misunderstanding and controversy. Christie notes that in modifying the 12 steps for MA, the word *God* was removed and replaced with *higher power*. Still, acceptance of spiritual faith as a guiding force in one's life is a sticking point for many addicted persons. McGonagle said:

> We suggest that the individual develop a concept of a 'power greater than themselves.' Sometimes a newcomer will use the group as a Higher Power. The important idea is to get MA members 'out of themselves' and away from any notion that they are the Higher Power and totally in control of their addictions or their lives. ("Program update," 2001, p. 7)

The coming-together of people with common problems to share their experience, strength, and hope with each other can indeed be a powerful force on a spiritual plane. Some people, even avowed atheists, have succeeded by using the group as their higher power, at least initially.

MA and the Opioid Treatment Program

Before MA was founded, Joan Zweben noted, "Enhancing the partnership between 12-step programs and professional treatment is emerging as one of the most important therapeutic tasks today in the addictions field." Such partnership has been a goal of MM leaders. Enlightened OTP staff can serve vital supportive roles in working with patients to promote their participation in 12-step programs and acceptance of spiritual concepts. Doubts or fears expressed by patients can open many doors to therapeutically helpful interactions that benefit participation in both the MM treatment program and 12-step groups.

McGonagle (1994) has observed that once regular MA meetings get started at a clinic, the environment usually changes for the better. Patients seem to more fully realize the benefits of MM in terms of their more active participation in treatment, illicit drug use among patients decreases, interest in personal health increases, patients assume greater responsibility for taking care of their families, and patients generally improve the quality of their lives.

MMT clinic staff can do much to help organize MA programs and encourage patients who show an interest. First, staff can familiarize themselves with how MA and other 12-step groups operate by attending open meetings and talking with patients recovering with the support of these groups. Second, there also is a great deal of AA literature available, including helpful manuals on starting and running local groups. Furthermore, Christie, Sweeney, and McGonagle continue to be available to help answer questions and assist in starting MA groups. Although 12-step program participation may not be uniformly beneficial for everyone, it has withstood the test of time and proved invaluable for a great number of people.

Methadone Anonymous: How Does It Work?

A deeper understanding of MA can be gleaned through the literature used to educate new MA members. According to the MA Preamble:

> MA members believe that methadone is a therapeutic tool of recovery that may, or may not be discontinued in time, dependent on the needs of the individual. Participants believe that continued abstinence from illicit opiates and other chemicals is the foremost goal of recovery. It is the purpose of the fellowship to learn to develop a positive lifestyle, live in harmony with each other and with the rest of the world and to help those within our organization who still suffer from chemical dependency of any kind to achieve and maintain sobriety.

> Methadone Anonymous is a fellowship of men and women who share their experience, strength and hope with each other that they may solve their common problem and help others to recover from drug addiction. The only requirement for membership is a desire to stop drugging. There are no dues or fees for MA membership; the groups are self-supporting through group member contributions. The true and overriding purpose is to stay clean and sober and to help other addicts who are still suffering. (MA, 2012)

MA adheres to the principle of anonymity shared by all 12-step groups. As stated in MA literature:

> The 12-step philosophy states that anonymity is the spiritual foundation of all our traditions, ever reminding us to place principles before personalities. What that means is what you hear and what you see here, let it stay here. (Bruce Casey, personal communication, November 19, 2011)

MA utilizes a classic 12-step approach to recovery pioneered by AA. Members who faithfully pursue this approach are promised 12 outcomes:

1. We will attain and maintain sobriety.
2. We are going to know a new freedom and a new happiness.
3. We will not regret the past, nor wish to shut the door on it.
4. We will comprehend the word "serenity" and we will know peace.
5. No matter how far down the scale we have gone, we will see how our experiences can benefit others.
6. That feeling of uselessness and self-pity will disappear.
7. We will lose interest in selfish things and gain interest in our fellows.
8. Self-seeking will slip away.
9. Our whole attitude and outlook on life will change.
10. Fear of people and economic insecurity will leave us.
11. We will intuitively know how to handle situations which used to baffle us.
12. We will suddenly realize that a Power greater than ourselves is doing for us what we could not do for ourselves. (MA, 2012)

Most MA meetings follow a standard format that includes the following:

1. The chairperson opens the meeting and follows the meeting format.
2. A member reads the preamble.
3. A member reads the steps.
4. A member reads the promises (optional).
5. A member reads the anonymity statement.
6. Secretary break: make MA annoucements and read anniversary dates.
7. Chairperson celebrates clean time and makes suggestions.

8. Chairperson announces first speaker who shares their experiences, strength, and hope.
9. Coffee break (optional).
10. Chairperson announces second speaker (open meeting).
11. Closed Meeting: after one speaker qualifies, members share and speaker leads.
12. Close meeting: prayer of speaker's choice. Note: www.methadone anonymous.us/MeetingFormat.html states it is the tradition of MA to open a meeting with the Serenity Prayer. In *Methadone Anonymous Meeting Format* provided by MA Intergroup through Bruce Casey, the meeting is closed by a prayer of speaker choice.

When MA patients are asked, "How does MA work?" most group members, like AA and NA members when similarly asked, simply respond, "It works very well."

THE FUTURE OF RECOVERY SUPPORT FOR MM PATIENTS

To review, we've discussed the challenges faced by individuals involved in medication-assisted recovery (specifically MMT) as they seek participation in mainstream recovery mutual-aid groups, particularly NA. Additionally, we focused on the developmental history and the founding and program of MA as a recovery support alternative. Several significant changes are anticipated in the future of recovery support for people in medication-assisted recovery.

First, MA meetings will increasingly separate from OTPs and develop autonomy and maturity without reliance on the OTPs in which they were birthed. As MA comes of age, it will move beyond the original AFIRM model that called for meetings to be held within OTPs and to be cofacilitated by an OTP staff member.

Second, the name and focus of MA will change to reflect a wider span of medications used in the treatment of opioid addiction (e.g., buprenorphine, naltrexone, and other medications). Third, MA will be nested within a much larger menu of mutual-support resources available to people in medication-assisted treatment. In 2006, the NAMA, working in collaboration with Albert Einstein College of Medicine in Bronx, NY, received Center for Substance Abuse Treatment Recovery Community Services Program grant funding to create the Medication-Assisted Recovery Support (MARS) Project. MARS was built on two basic premises: First, patients receiving pharmacotherapy for opiate addiction at OTPs need to understand recovery in the context of such treatment and not as something that occurs only after such treatment has ended. At the MARS Project, that understanding is conveyed through core training that is offered to OTP patients. Second, it is believed that the same recovery support services that have proven effective at recovery centers around the United States will prove a boon to MM patients. The MARS Project's results to date have justified supplemental funding to train staff from 10 OTPs around the country to replicate the MARS model.

Finally, the number of patients being treated with methadone and buprenorphine who report a warm welcome from local AA, NA, and other mutual-aid programs suggests a possible day in the future where there will be no need for a specialty group for people in medication-assisted recovery. That day may be approaching more rapidly than could be expected.

REFERENCES

Gilman, S. M., Galanter, M., & Dermatis, H. (2001). Methadone Anonymous: A 12-step program for methadone maintained heroin addicts. *Substance Abuse, 22*(4), 247–256. doi:10.1023/A:1012200712300

Ginter, W. (2009). *Advocacy for medication-assisted recovery: An interview with Walter Ginter.* Retrieved from http://www.facesandvoicesofrecovery.org

Glickman, L., Galanter, M., Dermatis, H., & Dingle, S. (2006). Recovery and spiritual transformation among peer leaders of a modified Methadone Anonymous group. *Journal of Psychoactive Drugs, 38*(4), 531–533. doi:10.1080/02791072.2006.10400592

Hser, Y.-I. (2007). Predicting long-term stable recovery from heroin addiction: Findings from a 33-year follow-up study. *Journal of Addictive Diseases, 26*(1), 51–60. doi:10.1300/J069v26n01_07

McGonagle, D. (1994). Methadone Anonymous: A 12-step program. Reducing the stigma of methadone use. *Journal of Psychosocial Nursing, 32*(10), 5–12.

Methadone Anonymous. (2012). *The 12 steps.* Retrieved from http://www.methadonesupport.org/12-steps.html

Murphy, S., & Irwin, J. (1992). 'Living with the dirty secret': Problems of disclosure for methadone maintenance clients. *Journal of Psychoactive Drugs, 24*(3), 257–264. doi:10.1080/02791072.1992.10471646

National Consensus Development Panel on Effective Medical Treatment of Opiate Addiction. (1997). Effective medical treatment of opiate addiction. *Journal of the American Medical Association, 280*(22), 1936–1943. doi:10-1001/pubs.JAMA-ISSN-0098-7484-280-22-jcf71002

Obuchowsky, M., & Zweben, J. E. (1987). Bridging the gap: The methadone client in 12-step programs. *Journal of Psychoactive Drugs, 19*(3), 301–302. doi:10.1080/02791072.1987.10472416

Program update: Methadone Anonymous comes of age. (2001). *Addiction Treatment Forum, 10*(3).

Vigilant, L. G. (2005). 'I don't have another run left with it': Ontological security in illness narratives of recovery on methadone maintenance. *Deviant Behavior, 26*(5), 399–416. doi:10.1080/016396290931650

White, W. L. (2011). *Narcotics Anonymous and the pharmacotherapeutic treatment of opioid addiction.* Chicago, IL: Great Lakes Addiction Technology Transfer Center and Philadelphia Department of Behavioral Health and Intellectual Disability Services.

White, W. L., & Torres, L. (2010). *Recovery-oriented methadone maintenance*. Chicago, IL: Great Lakes Addiction Technology Transfer Center, Philadelphia Department of Behavioral Health and Mental Retardation Services, and North-east Addiction Technology Transfer Center.

Zweben, J. E., & Sorensen. J. L. (1988). Misunderstandings about methadone. *Journal of Psychoactive Drugs, 20*(3), 275–280. doi:10.1080/02791072.1988.10472498

Mutual-Help Groups for People With Co-Occurring Disorders

JOAN E. ZWEBEN
East Bay Community Recovery Project, Oakland, California, USA; Department of Psychiatry, University of California, San Francisco, California, USA

SARAH ASHBROOK
East Bay Community Recovery Project, Oakland, California, USA; Private Practice, Berkeley, California, USA

This article gives an overview of the development of mutual-help groups for addictive disorders, mental health disorders, and co-occurring disorders. It highlights the history and current status of each type of group, discusses some alternatives to 12-step programs, and describes current challenges and dilemmas. It reports on the limited research on groups for co-occurring disorders and highlights the research in the other areas. It also reviews some of the interventions designed to facilitate the use of mutual-help groups, including groups for individuals with severe mental illness.

INTRODUCTION

Individuals with co-occurring psychiatric and substance use disorders (CODs) often find themselves without a "home" within mutual-help groups in which they can share their specific experiences and concerns. The 12-step system is well developed for handling a wide range of substances and addictive behaviors, but those with comorbid mental health issues are generally discouraged from sharing this specific aspect of their challenges in mutual-help meetings as mental illness is often thought of as an "outside" issue. Over time, it is increasingly recognized that CODs are the norm, not the exception, and are best addressed in an integrated fashion in professional treatment settings. The incorporation of CODs as a topic in mutual-aid groups is limited as the mutual-help system changes without the incentives of funding or other public policy interventions accelerating the process. Nonetheless, there has been an evolution toward acknowledging that people with addiction issues often have other mental health problems, and open discussion is increasing within mutual-help group meetings with names like the Sober 5150s in Alcoholics Anonymous (AA) and Double Trouble in Narcotics Anonymous (NA).

In this article, we will review the evolution of mutual-help groups for substance use disorders, highlighting key events in their history and briefly discussing alternatives to 12-step programs. We will then review the history of these groups within the mental health system and how a combination of self-help/mutual-help groups blended with professionally led support groups. We will subsequently address the development of mutual-help groups for persons with coexisting disorders. We will review some landmarks in this evolution, discuss current opportunities and dilemmas, and describe interventions intended to facilitate the use of the mutual-help system by people with psychiatric conditions, including those with severe mental illness.

The 2009 National Survey on Drug Use and Health (Substance Abuse and Mental Health Services Administration [SAMHSA], 2010) shows significant prevalence rates for substance use and mental disorders in the United States, such as among adults aged 18 years or older, 20.8 million people were classified with a substance use disorder; 45.1 million people were classified with a mental health problem; and close to 9 million people have CODs. With such large numbers of adults in the United States experiencing COD issues, it is important to link them with networks of people who are in the process of recovery to help them acquire skills and support to help them manage both illnesses. Growing recognition of the importance of recovery-oriented systems of care (White, 2008a), in which professional treatment plays an important but not exclusive role, has increased interest in how to facilitate the use of mutual-help groups. Terminology has evolved over time. The term "dual diagnosis" was one of the first to be widely used but has been largely replaced by "co-occurring disorders," or "COD." This is due in part to the recognition that "dual diagnosis" literally means "two labels," and many persons in recovery have multiple conditions. We have not attempted to change the terminology of our sources when quoting their work but use the term "co-occurring disorders" when possible.

The idea that people who have shared certain types of difficult experiences can offer inspiration and guidance to others "has been well-documented since antiquity" (Davidson, Chinman, Sells, & Rowe, 2006, p. 443). Mutual-aid support groups today cover vast categories of topics and concerns and vary from strictly secular to explicitly spiritual, with seemingly everything in between. No two groups are alike as the demographics and attitudes of each group are unique. The overall goal of every support group is to improve the quality of life of its members through the recognition of similarities and the reduction of shame and stigma (Sheffield, 2003).

Despite the uniqueness of each group and variations in mutual-aid programs, there are some universally recognized psychosocial processes that transpire, such as acceptance, inclusion, instillation of hope, catharsis, role modeling, normalizing, learning new coping strategies, positive reinforcement, stigma reduction, self-disclosure, and more.

With the prevalence of 12-step programs offering readily available support, it is troubling that these individuals with CODs describe a lack of empathy and acceptance in traditional mutual-aid groups (Magura, 2008). Despite the availability and benefits of 12-step groups, people with CODs did not consistently attend single-focus recovery groups due to difficulty bonding with other members, failure to address medication issues, and other important issues of dual recovery (Villano et al., 2005; Vogel, Knight, Laudet, & Magura, 1998). One of the cofounders of AA, Bill Wilson, had a long, documented history of depression, and "when his depressions became severe and he sought relief from them through psychotherapy, many AA members were outraged. Bill was castigated for not working his own program. . . . accused of never having taken the AA Steps" (Hartigan, 2000, p. 6). Within AA literature and lore, the cofounder's COD is hardly touched upon likely to help safeguard the singleness of purpose, which states, "The only requirement for AA membership is a desire to stop drinking," (p. 139) and the primary purpose of the fellowship is "to carry its message to the alcoholic that still suffers" (p. 150; from *Twelve Steps and Twelve Traditions*). Bill Wilson suffered from CODs, but depression does not come in to play in AA's history just as the other AA cofounder Dr. Bob Smith's dependency on drugs other than alcohol is minimized.

HISTORY OF MUTUAL HELP FOR ADDICTIVE DISORDERS

Numerous support groups for people with alcohol and other drug problems are currently available utilizing a variety of formats, the most prevalent of which is 12-step. There is a long history of mutual help that predates the inception of AA in June 1935, which is chronicled comprehensively by William White (2008b) in "Recovery: Old Wine, Flavor of the Month or New Organizing Paradigm?" (see also Laudet, 2008; White & Kurtz, 2008). The spark that ignited the 12-step movement, and ultimately the growth of mutual-aid groups, came as a result of Bill Wilson and Dr. Bob Smith converging under a vision of one alcoholic helping another to achieve sobriety and a better way of life. In 1939, the first edition of the basic text *Alcoholics Anonymous* laid out the "single purpose" primary tenet: "the only requirement for membership is an honest desire to stop drinking. . . . We simply wish to be helpful to those who are afflicted" (AA, 1976, p. xiv). The decade that followed that fortuitous meeting was turbulent and fraught with friction and dissension: "every A.A. group had many membership rules" (AA, 1953). Challenges to the primary purpose surfaced and the program evolved (*Twelve Steps and*

Twelve Traditions, 1952, p. 139). "Group after group finally abandoned all membership regulations" and allowed new members to decide for themselves "whether they were an alcoholic and whether he should join" (*Twelve Steps and Twelve Traditions*, 1952, p. 141).

August 1937 heralded the admission of Florence R., the first female alcoholic in New York, and "the man with a double stigma" (AA, 1953, p. 143). The man asking for admittance described himself to Dr. Bob as "the victim of another addiction even worse stigmatized than alcoholism. . . . sex deviate." He was permitted to join, "plunged into Twelfth Step work. . . . Never did he trouble anyone with his other difficulty. A.A. had taken its first step in the formation of Tradition Three." In April 1945, "a [B]lack man who was an ex-convict with bleach-blond hair, wearing women's clothing and makeup" and who was an admitted "dope fiend" sought access to the group. When asked what to do about it, Bill posed the question, "Did you say he was a drunk?" When answered, "Yes," Bill replied, "Well, I think that's all we can ask" (Hartigan, 2000, p. 8; Silkworth.net). Yet, experiences such as these in those early years led to the formation of the 12 traditions, specifically Tradition 3, which codified, "The only requirement for membership is a desire to stop drinking."

In August 1946, Bill W. wrote a *Grapevine* article titled, "Who Is a Member of Alcoholics Anonymous?" He declared that the rules and requirements created by the members "are legion" and stated, "If all of these edicts had been in force . . . it would have been practically impossible for any alcoholic to have ever joined" (AA, 1988, p. 37). In the *Grapevine* article, he broached the subject of CODs and cited how "most of the early members of AA would have been thrown out . . . because they had mental as well as alcoholic difficulties" and how groups are confronted with "many alarming problems. . . . Those with mental difficulties throw depressions or break out in paranoid denunciations of fellow members" (AA, 1988, p. 37). The message was unambiguous and unmistakable: "[O]ur membership ought to include all who suffer alcoholism. Hence we may refuse none who wish to recover" (AA, 1988, p. 22). Other *Grapevine* articles followed over the years, repeating the inclusionary message of the third tradition, which "tells every alcoholic in the world that he may become, and remain, a member of Alcoholics Anonymous so long as he says so" (*Grapevine*, 1948, p. 79). The following AA Preamble first appeared in the *Grapevine* (June 1947), is compiled from phrasing in the forward to the orginal edition of Alcoholics Anonymous, and continues to be found throughout the literature and is consistently read at the opening of meetings:

> Alcoholics Anonymous is a fellowship of men and women who share their experience, strength and hope with each other that they may solve their common problem and help others to recover from alcoholism.
>
> The only requirement for membership is a desire to stop drinking.

> There are no dues or fees for AA membership; we are self-supporting through our own contributions. AA is not allied with any sect, denomination, politics, organization or institution; does not wish to engage in any controversy, neither endorses nor opposes any causes.
> Our primary purpose is to stay sober and help other alcoholics to achieve sobriety.

The dissemination of the "original" 12-step program AA led to "progressive growth in overall membership . . . , a diversification of A.A. member characteristics . . . , and a growing diversity of styles of recovery within A.A.," and it began to lead to the adaptation and creation of "anonymous recovery programs for those with other drug choices" (White, 2008a, pp. 3–4). Twelve-step recovery methods now address a wide range of substance use disorders, in a proliferation of self-help/mutual-aid organizations known by the moniker "anonymous" groups or fellowships. NA evolved out of the AA program in the late 1940s, and others for specific drugs have since followed. Other "anonymous" groups are nonspecific regarding the addictive substance, while still others deal with other problems, such as, gambling, food-related issues, debt, and various other issues. Modern alternatives to 12-step programs began in the mid-1970s and have grown rapidly to include non-12-step addiction-recovery group options, such as Celebrate Recovery, LifeRing Secular Recovery, Millati Islami, Men for Sobriety, Methods of Moderation and Management, Moderation Management, Narconon (Church of Scientology), Pagans in Recovery, Secular Organizations for Sobriety, and many others. Self-Management and Recovery Training is one of the more recognized alternatives.

THE RESEARCH LITERATURE

Studies of 12-step and alternative groups continue to grow and include a few studies of people with COD. Researchers have examined the rates of meeting attendance in 12-step groups by persons with COD and explored the association between diagnosis and meeting attendance (Jordan, Davidson, Herman, & BootsMiller, 2002). Results indicated similar attendance rates for those with substance use disorders without severe mental illness and those with COD. However, study participants with schizophrenia or schizoaffective disorders had notably fewer days of attendance in AA or NA groups. Villano and his colleagues (2005) looked at referral practices with clients and found the most frequently cited reason for suggesting 12-step participation to clients with COD was increased social support while the potential obstacles they might find in traditional 12-step groups cited by clinicians were "stigma because of mental illness" (21%), "getting misinformation about psychiatric medications" (18%), and "mental illness symptoms would interfere with functioning in the group" (14%; p. 67). It is quite difficult to ascertain the prevalence of the problem, although there is anecdotal evidence to support the idea that some individuals with COD have experienced various levels of prejudice and intolerance and may not have felt comfortable, or helped, by single-purpose groups. Bogenschutz (2007) conducted a comprehensive review and concluded that nonspecific change mechanisms such as self-efficacy and social support are similar to those found in the general AA literature. He notes that though attendance rates are comparable, further work is necessary to understand the process of recovery in persons with COD (Bogenschutz, 2007).

MUTUAL HELP WITHIN MENTAL HEALTH

The history of mutual-help groups within mental health contains more ambiguities, as many of these groups are more involved with and/or supported by outside organizations, including psychiatric institutions, government entities, and other community-based organizations. Membership need not consist exclusively of persons with psychiatric disorders, and some of these groups collect membership fees.

According to Mental Health America (http://www.nmha.org), intense stigma toward those with mental illness continued largely unchanged in this country until the start of the 20th century. A former psychiatric patient named Clifford W. Beers heralded the inception of the mental health mutual-aid reform movement 100 years ago with the establishment of the National Committee on Mental Hygiene (NCMH; later to become the National Mental Health Association, then Mental Health America in 2006). Beers wrote an autobiography called *A Mind That Found Itself* (1908) about his personal experience with mental illness and psychiatric hospitalizations, which served to increase awareness of the plight of individuals with severe mental illness. Yet, NCMH was a reform movement rather than a mutual-aid self-help group because membership consisted of concerned citizens and upstanding members of society rather than individuals with psychiatric histories similar to Beers's because he believed society was not ready to listen to prior patients. By the 1940s, small groups of individuals with mental health issues had begun forming to help themselves and each other. For example, there was an acknowledgment in the *Grapevine* (1947) that many alcoholics "have been state asylum inmates" and that AA "meetings are held within the walls" of mental health facilities (AA, 1988), and We Are Not Alone (WANA) was founded.

In the 1940s, a group of former Rockland State Hospital psychiatric patients led by Michael Obolensky began meeting at the YMCA, in cafeterias, and on the steps of the New York Public Library to help others with similar histories with their transition back into the community and for socializing and fellowship. Calling the group We Are Not Alone, or WANA, was a deliberate attempt to avoid references to the mental illnesses and hospitalizations that brought them together. The group met on a regular basis for mutual support, printed bulletins and pamphlets, visited institutionalized patients in psychiatric units, and assisted other psychiatric patients with their discharge from psychiatric hospitals. It was the meetings on the steps of the New York Public Library that attracted the attention of Hetty Richard, who together with Elizabeth Schermerhorn, helped to stabilize and expand WANA and form a club called Fountain House, where these former patients could come together in a more formal way and create a community consisting of people struggling with mental illness. Initially started as a mutual-aid/self-help organization, WANA evolved into a psychosocial rehabilitation clubhouse community in the mid-1950s with the addition of professional staff.

The development of effective psychiatric medications fueled the movement toward deinstitutionalization, setting the conditions for community support groups to flourish (Gronfein, 1985). The mental health field has seen significant progress during the past 60 years, resulting from advances in the conceptualization of mental disorders and the brain, which led to the introduction and use of typical antipsychotic medications in the 1950s. The first antipsychotic tranquilizer Thorazine was introduced in 1954. In 1955, it is estimated that state and county mental hospitals housed nearly 560,000 patients. Mass deinstitutionalization followed in the 1960s and 1970s. By 1977, the population had dramatically decreased to 160,000 institutionalized individuals (Gronfein, p. 437). The impetus to deinstitutionalize individuals with psychiatric disabilities in the decades that followed the arrival of neuroleptic medications came as a result of a complex set of conditions taking place in the United States. These included changes in public policies, shifting philosophies, the civil rights movement, and the increased use of psychiatric medications for individuals with psychiatric disabilities.

Many of these once-hospitalized individuals began to advocate and initiate progress in a movement that led to the simultaneous evolution of 12-step and other self-help mutual-aid groups, to help those suffering with mental health issues. This consumer movement and growth in mutual-aid groups has continued to evolve, expanding into the arena of peer support, which consists of the use of consumers as providers of services and supports. The U.S. SAMHSA (2010) reported that "groups, programs, and organizations run by and for people with serious mental illness and their families now outnumber traditional, professionally run, mental health organizations by an almost 2 to 1 ratio," and "Individuals with serious mental illnesses have provided each other support informally both inside and outside of treatment settings and, further, that this support has been viewed by researchers to be of some benefit" (Davidson et al., 2006, pp. 443–444). Participation in mutual-support/self-help groups, whereby individuals voluntarily come together to address similar concerns, offer people with mental illness and psychiatric disabilities positive social support and the ability to participate in meaningful activities. Peer identification and the shared experience helped to bond individuals together into supportive communities where reciprocity of benefits can take place at both the individual and collective levels. Regarding mutual-aid support groups specifically within mental health, there are a variety of groups available for a range of mental health problems. Many of these have been influenced by the 12-step model. Established self-help/mutual-support groups for single-topic issues include GROW (1957), Recovery International (previously known as Recovery Inc.), and Schizophrenics Anonymous (SA). Lesser-known mutual-aid groups for individuals with mental and emotional illness issues, following the 12-step model of recovery, include Emotional Health Anonymous (EHA), Emotions Anonymous (EA), and Neurotics Anonymous (NAIL), the precursor to EA.

Abraham Low, M.D., under the auspices of the Neuropsychiatric Institute of the University of Illinois Research and Education Hospitals, founded Recovery Inc., later known as Recovery International, in 1937. There were 30 former psychiatric patients in the first group. Arising out of a need for more structured support for patients released from the Psychiatric Institute, Low oversaw the development of a program intended to reduce the negative consequences of habituated thoughts and behaviors and to prevent relapses leading to rehospitalization. The approach is an early precursor to cognitive-behavioral therapy and consists of a system of cognitive-behavioral self-help techniques, but "because Recovery International is a peer-to-peer self-help program, it is not therapy, but rather a method of peer-based training and support on how to adapt the Recovery International tools to everyday life" (Abraham Low Self-Help Systems Website, 2012). Membership in the non-profit organization has five levels (e.g., Regular, $30; Contributing, $50; Supporting, $100; Sustaining, $200; and Life, $1,000). Trained peer facilitators with Abraham Low Self-Help Systems lead groups, and suggested donations for each group are $4 per meeting while online forums are free. Participants are encouraged to comply with health care professionals and to continue receiving support through 12-step programs in conjunction with their Recovery International membership. Recovery International currently provides more than 600 peer-led community-based meetings in the United States and globally, including Canada, Ireland, Israel, India, Puerto Rico, Spain, and the United Kingdom. According to the *Recovery International Group Meeting Evaluation: Final Report* by the University of Illinois at Chicago, Department of Psychiatry (Pickett, Phillips, & Kraus, 2011), the following benefits have been associated with participation in Recovery International: decreased severity of mental health symptoms and a reduction in the use of mental health and social services. Additionally, the study found improved self-esteem, confidence in one's own ability to achieve mental health recovery, and the willingness to ask others for help and support as additional benefits. Lastly, participants showed increased social connectedness/support, feelings of hope, coping mastery ability, and overall mental health recovery.

Ex-psychiatric patients—including Father Cornelius Keogh—who had originally sought help through AA in the Sydney area of Australia but found that their psychiatric problems were more exclusive, founded their own mutual-support group and called it Recovery. The focus of those original groups was recovery from mental illness, and the early program became an amalgamation of the 12-step model and Abraham Low's Recovery Inc. program, designed to increase the determination to act, self-confidence, and self-control. The original literature included the 12 Stages of Decline and the 12 Steps of Recovery and Personal Growth. Over time, the program continued to attract people, many of whom did not identify with mental illness but struggled with life problems, who sought a connection with others seeking prevention and personal growth. In 1975, Recovery changed its name to GROW to reflect the broadening mutual-support membership, as 30% to 40% of current participants do not have a mental health diagnosis. These mutual-aid self-help support groups are run by their own members and are open to adults who are having mental or emotional problems. While GROW is open to anyone seeking help, people who have been in psychiatric hospitals or who are socioeconomically disadvantaged are reportedly actively recruited. GROW's approach toward the use of medication is an assurance of no interference from GROW or its representatives, and the program specifically states, "Members who are still under treatment are urged to obey carefully their doctor's instructions." The stated mission of GROW "is to nurture mental health, personal growth, prevention and full recovery from all kinds of mental illness" (http://www.grow.ie). GROW has a presence in Australia and Ireland.

Other mutual-aid groups for individuals with mental and emotional illness issues, which follow the 12-step model of recovery, include Depressed Anonymous (DA), EHA, EA, and NAIL, the precursor to EA.

EA adapted AA's 12 steps to create a program for people suffering from mental or emotional illness and replaced the word "alcohol" with "our emotions" in the 1st step. Originally founded in St. Paul, MN, in 1971, by 2004, there were estimated to be 1,100 active groups in the United States alone, making it the largest organization intended to help individuals who have difficulty coping with the stresses of daily life. "Emotions Anonymous is not a replacement for varied professional therapies but rather a complementary support activity as recommended by many mental health care professionals" (www.emotionsanonymous.org/HealthCareProf.pdf, 2011). Members come together regularly for the purpose of working toward recovery from emotional difficulties through the adapted version of AA's 12 steps. Within program literature, *AN INVITATION: You Are Not Alone,* there is a direct acknowledgment that AA granted EA permission to adapt their steps yet required that

EA retain certain nuances. While EA uses gender-neutral language in its publications, in the 12 steps and 12 traditions, God continues to be referenced in masculine terms because AA views the steps and traditions as historic writings that should remain unchanged. EA is the successor organization of NAIL, which was created by an AA member, Grover Boydston, on February 3, 1964, in Washington, DC. The creation of a program for neurotics was alluded to by Bill Wilson, one of the founders of AA, as early as 1956.

DA is a mutual-aid group that began holding meetings as early as 1986 but did not formalize until the late 1990s in the Louisville, KY, area. The stated purpose of DA is to support depressed individuals and to empower people into a therapeutic healing force "to help ourselves and others escape the prison of depression" (http://www.depressedanon.com, p. 2). The program reportedly aids in the prevention of depression relapse or recurrence by promoting information and resources; advocates for depressed persons and their families; and informs mental health and medical care professionals of the availability of support groups for persons with depression. Medication is not discussed at the meetings, nor is religion. Similar in methodology to AA, DA members are taught about having a choice of staying depressed or taking responsibility through the practice of the DA program of recovery, and the organization has many DA publications available online for purchase. The 12 steps are nearly identical, with the exception of the phrase, "we admitted we were powerless over depression although it appears DA does not utilize AA literature." DA hosts a "closed" online Google group intended "for persons serious about using the 12 steps to overcome depression. ... No religion/medications talk allowed" (http://groups.google.com/group/depressed-anonymous?hl=en&lnk=). With small pockets of members and minimal face-to-face groups in Alaska, Iowa, Kentucky, Massachusetts, Nevada, Oregon, Pennsylvania, Washington, West Virginia, and internationally in Canada, France, Israel, Poland, and the United Kingdom, DA is a limited resource for those with mental illness.

Founded in 1985, SA is a mutual-aid organization managed by members who have schizophrenia or a schizophrenia-related illness, and it is administered in partnership with the Schizophrenia and Related Disorders Alliance of America (SARDAA). SA has more than 150 groups that assemble throughout 31 states and in Australia, Brazil, Canada, France, India, Mexico, and Venezuela. Organized in 2008, SARDAA offers continuing support for SA while expanding its role to include the creation of a national toll-free hotline, provide information via http://www.sardaa.org, promote recovery, organize a speaker's bureau, and offer support for family and care professionals. SA works from the premise that there are six steps for recovery, encapsulated by an admission that the person needs help, chooses to be well, and believes they can help themselves and others; forgiveness; recognition that self-defeating thinking contributes to problems; and the decision and surrender to follow a spiritual path. The purpose of SA is to help restore dignity and increase a sense of purpose; offer fellowship, companionship, and positive support; improve members' attitudes and lives regarding their illness; disseminate the latest information regarding schizophrenia; and encourage members' recovery from mental illness (SARDAA, n.d.).

EHA is a mutual-aid program for people who suffer from emotional problems and/or mental illness not related to substance abuse, which segregates individuals with CODs. The organization specifically states, "Anyone who is an alcoholic, addict, overeater or who thinks they might be one is encouraged to attend the appropriate program for their problem. . . . We are not equipped to help people directly with a substance abuse problem, since that is not our direct experience" (http://www.emotionalhealthanonymous.org/faqs). The program is limited and does not appear to have existed prior to 2004. Located primarily in the San Gabriel area of California, there is also a single meeting in Hollywood, FL, on Thursday nights and a weekly teleconference meeting on Sundays at 5:40 p.m. Solely utilizing the book *Alcoholics Anonymous,* the basic EHA program is an adapted version of the 12 steps of AA without the substance abuse component. Specific pages of the "Big Book" have been tailored to fit emotionally and mentally ill persons rather than alcoholics through the replacement of the word alcoholic with the phrase "emotional problems." Regarding medications, EHA states it has no position on medication, while it encourages newcomers to work with medical professionals and attend meetings.

Pistrang, Barker, and Humphreys (2008) reviewed empirical studies on the effectiveness of mutual-aid self-help participation for individuals with mental health issues to determine whether involvement in mutual-aid groups led to improved psychological and social functioning. Out of 12 studies that met the criteria for group characteristics, target problems, outcome measures, and research design, Pistrang et al. reported promising evidence that mutual-help groups benefit people with chronic mental illness, depression/anxiety, and bereavement. Seven of the studies showed positive changes for those attending support groups. The authors commented on the variability of the design quality, and reporting of results recommended more high-quality research on this topic to evaluate the effectiveness of these groups for a range of mental disorders (Pistrang et al.).

While there are a variety of groups available for persons with mental and emotional problems, there are concerns that complicate the use of single-purpose recovery groups for individuals with CODs. These concerns include: symptoms impeding regular attendance and participation; tension and controversy over the use of prescribed medications; traditional, single-purpose 12-step programs not addressing the challenges posed by mental illness; stigma; and co-occurring disordered individuals may be treated differently and feel alienated (Bogenschutz & Akin, 2000; Jordan et al., 2002). According to Bogenschutz (2005), there is some dispute regarding the magnitude of these issues, but they are likely larger for those with severe mental illness, particularly within the schizophrenic spectrum.

INTEGRATED MUTUAL-SUPPORT GROUPS FOR PEOPLE WITH CO-OCCURRING DISORDERS

While mutual-support groups for alcoholics have been around for at least the past 100 years, the concept of CODs did not begin to emerge until the late 1980s and the growth in mutual-aid support groups specifically intended for individuals self-identifying with co-occurring issues was slow to follow. There are limited COD groups available through AA, which are found by word of mouth as they are infrequently listed in meeting directories. During AA's 20th Annual Intergroup Seminar in Charlotte, NC (2005), the topic of compiling meeting lists and the omission of COD groups came up for discussion. "Our heart goes out to them, and we wish them well, but we do not list them," as one attendee said. In AA parlance, meetings for people with COD are considered special-interest meetings.

Nonetheless, support groups for those individuals with mental health and substance abuse have gradually appeared. Perhaps the most effective may be those that have broken off from traditional single-purpose groups and adapted to the multifaceted needs of people with comorbid disorders. These include Double Trouble in Recovery (DTR), Dual Diagnosis Anonymous (DDA), Dual Disorders Anonymous, and Dual Recovery Anonymous (DRA). With nearly 50% of persons with serious mental illness experiencing co-occurring alcohol or drug abuse issues, there are many who could potentially benefit from these groups. However, those with CODs are a heterogeneous population on a broad continuum of psychiatric disorders and may have mild-to-moderate as well as high severity. Thus, participants may have very different needs, and researchers have to contend with a variety of variables in their investigations.

COD Groups in the Community

Currently there are still limited mutual-aid groups in most communities. The better-known mutual-support groups for individuals with both substance use disorders and mental health issues are DDA, DRA, and DTR. Best known in Oregon, Dual Diagnosis Anonymous meetings arose out of the collaborative process between a mental health professional and 12-step group members in the formation of a specialized meeting intended to assist persons with CODs in areas where there is no DDA, DRA, or DTR group functioning. DDA is grounded in the 12 steps of AA plus 5 additional "steps that focus on Dual Diagnosis (mental illness and substance abuse). [Dual Diagnosis of Oregon's] unique 12 Steps Plus 5 Program offers hope for achieving the promise of recovery" (http://www.ddaoforegon.com/index.htm).

DRA (http://draonline.org) is based on the principles of AA and the 12 steps, with an emphasis on accepting differences of members and that "a variety of symptoms are possible with a dual illness." DRA began to form in Kansas City, KS, in 1989 when it held its first meeting in a church setting followed by a second meeting, which was held in a mental health facility, under the principles of the 12 steps, experiences of dual recovery, and a belief in personal freedom and choice. By 1991, a 4-point program had begun to form, and by 1993, the first DRA Central Office was established. In 1994, the basic text for DRA, 12 Steps and Dual Disorders, was published and the first intergroup office was formed in Vancouver, WA. By 2001, international groups had begun to form, and there are now meetings held throughout the United States, Canada, Iceland, India, and New Zealand.

DRA honors how members are affected by a variety of "no-fault illnesses whose symptoms can disrupt the ability to function and relate to others effectively" (http://draonline.org, Accepting Differences). The Web site states there are two requirements for membership: "a desire to stop using alcohol or other intoxicating drugs" and the "desire to manage our emotional or psychiatric illness in a healthy and constructive way." Although the fellowship supports building a strong recovery network, which includes support from treatment facilities, professionals, spiritual affiliations, and other 12-step and/or self-help programs, the program is clear that DRA 12-step meetings be chaired and run by DRA members and that the meetings are a function of autonomous DRA groups. There is no formal affiliation with other organizations. However, DRA specifically addresses member concerns "that they have received misguided advice about their diagnosis and the use of medication at other Twelve Step meetings" (DRA, n.d.) and cites AA and NA literature specifically: "Though we can not speak for other organizations, their literature makes clear that these types of statements are not the official position of A.A., N.A., or any other Twelve Step recovery groups that we are aware of" (DRA, n.d.).

DTR is likely the best known of the three COD programs. According to Humphreys (2004), DTR has often been confused with another organization, Double Trouble, which was founded in Philadelphia in 1987 by a substance-dependent man who also had co-occurring psychiatric problems. While Double Trouble meetings were initially run by peers, mental health professionals reportedly acted as advisors at the inception and later began running many of groups, moving into New Jersey and taking more organizational control as Double Trouble expanded. Double Trouble shifted away from the self-help movement and grew into an agency providing psychiatric services. In its writings, it is explicitly and implicitly conceptualized as a component of professional treatment services rather than an autonomous alternative.

DTR started as a mutual-help group but also moved toward greater control by professional organizations. Howard Vogel, the founder of DTR, attended Double Trouble groups in 1989 to help address his own comorbid drug and psychiatric problems but quickly became disheartened by the professional treatment orientation (Humphreys, 2004). In 1989, he founded DTR in New York as an adaptation of 12-step programs intended for individuals who did not fit well under the traditional "one disease, one recovery" format. DTR welcomes those who self-identify as having substance abuse/dependency and psychiatric disabilities. Vogel et al. (1998) report that DTR developed out of Vogel's own personal understanding and experiences with CODs and his participation in "traditional 12-step meetings for his addictions. He found that existing groups were not suitable for those with added psychiatric disabilities who have problems unaddressed and often stigmatized in traditional 12-step programs, such as psychiatric symptoms, medications and their side effects" (Vogel et al., p. 4). Financial assistance was provided by the Mental Health Empowerment Project of the New York State Office of Mental Health (especially Edward Knight) to foster greater control by consumers of the mental health system. DTR formed and began to systematically train peer-group leaders, which contributed to the growth of the program (Humphreys, 2004). It is estimated there are between 200 and 250 DTR groups in the United States, with the majority located in the New York area. Consumers and/or professionals, many of whom are from agencies within the mental health field, continue to initiate new groups, and DTR trains consumers to start and conduct groups and provides ongoing support to existing groups. Some of these groups are open to the public, while others are not (Laudet, Magura, Vogel, & Knight, 2000).

As DTR spread during the last 20 years, it has become more difficult to ascertain the degree of separation and the level of support provided by federal, state, and local agencies. By holding meetings in a variety of venues, including treatment programs, which often intertwined DTR with state and local agencies in the provision of services, the boundary has become steadily blurred. While the majority of 12-step-style recovery groups are fully self-supporting, DTR does not appear to adhere to the seventh tradition, which states that every DTR group ought to be self-supporting, declining outside contributions. There is evidence that DTR has received the benefit of a SAMHSA systems change grant (DTR, n.d.). The Georgia Mental Health Consumer Network, Inc., an organization funded by grants, contracts, donations, and membership fees, is linked through an official DTR director and statewide coordinator who oversee DTR meetings in the state (http://www.state.sc.us/dmh/client_affairs/capss/2010_aug.pdf). The nonaffiliation clause that many mutual-aid self-help programs follow, quoted in the DTR Preamble, "Double Trouble in Recovery is not affiliated with any sect, denomination, political group, organization, or institution," does not appear to be respected as there are multiple examples of affiliation easily found on the Internet. Utilizing the DTR logo, the August 2010, Volume 4, Issue 4, quarterly publication from South Carolina Department of Mental Health, Office of Client Affairs, reports South Carolina SHARE, an independent advocacy organization, is launching a new DTR program, "for people who suffer from both addiction and mental illness. This program is the first of its kind in South Carolina, because it provides support for those who suffer from a combination of alcohol and/or drug addiction and mental illness" (p. 4). While elsewhere on the Web site (http://www.scshare.com), *Double Trouble in Recovery: A Collection of Dual-Diagnosis Mental Health Recovery Stories, Volume II,* described how a consumer named Michael "interviewed with the agency and was hired as their full-time Community Support Coordinator, and one of his primary responsibilities is overseeing the Double Trouble in Recovery program" and to "travel throughout the state to develop Double Trouble groups in different communities" (p. 16). The most striking example of the lack of adherence to the nonaffiliation policy is that Hazelden, a private, not-for-profit organization, has become the exclusive publisher of materials and supplies for DTR groups. Searches on the Internet for the DTR Web site (doubletroubleinrecovery.org) are fruitless or connect the seeker with Hazelden Behavioral Health Evolution (http://www.bhevolution.org/public/doubletroubleinrecovery.page). As of December 2011, Hazelden is the exclusive publisher of materials and supplies for DTR groups. At best, they appear to be a hybrid, a mutual-help group dependent on professional or corporate support.

Research on Dual Focus Groups

Relatively little systematic research has been done on mutual-help groups for those with CODs but there are a few studies on the barriers and benefits of participation. Havassy et al. (2009) reported that the overemphasis on abstinence and insufficient attention to mental health issues were obstacles to participation in single-topic 12-step groups. Additional barriers were discomfort with the emphasis on spirituality or fear that mutual-support groups are analogous with cults. Meissen et al. (1999) reported the majority of individuals with CODs do not attend local AA meetings even when encouraged to do so. Individuals with severe mental illness do not consistently attend 12-step groups for similar reasons, which also include stigma regarding mental illness, medication issues not being addressed, difficulty finding peers like themselves in single-topic groups, and decreased referrals from clinicians (Villano et al., 2005).

Enhanced engagement efforts appear to promote participation. In a pilot study, Bogenschutz (2005) reported that 10 seriously mentally ill patients who received a modified 12-step facilitation intervention (Nowinski, Baker, & Carroll, 1994) designed to engage them in a specialized 12-step program did in fact increase their attendance and decrease their substance use during the 12 weeks of treatment. In a subsequent report, Bogenschutz (2007) seeks to examine the process of change in such patients. In his review, he reported that those with COD attended 12-step meetings at rates comparable to those without COD, with the possible exception of those with psychotic disorders and social phobia. The benefits of attendance did not appear to be markedly different in the two groups. He concluded that the change mechanisms, such as self-efficacy and social support, are similar to those found in the general literature on AA. Timko, Sutkowi, Cronkite, Makin-Byrd, and Moos (2011) also found that an intensive referral intervention enhanced participation in both substance-focused and dual-focused groups and was associated with better 6-month outcomes. In the intensive referral condition, patients attended four additional outpatient sessions designed to familiarize them with dual-focused groups through information, discussion, and practice sessions, and a volunteer was made available to accompany them to a meeting. There was improvement in both alcohol and psychiatric outcomes (Timko et al.). Male veterans are often seen as reluctant to engage in mutual-help groups, partly due to the influence of the military culture. However, recent data suggest that with intensive referral efforts, those who were sexually abused and had severe problems were in fact willing to utilize such groups. Such involvement was predictive of greater abstinence from substances (Makin-Byrd, Cronkite, & Timko, 2011).

PREPARING PEOPLE WITH CO-OCCURRING DISORDERS TO ATTEND MEETINGS

Though specialized groups are available for people with CODs, the number of such groups is limited in any given area. Thus, it is useful to be able to "mainstream" patients to 12-step groups in addition to others they may be attending. The sheer number of meetings and geographical spread offers a great resource, and thus, it is useful to encourage patients to give these groups a fair try (Zweben, 1987).

A variety of manuals and other materials designed to facilitate the use of the mutual-help system are well suited for people with CODs (DTR, 1993; Gorski, 1989; Kaskutas & Oberste, 2002; Nowinski et al., 1994). They describe the history, culture, traditions, rituals, and other practices in a way that familiarizes potential participants with what is likely to occur. Programs may use discussions to encourage sharing of fears and concerns and to foster understanding of material in the workbook. Some use simulated meetings to provide an opportunity to practice appropriate behavior and role-play methods of handling feared situations. Case managers may take more severely disturbed clients to meetings or offer cell phone access if the client goes alone and is at risk for becoming overwhelmed. More functional clients can arrange with AA's or other such mutual aid programs' central offices to have a program participant take them there or meet them. It is common for clients in treatment groups to offer to accompany others to meetings. Although this has its hazards, it is not something clinicians can control and there are many benefits when such alliances are constructive.

Many elements of the meeting structure benefit clients with COD. Those who are highly anxious or depressed should be encouraged to ask for assistance in getting to a meeting and can often be linked with someone to bring them. The predictable structure of meetings across wide geographical areas serves as a container for anxiety, particularly as familiarity grows. The simplicity and redundancy that work so well for those who are newly abstinent is also beneficial for people with a wide range of psychiatric symptoms, including cognitive impairment from severe mental illness or traumatic brain injury. The rule of "no cross-talk" has an enormous protective function, reducing the urge for other members to "play therapist." In general, the practice of learning through sharing your own experiences, different from the feedback process in professionally led groups, creates a group dynamic that is relatively nonintrusive. However, the strong ethos of welcoming can produce anxiety for those who do not have good skills at setting boundaries.

For those with a severe mental illness (SMI), meetings are best selected carefully. Some meetings are more tolerant of eccentric behavior, and clients can be instructed on how to behave in meetings. People with SMI can be told it is inappropriate to discuss their delusions or hallucinations in meetings, and they benefit from a demonstration of the meeting rituals in the safety of their treatment program. This also provides the opportunity to practice in vitro in a simulated meeting. On occasion, the higher power will be incorporated into someone's delusional system, but this can presumably be managed by clinical staff.

All patients on medications should be coached on how to handle this issue in meetings. Although medication issues can be viewed as private, between patient and physician, not all meeting participants are comfortable with this stance. It is important to remember that "silence is the enemy of recovery," and the idea of concealing information can produce a conflict. Treatment program staff can set up role-plays for the client to practice addressing what they most fear about challenges to their medication use by meeting participants. Once the client has generated some responses, they can be reminded of AA slogans such as, "Work your own program." The AA pamphlet, *The AA Member and Medication*, outlines the history of the dangers of medication misuse, and also stresses, "No AA member should play doctor." It validates the view that medication is compatible with recovery.

Alternative mutual-help groups, such as those described earlier, may be preferred by some people with CODs. One key issue is the frequency and proximity of 12-step and other mutual-aid support meetings, which may not be adequate to provide a firm structure. Clinicians should work with their clients to define what level of intensity is appropriate given their level of recovery, and they should seek activities accordingly. Some clients attend alternative groups and 12-step meetings. Unfortunately, some of the alternative groups adopt a competitive stance and actively disparage the 12-step system, making it harder for participants to assemble a good structure from existing offerings.

CONCLUSION

In summary, the mutual-help system for people with CODs is less well developed than the one for alcohol and other drug use alone, but it has been in existence for a considerable period of time and is steadily growing in many parts of the country. Groups solely for mental health patients tend to be more closely connected with professional organizations or the mental health system but nonetheless can offer a community of peers that supports the recovery process in a wide variety of ways. Integrated groups that grew out of the 12-step system tend to put more emphasis on peer leadership. The research literature focuses on barriers to participation, ways to enhance participation, and outcomes for both psychiatric and substance use conditions. However, there are relatively few studies and there are large gaps. Much more work needs to be done on subpopulations (e.g., mood disorders, SMI) to specify key ingredients in the recovery process and whether they actually vary for participants with different disorders. It is hoped that researchers can examine the workings of these groups more extensively, to better define their distinct contribution to the recovery effort.

REFERENCES

Abraham Low Self-Help Systems, Recovery International, The Power to Change website (2012) http://www.lowselfhelpsystems.org/system/our-method-about-cbt.asp, accessed August 5, 2012.

Alcoholics Anonymous. (1952). *Twelve steps and twelve traditions*. New York, NY: Alcoholics Anonymous World Services, Inc.

Alcoholics Anonymous. (1988). *The language of the heart: Bill W's Grapevine writings*. New York, NY: The AA Grapevine, Inc.

Beers, C. (1910). *A Mind that Found Itself: An Autobiography*. New York, NY: Longmans, Green, and Co.

Bogenshutz, M. P., & Aikin, S. J. (2000). 12-Step participation and attitudes toward 12-step meetings in dual diagnosis patients. *Alcohol Treat Quarterly, 18*, 31–45.

Bogenschutz, M. P. (2005). Specialized 12-step programs and 12-step facilitation for the dually diagnosed. *Community Mental Health Journal, 41*(1), 7–20.

Bogenschutz, M. P. (2007). 12-step approaches for the dually diagnosed: Mechanisms of change. *Alcoholism: Clinical and Experimental Research*, *31*(Suppl. 10), 64s–66s.

CAPSS NEWS (August 2010). Client Affairs/Peer Support Services A Quarterly Publication from the SCDMH Office of Client Affairs. Vol. 4 Issue 4 Retrieved 8/5/2012 from the Official Web Site of the State of South Carolina http://www.state.sc.us/dmh/client_affairs/capss/2010_aug.pdf

Davidson, L., Chinman, M., Sells, D., & Rowe, M. (2006). Peer support among adults with serious mental illness: A report from the field. *Schizophrenia Bulletin*, *32*(3), 443–450.

Double Trouble in Recovery. (1993). *The dual disorders recovery book: A twelve step program for those of us with addiction and an emotional or psychiatric illness.* Center City, MN: Hazelden Foundation.

Double Trouble in Recovery. (n.d.). *Welcome to Double Trouble in Recovery pamphlet.* Retrieved from http://www.scshare.com/downloads/DTR_Brochure.pdf

Editor (reissued 2006) Depressed Anonymous: A Spiritual Program for Personal Recovery and Serenity. The Antidepressant Tablet, an Internet sample edition! http://www.depressedanon.com/PDF%20Files/The%20Antidepressant%20Tablet.pdf Accessed August 5, 2012.

Emotional Health Anonymous website (2011) http://www.emotionalhealthanonymous.org accessed November 13, 2011 and 8/5/2012

Dual Recovery Anonymous. (n.d.). *Medications and recovery*. Retrieved from http://draonline.org/medications.html

Gorski, T. T. (1989). *Understanding the twelve steps: An interpretation and guide for recovering people.* New York, NY: Prentice Hall/Parkside Recovery Book.

Gronfein, W. (1985). Psychotropic drugs and the origins of deinstitutionalization. *Social Problems*, *32*(5), 437–454.

Hamilton, T. (1994). *The Twelve Steps and Dual Disorders: A Framework of Recovery for Those of us with Addiction and an Emotional or Psychiatric Illness.* Center City, Minnesota: Hazelden

Hartigan, F. (2000). *Bill W: A biography of Alcoholics Anonymous cofounder Bill Wilson*. New York, NY: St. Martin's Press.

Havassy, B. E., Alvidrez, J., & Mericle, A. A. (2009). Disparities in use of mental health and substance abuse services by persons with co-occurring disorders. *Psychiatric Services*, *60*(2), 217–223.

Humphreys, K. (2004). *Circles of recovery: Self-help organizations for addictions.* Cambridge, UK: Cambridge University Press.

Jordan, L. C., Davidson, W. S., Herman, S. E., & BootsMiller, B. J. (2002). Involvement in 12-step programs among persons with dual diagnoses. *Psychiatric Services*, *53*(7), 894–896.

Kaskutas, L., & Oberste, E. (2002). MAA*EZ: Making Alcoholics Anonymous easier. Berkeley, CA: Public Health Institute.

Laudet, A. (2008). The impact of Alcoholics Anonymous on other substance abuse-related twelve-step programs. *Recent Developments in Alcoholism*, *18*, 71–89.

Laudet, A., Magura, S., Vogel, H., & Knight, E. (2000). Support, mutual aid and recovery from dual diagnosis. *Community Mental Health Journal*, *36*(5), 457–476.

Magura, S. (2008). Effectiveness of dual focus mutual aid for co-occurring substance use and mental health disorders: A review and synthesis of the 'Double Trouble' in Recovery evaluation. *Substance Use & Misuse, 43*(12/13), 1904–1926.

Makin-Byrd, K., Cronkite, R. C., & Timko, C. (2011). The influence of abuse victimization on attendance and involvement in mutual-help groups among dually diagnosed male veterans. *Journal of Substance Abuse Treatment, 41*(1), 78–87.

Meissen, G., Powell, T. J., Wituk, S. A., Girrens, K., & Arteaga, S. (1999). Attitudes of AA contact persons toward group participation by persons with a mental illness. *Psychiatr Serv, 50*(8), 1079–1081.

No author. (Reissued 2006). The Twelve Steps of Depressed Anonymous. The Antidepressant Tablet, an Internet sample edition! p. 10. http://www.depressedanon.com/PDF%20Files/The%20Antidepressant%20Tablet.pdf Accessed August 5, 2011.

Nowinski, J., Baker, S., & Carroll, K. (1994). *Twelve step facilitation therapy manual* (Vol. 1). Rockville, MD: U.S. Department of Health and Human Services.

Pickett, Phillips, & Kraus. (2011). *Recovery International group meeting evaluation: Final report.* Chicago, IL: University of Illinois at Chicago, Department of Psychiatry. Retrieved from http://www.lowselfhelpsystems.org

Pistrang, N., Barker, C., & Humphreys, K. (2008). Mutual help groups for mental health problems: A review of effectiveness studies. *American Journal of Community Psychology, 42*(1/2), 110–121.

Schizophrenia and Related Disorders Alliance of America. (n.d.). *Schizophrenics Anonymous guiding principles.* Retrieved from http://www.sardaa.org/schizophrenics-anonymous/sa-guiding-principles

Sheffield, A. (2003). Referral to a peer-led support group: An effective aid for mood disorder patients. *Primary Psychiatry, 10*(5), 89–94.

Substance Abuse and Mental Health Services Administration. (2010). *Results from the 2009 National Survey on Drug Use and Health: Vol. I. Summary of national findings.* Rockville, MD: Office of Applied Studies, National Survey on Drug Use and Health Series H-38A.

Thomas, M. (2008). *Double Trouble in Recovery: A Collection of Dual-Diagnosis Mental Health Recovery Stories, Volume II.* Retrieved from South Carolina SHARE http://www.scshare.com/downloads/Double_Trouble_Booklet.pdf

Timko, C., Sutkowi, A., Cronkite, R. C., Makin-Byrd, K., & Moos, R. H. (2011). Intensive referral to 12-step dual-focused mutual-help groups. *Drug and Alcohol Dependence, 118*(2/3), 194–201.

Villano, C., Rosenblum, A., Magura, S., Betzler, T., Vogel, H., & Knight, E. (2005). Mental health clinicians' 12-step referral practices with dually diagnosed clients. *International Journal of Self-Help & Self-Care, 3*(1/2), 63–71.

Vogel, H. S., Knight, E., Laudet, A. B., & Magura, S. (1998). Double Trouble in Recovery: Self-help for people with dual diagnoses. *Psychiatric Rehabilitation Journal, 21*(4), 356–364.

White, W. L. (2008a). *Recovery management and recovery-oriented systems of care: Scientific rationale and promising practices.* Pittsburg, PA: Northeast Addiction Technology Transfer Center; Chicago, IL: Great Lakes Addiction Technology

Transfer Center; Philadelphia Department of Behavioral Health/Mental Retardation.

White, W. (2008b). Recovery: Old wine, flavor of the month or new organizing paradigm? *Substance Use and Misuse, 43*, 1–14.

White, W., & Kurtz, E. (2008). Twelve defining moments in the history of Alcoholics Anonymous. In M. Galanter & L. Kaskutas (Eds.), *Recent developments in alcoholism* (Vol. 18, pp. 37–57). New York, NY: Plenum..

Zweben, J. E. (1987). Recovery-oriented psychotherapy: Facilitating the use of 12-step programs. *Journal of Psychoactive Drugs, 19*(3), 243–251.

Giving Back and Getting Something Back: The Role of Mutual-Aid Groups for Individuals in Recovery From Incarceration, Addiction, and Mental Illness

CHYRELL D. BELLAMY, MICHAEL ROWE, PATRICIA BENEDICT, and LARRY DAVIDSON

Program for Recovery and Community Health, Department of Psychiatry, Yale University School of Medicine, New Haven, Connecticut, USA

Mutual-aid groups for people in recovery from mental illness, addictions, and former incarceration are virtually nonexistent. This article provides a review of the literature on mutual-aid groups for people who have previous incarceration histories and a review of groups for people with mental illness and multiple concerns (i.e., co-occurring diagnoses). Next, we present the "What's Up?" group, a component of the Citizenship Community Enhancement Project, as an example of a mutual-aid group that was developed to better address these multiple concerns. The "What's Up?" group was designed as a mutual-aid component for individuals living with mental illness and/or co-occurring substance abuse concerns who also have a history of previous involvement with the criminal justice system. Experiences of participants highlight ways in which the "What's Up?" group provided opportunities for its members to not only "give back" but to "get something back" from the sharing of experiences and feedback offered from their peers.

INTRODUCTION

> We just want to give back . . .

The concept of "giving back" is a common theme in the community narrative of individuals who are in recovery from former incarcerations (as well as other concerns such as addictions and mental illness). Maruna, LeBel, Mitchell, and Naples (2004) suggest that these individuals " . . . have to feel that this reintegration has been justified by their own efforts to 'make good and redress past crimes'" (p. 272). By giving back, people are able to make something good come out of their former difficult situations. But what about the response of a peer-support staff member in relation to the importance of giving back?

> Why is it that we are always the ones that have to give back? Perhaps that's part of the problem; some of us have been giving so much of ourselves for too long. (peer supporter, 2012)

Giving back is one part of the mutual-aid process, but as this person suggests, it is only one part. What about the "getting something back part"? The process of developing mutual relationships involves people being able to give and to receive support or to learn from each other. The "getting something back" part, although it may be implicit in the notion of a self-help or mutual-aid group, has been less a part of the community narrative. In this article, we discuss the concepts of giving and getting something back within the framework of a mutual-aid group called "What's Up?"—a mutual-aid group component of the Citizens Community Enhancement Project (CCEP) for people with mental illness and substance use who also are recovering from incarceration. We first begin by reviewing the literature on mutual-aid groups for those who were formerly incarcerated; we then review the literature on groups for people with mental illness and addiction (including a discussion of challenges for members with multiple concerns), and then provide an overview of the "What's Up?" group and experiences of former members of the group.

THEORETICAL UNDERPINNINGS

Mutual Aid—Strengths-Based Versus Control-Based Narratives

There are several narratives common in criminal justice and particular to restoration and recovery. Maruna and LeBel (2003) describe these as control narratives, support- or needs-based narratives, and strengths-based narratives. In brief, control narratives suggest that people formerly incarcerated are seen as "risky until proven guilty" (Maruna et al., 2004, p. 272). Use of this narrative invites a host of sanctions that are then applied with the expectation that these efforts can "thwart an offender's criminal instincts" (Maruna & LeBel, p. 94). According to Maruna and LeBel: "Strengths-based or restorative approaches ask not what a person's deficits are, but rather what positive contribution the person can make" (p. 97). The strengths-based perspective emphasizes that stigma, and its consequences are at the root of what makes the individuals reoffend, not internal deficits. To combat social exclusion, the strengths-based or restorative paradigm calls for opportunities for those formerly incarcerated to make amends, demonstrate their value and potential, and make positive contributions to their communities (Maruna & LeBel, p. 97). Maruna and colleagues' work in this area, while focused on the concerns of individuals with a history of incarceration, builds on the strengths-based perspective that is currently offered in self-help and mutual-aid approaches across various concerns in the behavioral health field, specifically for those experiencing mental illness and substance abuse issues. More specifically, the strengths-based paradigm has included an orientation toward the helper-therapy (Riessman, 1965) and the wounded healer (White, 2000) principles as valued and necessary additions to the work—that is, that people in recovery can provide supports to others facing similar concerns because they "have been there."

The Helper/Wounded Healer Principle for People With Former Incarcerations

To understand the significance of the concepts of the helper-therapy and wounded healer principles for people with former incarcerations, LeBel (2007) conducted a study to explore whether having the helper/wounded healer orientation has an effect on incarceration recidivism and other psychological and community factors. The study was conducted among 228 formerly incarcerated individuals in New York. Results suggest that recidivism rates declined for individuals who were involved in activities oriented toward helping or "giving back" (LeBel). The findings suggest that people who have been formerly incarcerated want to give back, to become mentors and wounded healers. LeBel also found that identification with others who had former incarcerations had a strong association with "living a law-abiding life" and that having feelings of remorse was a strong predictor of the helper orientation. It should be noted that for people that were under current community supervision, there were fewer tendencies to help others. LeBel hypothesized that this could be the result of supervision restraints on ex-offenders, some of whom were not permitted to fraternize with formerly incarcerated individuals. LeBel's findings suggest the opposite—having group identification and a helper/wounded healer orientation was unrelated to criminal attitude, thus suggesting that individuals with former incarcerations can form positive relationships with their peers. In addition, having stronger social bonds with similar others was positively correlated with psychological well-being. Perceptions of personal stigma, on the other hand, were negatively related to psychological well-being and were related positively to having a criminal attitude (LeBel). These results are limited, yet provide support for strengths-based approaches like mutual aid and the helper/wounded healer orientation as a way for people with former incarcerations to experience "giving back" through sharing and learning from others.

The literature in this area is limited. More studies are needed that focus on the use of the helper/wounded healer orientation with people who have been formerly incarcerated so that LeBel's (2007) findings can be replicated and/or expanded upon and hopefully lend credence to advancing the field toward a more strengths-based discourse for individuals with former incarcerations. In addition, although there have been some mutual-aid groups specifically developed for people with former incarcerations, there is a dearth of research studies on these mutual-aid/self-help groups in the literature. In the next section, we provide an overview of mutual-aids groups as described in the literature both for formerly incarcerated individuals as well as for people with multiple concerns such as mental illness and substance abuse experiences.

MUTUAL-AID GROUPS

Mutual Aid for Individuals Formerly Incarcerated

Self-help groups for individuals formerly incarcerated have been documented in the literature dating back to the 1950s and 1960s (Hamm, 1988; Mcanany & Tromanhauser, 1977). Individuals upon return from prison would go back to their communities and form "rap sessions" with other ex-offenders. Mcanany and Tromanhauser report that the groups became more popular in the 1970s, with several unsuccessful attempts to create national or local mutual-aid organizations and groups but with success at local levels with groups such as the Seventh Step and Fortune Society and groups formed through the American Friends Service Committee. More recent organizations include: the Osbourne Association in New York City, The Ordinary People Society in Alabama, All of Us None of Us primarily in California, Women on the Rise Telling Herstory in New York City, and the Winners Circle Program sponsored by the Treatment Alternatives for Safe Communities.

The Winners Circle Program consists of groups for people returning from incarceration, modeled after 12-step programs. However, one difference is that "cross-talk" is permitted and outsiders often are used to provide lectures for the groups. Lyons and Lurigio (2010) report that the Winners Circle is an example of a group that builds recovery capital among the members by providing information about employment, reducing stigma, and providing connections for individuals to the community.

Although there has been a growth of organizations and programs, there remains a gap in addressing the increase in numbers of individuals returning home each year from prisons, often estimated at approximately 700,000 people (Leary, 2011). Programs and organizations, whether identified as mutual aid or community reentry, should consider the initial evidence from LeBel (2007), which suggests ways in which the mutual-aid/self-help process can impact recidivism and psychological well-being and ways in which society can, in turn, benefit from these individuals who want to give back to their communities. In addition, the literature on mutual-aid groups with individuals experiencing other concerns also provides support for mutual-aid groups.

Mutual-Aid Groups for Individuals With Mental Illness and Addiction

There is an expansive literature on the use and benefits of self-help groups for people in recovery from mental health concerns (Armstrong, 1995; Bellamy et al., 2006; Corrigan et al., 2002; Garvin, 1992; Kurtz, 2004; Mowbray, Robinson, & Holter, 2002; Phillips, Lakin, & Pargament, 2002; Rappaport, Reischl, & Zimmerman, 1992; Roberts, Salem, Rappaport, Luke, Toro, & Seidman, 1997). Some of the internationally known self-help groups include: Schizophrenics Anonymous, Depression and Bipolar Support Alliance, GROW, and Recovery International (formerly, Recovery, Inc.).

For individuals with co-occurring substance use, the options available for other more "identifiable" self-help groups are reduced significantly. Some prefer to attend Alcoholics Anonymous (AA), Narcotics Anonymous (NA), or other self-help groups, either using a combination of self-help approaches for mental illness and addiction or one or the other. It is not our attempt to "bash or discredit" the members of AA or NA groups; however, it is important to discuss the concerns that some persons with mental illness have reported in part because of stigma (actual or perceived) related to their psychiatric symptoms; their reduced or limited social skills; or the strong antimedication stance historically taken by some AA and NA groups (Polcin & Zemore, 2004). It should be noted that the authors of this article recognize the importance of AA and NA groups for individuals with mental illness and substance abuse concerns and are aware that for the majority, these groups in some areas of the United States may be the only choices available for self-help groups.

The Experiences of People With Multiple Conditions in Existing Mutual-Aid Groups

Moos and Moos (2005) surmise that individuals not having relative success with their first encounter with AA or other self-help groups, may be at a higher risk for developing long-term problems (Moos & Moos). To address this concern, self-help groups for persons with co-occurring disorders have been developed such as Double Trouble in Recovery (DTR; Laudet, Magura, Vogel, & Knight, 2000; Magura, Laudet, Mahmood, Rosenblum, Vogel, & Knight, 2003). In DTR groups, individuals are free to discuss their mental health issues, including their symptoms. DTR groups are becoming more widespread. For example, the Connecticut Community for Addiction Recovery, a mutual-aid organization, provides trainings for individuals in the state of Connecticut on how to start DTR groups.

Our own experience has also highlighted the challenges faced by persons with multiple conditions when accessing existing mutual-support organizations. Institutional review board approval was obtained to conduct a focus group with members of the CCEP who had attended AA, NA, and/or DTR groups. Four themes emerged that spoke to the challenges people face and the strategies they used in such groups: (1) feeling different; (2) fitting in; (3) taking it for what it is; and, (4) it is not for everyone.

Feeling Different

Several participants spoke about feeling different at AA or NA meetings. One said: "I did not look 'right' (when coming back to AA after a psychiatric relapse). Sometimes I felt ostracized because I looked peculiar. My symptoms stood out. My sponsor did not want to deal with me—his only response was, 'do the 5th step.'"

Fitting In

Most participants said that "fitting in" in 12-step meetings was difficult for them, especially regarding trust in others' intentions: "I was told to shut up when talking about my mental illness. Someone called me a mental case and told me I should be hospitalized. I was even told not to come back to the meeting. If you are not part of their clique, you do not feel like you belong."

Taking It for What It Is

Several participants learned to accept AA and NA for what they could do for them. Said one participant:

> Even with AA, it was uncomfortable for me to trust and be vulnerable. At first, I was turned off by the stories of others. I felt uncomfortable opening up because I didn't know whether they were telling the truth. But then by listening, I could hear their stories and I felt that I was not that bad.

One peer mentor mentioned that he took several participants with him to AA meetings but that they would get up and leave. He encouraged them to come back: "Let them have enough time to hear what is being said." Several participants mentioned that people in AA are not familiar with mental illness: "They operate on a feeling level. They are better able to deal with, 'I did not feel well today.'" Learning to talk about his problems in a more "generic" way helped this person to stay long enough to hear what others had to say. Others spoke of negative experiences, but said that when they returned, they were eventually welcomed.

It is Not for Everyone

Some participants said that because of their negative encounters, they will never go back to AA or NA. Others simply said it is not for everyone. Three chose to attend AA and/or a DTR group, stating they felt more comfortable being able to talk about their complete experiences, not just the alcohol or drug problems.

To better understand some of the challenges discussed by the focus-group members described here, we also held a focus group with AA members recruited from the community who did *not* have a history of mental illness to ask about their experiences of having people with disclosed mental illnesses in AA meetings. Overall, focus-group participants felt that AA groups were generally receptive to the participation of persons with mental illness. They acknowledged that this was not the case for all AA groups or members, however. Regarding our question about participation in AA meetings while taking psychiatric medications, participants thought this was not a major issue in AA as a whole at present but acknowledged that it crops up in some meetings. Regarding recommendations and tips for persons with mental illness trying to "make it" in AA, participants had a number of concrete suggestions, including:

1. Going to beginners' meetings, where beginners speak first;
2. Going early and leaving late to meet people individually and informally;
3. Trying different meetings until you find one you like;
4. Going to a speakers meeting—most of the meeting is taken up with speeches and you can say, "I'm just here to listen tonight," if you are uncomfortable speaking;
5. Finding a sponsor who has something in common with you (one person acknowledged that it did not work for him one time when he sponsored a person with mental illness and suggested that matchup is important. He said: "Mental illness is not my field; I'm here to help you stay sober");
6. Finding others, not only a sponsor, you can call upon when you need them;
7. Reaching out and asking for help ("There is great camaraderie if you reach out"); and

8. Taking on a valued role, such as "coffee commitment" ("I had to be there. People depended on me").

These suggestions are beneficial for anyone attending self-help groups, but especially for individuals with multiple concerns so that perhaps they can attend and benefit from these more traditional self-help approaches. However, these experiences also point to the need for individuals with multiple concerns to have other mutual-aid and self-help options available where they can discuss their multiple concerns and challenges. In addition, a suggestion for programmatic assistance should be made available for people with mental illness that can facilitate their transition into these more traditional addiction-based self-help groups (Hatfield, 1993; Herman, Frank, Mowbray, Ribisl, & Davidson, 2000; Kurtz, 1997; Moos & Moos, 2005).

There are limits to the focus-group data we described, including that only one focus group was done with each group and that the focus-group participants focused on their own personal experiences with these more traditional self-help approaches. In addition, we did not conduct a focus group with an NA group, which tended to be the self-help group that was more often referred to in the examples described by our CCEP focus-group participants. There is not a "one size fits all" with any self-help or mutual-aid group. However, these findings lend some initial support to the creation of mutual-aid groups for individuals with multiple concerns.

WHAT'S UP: A MUTUAL-AID GROUP FOR PEOPLE WITH CO-OCCURRING CONDITIONS AND A CRIMINAL JUSTICE HISTORY

Self-help/mutual-aid groups for people in recovery from mental illness, addiction, and former incarcerations are virtually nonexistent. To address this need, we developed the CCEP, a 16-week group that consists of citizenship-based nontraditional classroom learning, a mutual-aid group called "What's Up," a valued role project, and a wraparound peer-mentoring component. Citizenship classes enhance participants' knowledge of available community resources; their problem-solving and other life skills for daily living; knowledge of their criminal justice-related rights and responsibilities and assistance in developing the social skills, hope, and resilience to meet them; and their ability to establish social networks based on mutual trust and shared interests. The valued role projects encourage participants to contribute to their communities by drawing on their life experiences and skills they gained through mutual aid, class work, and contacts with community presenters. The peer mentors for CCEP encourage participants to maintain their sobriety by offering examples of their own struggles and community reintegration work and providing social support, referral to mental health and addictions treatment, and practical advice to them (see Rowe et al., 2009, for a more extensive overview of the project). Results from a randomized study on the citizenship intervention show that it facilitated participants' decreased alcohol use (Rowe et al., 2007) and decreased drug use (Clayton, O'Connell, Bellamy, Benedict, & Rowe, 2012) compared with those receiving usual services.

The "What's Up" mutual-aid group was developed in response to a need that participants of CCEP expressed to have a portion of time set aside for them to talk with their peers about what was happening in their lives outside the context of the classroom discussion. "What's Up?" meets an hour prior to the 1-hour instructional class. The mutual-aid group format consists of participants sharing what is going on for them in their lives and then accepting/receiving feedback and suggestions from others. A participant gets to listen but does not get to respond during the course of receiving the feedback (participants do often talk to each other outside of the group to obtain further information). The premise of feedback is based on participants developing the ability to give back to other students by providing suggestions of other ways to address challenges. It is also based on the ability to "get something back," to be able to hear from their peers' suggestions on how to manage situations or circumstances differently, and to hear encouragement when things are going well or not so well. Participants give hope to each other and often "ride" off the hope of another until they begin to embrace it for themselves.

For people with a history of incarceration (without a diagnosed mental health disorder), the framework can provide skill building that blends "self-advocacy with empathic sensitivities ... and provide positive tools for making and maintaining meaningful relationships in multiple aspects of life in the community" (Wolff & Draine, 2004, p. 474). Wolff and Draine advocate for programs and groups that build on "positive self-image, self-esteem, and mastery, the ability to effectively manage and rebound from disappointments and setbacks, and appropriately self-regulate behaviors and reactions" (p. 474). Stigma is met head on as participants learn to explore themselves, their relationships with others (such as family members), their relationships in the community, and how it all fits in within the larger society (often within a race- and class-based discussion).

"What's Up?" provides a vehicle by which participants discuss and put into practice the Five Rs of citizenship: rights, responsibility, roles, resources, and relationships (Rowe et al., 2009). Participants learn from each other that they have a *right* to their feelings and opinions and an expectation that they will be treated with dignity and respect. Personal and community *responsibility* is learned by participants feeling a collective responsibility to their fellow members and then learning to extend that sense of connection and responsibility to their families, friends, and the broader community. *Roles* are offered to participants as facilitators of the group process in addition to the role they play in giving back to the other participants through feedback. Learning how to give feedback takes time for some people, but by observing the process from other members, they quickly jump into the role. In addition, roles are explored by participants discussing various possibilities of identities outside the context of the group, such as family members, community members, employees, friends, etc. Getting feedback and support on how to manage and/or negotiate these roles from each other helps the participants to know that they are not the only ones with those experiences. *Resources* are shared among the participants during feedback. We often find that collectively, participants have a wealth of knowledge about resources in the community, probably even more so than formal service providers. Finally, by learning and practicing the skills of giving and getting something back, participants are able to better maintain *relationships* with each other and in the community (Rowe et al., 2009).

Participants' Experiences

Another study was done that involved interviewing participants from CCEP (institutional review board approval was obtained) about their experiences in the "What's Up" group (Schmidt, 2009). Some participants mentioned their lack of trust at the beginning, when they first joined the group, and spoke of a sense of relief by sharing with others and of learning to trust the group process:

> When I first showed up to the program, I was like, I don't know these people. I'm not going to open my door, tell them my personal business, tell them what I'm about, tell them what I am, or who I am. . . . But then I felt like I was relieving a whole bunch of pressure and pain off my back. All the weight was lifted when I did this. And ever since then, I've been feeling free. I felt good. I felt good about myself. . . . I talked about everything. I talked about a lot of stuff that I never talked to other people about. . . . I mentioned a lot of personal stuff, a lot of personal business, my personal lifestyle, that I don't tell other people. And I opened up. That was the first wall I knocked down. That brick wall right there. Once I knocked that brick wall down, all the other walls started stumbling. Bricks started falling slowly but surely. . . . Because I felt like I could trust these people. These people is the type of people that says what stays in the group stays in the group. What goes on in group, what's being mentioned in group don't go out of group. . . . When I spoke out, nothing ever came back to me. It never was spoken. It never came back and hit the streets. And I felt good about it. I felt free and comfortable about it.

Another person spoke to the challenges of learning how to "get something back":

> The feedback, they was to help me, not to hurt me. Even sometimes when you don't want to hear what they got to say—and I do, I listen to

> them—and 9 out of 10 they right. Even though I don't want to hear it, I listened anyway. I took the cotton out of my ears and I listened. I listened to what they had to say, and it was up to me to take their advice. So I wind up taking their advice, and it ended up 9 out of 10 working for me.

Through the "What's Up" process, participants were able to benefit from the experiences of others who had gone through similar experiences, and over time, they were able to accept the advice as a gift from their peers. Participants also shared in the interviews about learning new ways to deal with stress while remaining focused on their recovery:

> So, I found my sister dead, and that was very hard for me. ... I used to use drugs in place of feeling things. So when I came into [the] program ... [they] said '___, listen, this is what we're going to do.' On the days like, you know, the anniversaries, the birthdays, those days were very hard for me and those were the days that I would use the most. So, they said, 'Listen, you're clean now. What area of your life is important to you?' They asked me that question. And I said, 'Oh, I'd have to think about that.' And then they asked me, 'What would you like to do instead of getting high?' And I was like, 'Hmm,' because I didn't know anything else but getting high. So I said, 'Wow! I would like to go to the park and build a big sand castle.' She said, 'Now that's something that you can think about doing on those days, their anniversaries and their birthdays and stuff like that.' And then I had someone else in the group said, '____, listen, we will come with you.' And we went to Lighthouse Park, and we built a sandcastle. And it was great. And I didn't get high. These are things that they taught me that help me. You know, and today, I am so grateful to them because of it, you know?

One person spoke specifically to the experience of being built up rather than feeling the need to be broken down, something that she had experienced in NA/AA groups:

> In the beginning, it was very, very hard for me, because like I said, I came in and I was a bag of shambles, and I didn't know how to piece my life together. I had been recently incarcerated and I had just been released. ... So I started attending. And I wasn't at all doing well. I had been, man, the drugs, the alcohol. I had been cutting. I was a cutter. And all these things I have under control now. I can even show you some of the cut marks that I used to cut myself. ... But today, I'm a new person. You know? You know how they say in NA and AA programs that they'll break you down and build you back up? I was already broke down, and they allowed me to build myself back up. And I appreciate that today.

The participants' comments captured the essence of the "What's Up?" experience. It is a familiar story that has been described anecdotally by many CCEP participants during the past 8 years: (a) an initial reluctance to being a part of the group because of trust and previous experiences with other self-help groups; (b) an awareness of having similarities with other participants by hearing their stories and providing feedback; and (c) an acceptance of their new role as someone who both gives back to others and learns to appreciate and embrace what it means to receive from others. We hope to explore these processes more specifically particularly to measure how the "giving back" and "getting back" process influences community-related outcomes for people in recovery from mental illness, and/or co-occurring diagnoses, and former incarceration.

DISCUSSION

Although there are limited numbers of groups for people in recovery from mental illness and incarceration, the literature and participants' examples provided here give some evidence of the ways in which mutual-aid groups can support the recovery of people with criminal justice histories who, in addition, have psychiatric and/or substance use diagnoses. Mutual aid as a strengths-based approach allows for the development of individuals' ability to practice giving back and learning more about what it means to give back and to get something back. These instrumental interpersonal skills are essential toward the goal of community reentry and reintegration.

The "What's Up?" group is one model of a mutual-aid group that provides this opportunity, the Winners Circle is another, and others are emerging in small pockets around the country. There is a need for the creation and development of additional groups for this population. Recovery and restoration experiences of individuals using these mutual-aid groups need to be further examined, particularly in regard to long-term outcomes and how the group process may facilitate community reentry. Additionally, community reentry outcomes need to be examined for self-help/mutual-aid approaches compared with outcomes for people attending the traditional programs being offered for community reentry for people returning home from incarceration.

REFERENCES

Armstrong, M. L., Korba, A. M., & Emard, R. (1995). Of mutual benefit: the reciprocal relationship between consumer volunteers and the clients they serve. *Psychiatric Rehabilitation Journal, 19*(2), 45–49.

Bellamy, C. D., Garvin, C., MacFarlane, P., Mowbray, O. P., Mowbray, C. T., & Holter, M. C. (2006). An analysis of groups in consumer-centered programs. *American Journal of Psychiatric Rehabilitation, 9*(3), 219–240.

Clayton, A., O'Connell, M. J., Bellamy, C., Benedict, P., & Rowe, M. (2012). The Citizenship Project Part II: Impact of a Citizenship Intervention on Clinical and Community Outcomes for Persons with Mental Illness and Criminal Justice Involvement. *American Journal of Community Psychology, 45*(1/2), DOI 10.1007/s10464-012-9549-z

Corrigan, P. W., Calabrese, J. D., Diwan, S. E., Keogh, C. B., Keck, L., & Mussey, C. (2002). Some recovery processes in mutual-help groups for persons with mental illness: I. Qualitative analysis of program materials and testimonials. *Community Mental Health Journal, 38*(4), 287–301.

Garvin, C. D. (1992). A task-centered group approach to work with the chronically mentally ill. *Social Work with Groups, 15*(2/3), 67–80.

Hamm, M. S. (1988). Current perspectives on the prisoner self-help movement. *Federal Probation, 52*, 49–56.

Hatfield, A. B. (1993). *Dual diagnosis and mental illness (schizophrenia and drug or alcohol dependence).* National Alliance for the Mentally Ill. Retrieved from http://www.schizophrenia.com/family/dualdiag.html

Herman, S. E., Frank, K. A., Mowbray, C. T., Ribisl, K. M., & Davidson, W. S. (2000). Longitudinal effects of integrated treatment on alcohol use for persons with serious mental illness and substance use disorders. *The Journal of Behavioral Health Services and Research, 27*, 286–302.

Kurtz, L. F. (1997). *Self-help and support groups: A handbook for practitioners*. Thousand Oaks, CA: Sage.

Laudet, A. B., Magura, S., Vogel, H. S., & Knight, E. (2000). Support, mutual aid and recovery from dual diagnosis. *Community Mental Health Journal, 36*, 457–476.

Leary, M. L. (2011, November). *Remarks of Mary Lou Leary, principal deputy assistant attorney general, Office of Justice Programs*. Presented at Tucson/Phoenix Criminal Law Seminar, Tucson and Phoenix, AZ. Retrieved from http://www.ojp.usdoj.gov/newsroom/speeches/2011/11_1116mleary.htm

LeBel, T. P. (2007). An examination of the impact of formerly incarcerated persons helping others. *Journal of Offender Rehabilitation, 46*(1/2), 1–24.

Lyons, T., & Lurigio, A. J. (2010). The role of recovery capital in the community reentry of prisoners with substance abuse disorders. *Journal of Offender Rehabilitation, 49*, 445–455.

Magura, S., Laudet, A. B., Mahmood, D., Rosenblum, A., Vogel, H. S., & Knight, E. L. (2003). Role of self-help processes in achieving abstinence among dually diagnosed persons. *Addictive Behaviors, 28*, 399–413.

Maruna, S., & LeBel, T. P. (2003). Welcome home? Examining the reentry court concept from a strengths-based perspective. *Western Criminology Review, 4*(2), 91–107.

Maruna, S., LeBel, T. P., Mitchell, N., & Naples, M. (2004). Pygmalion in the reintegration process: Desistance from crime through the looking glass. *Psychology, Crime & Law, 10*(3), 271–281.

Mcanany, P. D., & Tromanhauser, E. (1977). Organizing the convicted self-help for prisoners and ex-prisoners. *Crime & Delinquency, 23*, 68–74.

Moos, R. H., & Moos, B. S. (2005). Sixteen-year changes and stable remission among treated and untreated individuals with alcohol use disorders. *Drug and Alcohol Dependence, 80*, 337–347.

Mowbray, C. T., Robinson, E. A., & Holter, M. C. (2002). Consumer drop-in centers: Operations, services, and consumer involvement. *Health & Social Work, 27*(4), 248–261.

Phillips, R. E., Lakin, R., & Pargament, K. I. (2002). Brief report: Development and implementation of a spiritual issues psychoeducational group for those with serious mental illness. *Community Mental Health Journal, 38*(6), 487–495.

Polcin, D. L., & Zemore, S. (2004). Psychiatric severity and spirituality, helping, and participation in Alcoholics Anonymous during recovery. *American Journal of Drug and Alcohol Abuse, 30*, 577–592.

Rappaport, J., Reischl, T. M., & Zimmerman, M. A. (1992). Mutual help mechanisms in the empowerment of former mental health patients. In D. Saleeby (Ed.), *The strengths perspective in social work practice* (pp. 84–97). New York, NY: Longman.

Riessman, F. (1965). The 'helper' therapy principle. *Social Work, 10*(2), 27–32.

Roberts, L., Salem, D., Rappaport, J., Toro, P., Luke, D., & Seidman, E. (1999). Giving and receiving help: Interpersonal transactions in mutual-help meetings and psychosocial adjustment of members. *American Journal of Community Psychology, 27*(6), 841–868.

Rowe, M., Benedict, P., Sells, D., Dinzeo, T., Garvin, C., Schwab, L., Baranoski, M., Girard, V., & Bellamy, C. (2007). A peer-support, group intervention to reduce substance use and criminality among persons with severe mental illness. *Psychiatric Services, 58*, 955–961.

Rowe, M., Bellamy, C., Baranoski, M., Wieland, M., O'Connell, M. J., Benedict, P., Davidson, L., Buchanan, J., & Sells, D. (2009). Citizenship, community, and recovery: A group- and peer- based intervention for persons with co-occurring disorders and criminal justice histories. *Journal of Groups in Addiction & Recovery, 4*, 224–244.

Schmidt, B. (2009). *Building a sandcastle from a 'bag of shambles': A qualitative analysis of the jail diversion process (Unpublished master's thesis).* New Haven, CT: Yale University.

White, W. L. (2000). The history of recovered people as wounded healers: 11. The era of professionalization and specialization. *Alcoholism Treatment Quarterly, 18*(2), 1–25.

Wolff, N., & Draine, J. (2004). Dynamics of social capital of prisoners and community reentry: Ties that bind? *Journal of Correctional Health Care, 10*(3), 457–490.

Part III: Mutual Support Groups for Addiction – Generalizing the Principles

Use of Mutual Support to Counteract the Effects of Socially Constructed Stigma: Gender and Drug Addiction

JOLENE M. SANDERS
Department of Sociology & Social Work, Hood College, Frederick, Maryland, USA

This article describes the stigma women perceive as drug addicts and the strategies used to confront that stigma once they become members of a mutual support group, Narcotics Anonymous (NA). Stigma is heavily associated with being a drug addict and even more pronounced for the female drug addict. Public policy and media continue to focus on women's reproductive roles, igniting and perpetuating the stigmata associated with being female and addicted. The heavy emphasis on women's reproductive roles contributes to a double standard that women perceive it as unique to them as compared with their male counterparts. This study surveys a sample of women in NA that represents a potentially highly stigmatized group by race and class and uncovers the extent to which women perceive stigma both in their active addiction and once in recovery. Unexpectedly, women from a more socially disadvantaged background do not necessarily experience more stigma than their more privileged White, middle-class counterparts. Not surprisingly, women who have been involved in NA for longer periods of time and have completed the 12 steps perceive the least amount of stigma.

INTRODUCTION

Women seeking recovery from addiction bring with them feelings of guilt and shame that arise, in large part, from the stigma associated with overconsumption of substances. Although men are also stigmatized for their affliction, women experience a double standard applied to them, and this alone deters some women from seeking treatment for their addiction. Sustained cultural emphasis on gender roles, especially women's reproductive roles, contributes to the double standard for which women perceive they are judged. Additionally, stigma can be considered a social construction that exists in a larger cultural and political framework that women both conform to and challenge in their recovery from addiction. This article looks at the role mutual-support groups play in helping women to confront the social construction of the double standard as they seek recovery through affiliation and participation in a mutual-support group. Mutual-support groups offer an alternative to formal treatment and attempt to address the issue of stigma in their respective approaches to recovery. Mutual-support venues designed specifically for women allow them to acknowledge their perceptions and feelings associated with stigma, whether alcoholic or addicted to other drugs. Additionally, mutual-support groups that address drug addiction rather than alcohol addiction, solely, attract a more diverse membership including those women who have historically been the most socially marginalized, as well as addicted. It is the argument of this study that women in Narcotics Anonymous (NA) are likely to be highly stigmatized due to their social marginality and their addiction to illicit drugs. Therefore, particular attention is given to a sample of women seeking mutual support in NA. NA attracts a diverse population and is inclusive of all substance abuse including licit and illicit drug abuse as well as alcohol abuse.

Defining Stigma

A stigma is an attribute, behavior, or reputation that is socially discrediting in a particular way, leading to social disapproval by others (Goffman, 1963). A more expanded view of stigma points to negative stereotypes that result from stigmata that can, in turn, be generalized to an entire group of people. Individuals are labeled, classified, and in some way perceived as different from the normative group. The purpose of stigma is to make a clear distinction between the "in" and the "out" crowd to reinforce appropriate behavior or that which is perceived as moral.

However, social views differ over time and are shaped by various forces. The in-crowd is often defined by what group is in power, a political distinction, and the out-crowd can be more easily labeled as deviant. If certain moral views are shared by the elite, but not by the outsiders, stigma becomes a viable tool to mandate conformity. Of course, social revolutions, movements, and protests facilitate change in who occupies the in-crowd and what is held up as moral. Therefore, the designation of in-crowd and out-crowd is not static or fixed. Consequently, stigma, itself, is a socially constructed phenomenon. It is this social construction that this work focuses on, particularly as it relates to the female drug addict. Additionally, stigma and corresponding stereotypes re-create prejudice against minority groups, as well as other alleged deviant groups such as drug addicts. The manipulation of stigmata and stereotypes is well documented in the critique of social policy designed to prevent drug use and abuse, of propaganda campaigns that advocate the criminalization of drugs, and of the "war on drugs" that seeks to incarcerate rather than rehabilitate substance abusers (Belenko, 2000; Burton-Rose, 1998; Johns, 1992; Robinson & Scherlen, 2007; Shoemaker, 1989).

A significant social force in creating stereotypes is the media. Reality TV shows, cable channels dedicated to recovery, and the ever-present 24-hour news cycle actively seek to sensationalize substance abuse and addiction among the rich and the famous and in turn create a spectacle, a commodity to be consumed. Whether referred to as entertainment or news, the effect is the same—public humiliation. Although this emotion may not be directly felt by the individual who has agreed to participate in such a public forum, or because of their celebrity status they have come to tolerate public scrutiny, the stigmata associated with addiction are propagated, nonetheless, and this, in turn, reinforces the negative stereotypes about all those who are addicted. As a result, the everyday addict whose life-world is completely opposite of that of a Hollywood celebrity does not have the protective shield of wealth and fame and is consequently tarnished, branded, and humiliated by the public depiction. In this process of constructing stigma, the media is complicit in recasting negative images of the addicted.

Mutual Support Groups for Women

One significant response to stigma and in particular women's experience of it in relationship to substance use disorder has been the formation of gender-specific mutual-support groups. Three groups in particular—Women for Sobriety (WFS), women-only meetings of Alcoholics Anonymous (AA), and women-only meetings of NA—offer a recovery venue that acknowledges the role of stigma in addiction. WFS, discussed by Fenner and Gifford in this issue, began as an alternative to AA and specifically targets female alcoholics. Its founder, Jean Kirkpatrick, sought a cognitive rather than a spiritual approach toward recovery from her own alcoholism and started WFS in 1975. Unique to WFS, Kirkpatrick sought to enhance women's self-esteem through her 13 affirmations. She, a sociologist, acknowledged women's disadvantaged position within the social structure and linked this to women's low self-esteem. In addition to the deliberate focus on self-esteem, the WFS program philosophy recognizes the guilt women harbor over their drinking and works to help women overcome this guilt. In fact, it has been argued by others, as well, that the guilt women as recovering alcoholics feel is largely attributed to stigma. Downing (1991) wrote of triple stigmatization of the female alcoholic, which incorporates the double standard as applied to women. Women are initially branded as part of the inebriant class, are further branded due to the perception that they are not conforming to the traditional views of how women are supposed to behave in society, and thirdly, are subject to the perception that women who drink too much are inevitably sexually promiscuous (Sandmaier, 1980).

Given its WFS's explicitly gendered approach, Kaskutas (1996) sought to find out why WFS as an organization is not more widely known and why women do not publically disclose their affiliation with the organization. Unlike AA and its tradition of anonymity, WFS has no such code. In fact, it has to work against the dominant mutual-support paradigm of AA and needs some form of publicity to grow. Kaskutas (1996) offered that stigma accounts for some of the "invisibility" of WFS. Related to WFS's limited reach, too, may be that it attracts a particular demographic that may choose to stay invisible. In 1992, Kaskutas found that WFS membership was predominantly White, middle-aged, well educated, and of the upper socioeconomic class. Anonymity may remain a preferred mutual-support strategy even in groups that do not endorse it due more to the stigma perceived by female participants than to any organizational norm.

The reasons women cite for attending the various mutual-help groups designed specifically for women expose elements of the double standard women perceive. The same survey of women in WFS conducted in 1992 and cited above reports that women attend WFS for four overarching reasons. These include receiving support from others, attraction to the program philosophy, welcoming an all-women forum, and perceiving WFS as a safe environment. Among those who also attend AA meetings (about one third of the WFS sample), they reported doing so primarily out of the belief that it is necessary for them to stay sober, because they like the program philosophy, and because they receive general support via fellowship, sharing, and learning from others in the program (Kaskutas, 1994). Alternatively, for those WFS members who did not attend AA meetings, 10% attribute lack of attendance to not feeling comfortable or because they felt they did not "fit in." When comparing WFS to AA, Kaskutas finds that women enjoy the supportive, safe, nurturing, and intimate environment of the all-women's forum of WFS (1994). These findings, together, call for the consideration of an all-women's forum in AA that may combine what appear to be disparate reasons to attend either WFS or AA.

Similar to WFS, women-only groups of AA have evolved as a response to what has been perceived as a male-dominated culture of recovery. While not explicitly focused on women's self-esteem, reference to women's issues and more specific dialogue to women's everyday experiences can be heard at these meetings. Sticking to the original 12 steps, women ascribe to a spiritual-based program as do all members of AA, but they have carved out their own gendered environment. Women attend women-only meetings because they feel safer, they can talk about issues specific to women, and in general, they feel more comfortable (Sanders, 2010, p. 24). It is within this gendered space that women are able to confront issues related to stigma.

For many of the same reasons women attend women-only AA meetings, so do women recovering from a drug (other than alcohol) addiction attend women-only NA meetings. Sometimes referred to as "Women's Rap" meetings, women in NA report that they can be more honest in women-only meetings, that they can learn from other women who have been through similar things, that they do not feel judged, and that they are more comfortable, in general, talking about themselves. These reasons suggest a double standard could persist in NA, as well as in AA. Moreover, given the expanded reach of the media, social policy, and even treatment programs (Chavkin & Breitbart, 1997; Chavkin, Elman, & Wise, 1998) in contributing to stigma, it is to be expected that women in NA will experience stigma across multiple dimensions—gender, race, class, and drug of abuse. While all three of these mutual-support groups either directly or indirectly address the issue of stigma, NA as a mutual-support group explicitly acknowledges stigma in its organizational literature and recognizes that addicts have lived a lifestyle that is perceived by outsiders as worthy of that stigma. Moreover, NA's membership is more diverse than either AA or WFS, and NA addresses illicit drug abuse rather than solely alcohol abuse. Therefore, this study looks specifically at a sample of women in NA to gauge their level of perceived stigma as recovering addicts.

METHODOLOGY

A survey was conducted among women attending NA meetings in the summer of 2010. The survey instrument and data collection methodology received institutional review board approval, and a student research assistant helped to facilitate data collection. A letter of introduction and consent accompanied each questionnaire. Questionnaires were disseminated at women-only meetings just after the meetings, and respondents were asked to complete the four-page questionnaire and return it in the self-addressed, prestamped envelope. Qualitative data were gained by attending open NA meetings, which allow for nonmembers to attend. Notes were taken just afterward. Response rate was low (30%), even given that the research assistant matched the demographic profile (African American and female) of much of the sample and resides in the same community. A laminated meditation card inscribed with a recovery message was attached to each questionnaire as an incentive. Additionally, $5 gift cards were given out in some instances to increase the response rate. Ultimately, due to low response and a small pool of women-only meetings, the sample frame was extended to include women attending regular, mixed-gender meetings of NA as well. The final survey consisted of 92 completed questionnaires.

The survey instrument was carefully designed to capture data elements that would be meaningful for public policy analysts, as well as for those who directly work with the female substance abuser. To this end, familiar demographic survey questions were included as were more specific questions about substance abuse and participation in NA. Questions to measure stigma were adapted from a stigma scale applied to those with mental illness (King et al., 2007) and from a questionnaire designed to measure perceived discrimination and devaluation (Link, Struening, Rahav, Phelan, & Nuttbrock, 1997). Both categorical questions (yes/no) and Likert-scale responses were gathered.

Approximately 44 NA meetings were attended to gather both quantitative and qualitative data about women in NA. In addition to distributing a survey, notes taken after each meeting provided supplemental information about how women perceive the stigma associated with their addiction. One third of the meetings attended were women-only meetings, and these provide the context from which much of the personal narrative is derived. Quantitative data that measure women's responses to various forms of stigma are analyzed and presented in tables as well as in a narrative format. Descriptive data analyses are conducted of the quantitative data, as is a *t*-test to compare group means and a correlation table to observe associations between variables. Qualitative data presented are primarily excerpts from personal stories that highlight women's experience with stigma both before and after they seek mutual support in NA. Additionally, reference made to some qualitative data gathered in a previous sample of women in AA (Sanders, 2003) offers a comparative reference in the "Discussion" section of this article.

FINDINGS

The Sample

This sample of women in NA is unique and is not reflective of NA in general but matches more closely the geographic location in which NA meetings were attended. The NA meetings attended were located in the inner city and surrounding working-class suburbs of a major metropolitan area on the East Coast. The racial composition of this survey consists of either Caucasian or African American identity. More than half were White and more than two fifths were African American. Only 2% do not fit into either of these two categories. More than three quarters are between 30 and 60 years of age and slightly more than one fifth are younger than 30 years of age. In reference to marital status, almost half of the women surveyed have never married and slightly more than 10% are married. Sixty-three percent hold a high school diploma or its equivalency, while equal proportions (18.5%) either did not complete high school or have completed college. Turning to employment

TABLE 1 Demographics

Demographic	%	Demographic	%
Age (years)		Education	
18–24	20.8	< High school	18.5
25–44	44.8	High school diploma	31.5
45–64	43.6	Some college	31.5
65 and older	1.1	College degree	18.5
Race		Employment Status	
White	54.3	Employed	54.4
African American	43.5	Unemployed	16.7
Other	2.2	Disabled	16.7
		Homemaker/student	12.2
Marital Status		Personal Income	
Married	11.1	< $20,000	56.6
Living with a partner	17.8	$20,000–$49,000	31.2
Separated/divorced	16.6	$50,000–$79,000	8.9
Never married	47.8	> $80,000	3.3
Widowed/other	6.6		
Drug of Choice (top three)		Addicted to Alcohol	47.3
Cocaine	32.2		
Heroin	28.9		
Cocaine & Heroin	17.		

Total $N = 92$.

status, just more than half were employed at the time of the survey, and 17%, each, were either unemployed or disabled. Finally, personal income of less than $20,000 per year was reported by almost three fifths, and another 31% had a personal income between $20,000 and $49,000 per year. Only 12% earn $50,000 or more, annually. Given that the majority of women are not married, personal income is likely their primary source of household income. This demographic picture suggests that this sample of women is disadvantaged or struggling measured by socioeconomic indicators (see Table 1).

In reference to their drug use, the majority of women were addicted to cocaine, heroin, or both. Slightly less than one third reported cocaine as their primary drug of choice. Another 29% reported heroin as their drug of choice, and 17% claimed both. This trend is consistent with the treatment admissions data for this metropolitan area, and historically, this region has had high rates of both cocaine and heroin abuse. Additionally, almost half reported addiction to alcohol in addition to their primary drug of choice. Almost two fifths have had either less than 1 year in NA without drug use or between 1 and 5 years in NA clean and sober.

Perceived Stigmata

The pervasive view that addicts are dishonest and cannot be trusted as well as selfish and take advantage of others was the most challenging for these

TABLE 2 Perceived Stigmata

Question	% strongly disagree or disagree	Question	% strongly disagree or disagree
1) Stigmata to overcome:		*2) Other negative images:*	
Dishonest	64.8	Criminal	34.1
Selfish	62.6	Mentally Ill	33
Unclean	51.6	Incest Survivor	14.3
Bad Mother	40.7	HIV/AIDS/HEP	12.1
Promiscuous	40.7	Lesbian	12.1
		Pregnant	10.9
3) *Negative treatment by others:*		*4) Lack of understanding:*	
Family	50.9	General public	74.5
Friends	48.3	Community	72.6
Work	18.4	Media	64.7
School	11.5	Family	59.6

Notes. Total *N* is 91. Respondents were asked to check all that apply to questions 1, 2, and 3 and to respond to a Likert scale to Question 4. Question 4 reads: "*I believe ... has a fair and realistic understanding of what it is like to be a female addict.*" Responses reflect strongly disagree & disagree.

women. Almost two thirds of this sample reported difficulty overcoming the perception of personal attributes thought to be directly associated with the addict (see Table 2). Given that a majority of these women were heroin or crack addicts, this finding is not a surprise even if it does not directly reflect an obvious gendered effect. In direct support of the gendered argument that female addicts are being judged based on a double standard, these women perceive that others view them as bad mothers as well as promiscuous. Fully two fifths of the women in this sample believe they are being held accountable for their reproductive roles, a traditional gendered orientation, and the stigma attributed to them is difficult to surmount. This finding, alone, makes credible the argument that the double standard exists at least as perceived by female addicts in NA.

Beyond individual personality attributes attributed to the addict and the obvious gendered identities are the various other social identities associated with being an addict. The number-one stigmatized identity for these women is that of being a criminal. Slightly more than a third of this sample has found or finds it difficult to overcome the label of criminal, felon, or ex-convict. Women who have been caught up in the war on drugs experience double jeopardy, deviance based on two identities, addict and criminal. For these women, the two forms of deviance are most likely related by drug addiction preceding the criminal behavior.

The following examples illustrate the intersection between gender, drug abuse, and taking the label of "criminal." An African American in her late 50s led a women's meeting and told her story about drug addiction, domestic violence, incarceration, and recovery. This woman had just more than a year of clean time, mentioned that she has struggled with addiction for 26 years, and said that early in her drug use, she was with an abusive husband. She described that one night to protect her children and herself, she shot her husband and consequently served 5 years for this crime. During the course of her addiction, she has been in and out of jail several times but reports that she is doing well today.

Another woman, a White woman who appeared to be in her 40s, spoke up at an open mixed-gender meeting of NA and shared her concern that she was recently released from prison after several years. She expressed having trouble getting back into NA and connected to other women. She told the group that she wants to stay clean and sober but that it has been difficult. She responded to the topic of the meeting and said, "I can relate to having low self-esteem especially as an ex-felon." She told of the difficulty in getting a job because she is an "ex-con," and after 4 months of struggling, she was just offered a job. She remarked that she was honest and told the employer she was an ex-convict, but did this only because she knew the employer had a record of hiring ex-cons.

Second only to being labeled a criminal is that of being mentally ill. A third of these women, too, feel stigmatized based on having a mental illness. In spite of efforts during the past 30 years to treat mental illness as any other somatic illness, a double standard (based on diagnosis) clearly persists. At least these women perceive this to be so. In spite of much growth in the neurobiological understanding of mental illness and equity toward the treatment of mental illness, the shared perception is that others do not accept mental illness as they do other chronic diseases. The acknowledgement of dealing with both mental illness and substance abuse was seen at a women's meeting as a woman sharing mentioned being diagnosed as bipolar and taking medication. She said in the past that she had been treated for depression, but said her current diagnosis and treatment were working better. Both her counselor and others have said "don't stop taking your medication because you will use again if you do." This same woman told how she thought everyone had racing thoughts, that she has had them since she was young, and that she did not know you could focus on just one thing at a time. She is now learning this while going back to school. She also stated that she has to memorize things because she will not remember. She ends by recalling that even as a small child, she felt she was not good enough and spoke of coping with this same feeling today.

Although no other label has as much negative resonance with these women than that of being either a criminal or mentally ill, a few other identities need to be noted. Women who are either lesbian or incest survivors, have HIV/AIDS or human papillomavirus, or who have used while pregnant (see Table 2) share some difficulty overcoming the negative images associated with these labels. Although negative images of all of the identities would be expected, it is interesting that only 1 in 10 women reported difficulty with stigma due to being a pregnant addict. However, it is not known how many women have actually been pregnant while using, but it is known that 70% of the women have at least one child. Given that most of these women do not have long-term sobriety—less than a year in NA—it is likely that more than 10% have used drugs while pregnant or at least have been pregnant during the course of their drug addiction. Other specific substance abuse identities such as being a methadone user are not perceived as heavily stigmatized. Only 5.5% reported difficulty with this. However, it is not known how many women actually use methadone or other medically assisted treatment. Also, slightly more than 5% denoted that being a minority is viewed as a stigma that is a challenge to overcome.

In addition to the perceived characteristics and roles associated with being an addict, these women have experienced what they perceive as negative treatment and lack of understanding by others. According to this survey of addicted women, the perception that others have of them matters a great deal (see Table 2). More specifically, between 60% and 75% of the women in this sample strongly disagree or disagree with the statement, "I believe . . . the general public; community; media; and family has a fair and realistic understanding of what it is like to be a female addict." The larger public and social institutions in which these women live their lives continue to have an impact on how these women perceive themselves in relationship to their addiction.

Finally and perhaps most importantly is the perception that family members have treated the addict negatively or simply do not understand the addict. Responses to two different statements make clear that these women are concerned about the failed relationships they have had with family members. This could be a result of either what their own families project onto them as addicts or what they have indeed earned due to their addict behavior. Given either interpretation, more than 50% report that they have been treated negatively by their families due to their addiction (see Table 2). Similarly, just shy of 60% believe that their families do not have a realistic understanding of what it is like to be a female addict (see Table 2). For women, drug addiction is not an isolated problem as they remain significantly tied to their families of origin and families of procreation. Women who have been raised in dysfunctional families—in this case, a family harmed emotionally, psychologically, and spiritually by addictions—often repeat patterns of dysfunctional behaviors within their own families of procreation, perpetuating the cycle of addiction. Stigma resulting from the double standard, again, defined in terms of women's reproductive roles can also be extended to include parenting and family relations in general.

Statistical Associations

To further test the relationships between demographic and other variables, a cumulative stigma scale was created by combining the four generalized statements referenced as "lack of understanding by others." The scale reflects the totality of these women's responses collapsed into one measure. First, a *t*-test was run to compare group means between the White and Black women. It is likely that these groups differ (.019 *p*-value at the 95% confidence interval) in terms of the cumulative stigma they perceive. The White subgroup has a mean of 12.20 and the Black subgroup has a mean of 10.75 on a scale with a range between 4 and 16. Therefore, the White women perceive greater stigma (or lack of understanding by others) than do the Black women. Next, a test to measure correlation was conducted and only the demographic variable, level of education, was significantly associated with the cumulative negative perception of stigma these women feel. The Pearson correlation coefficient reflects that education and cumulative stigma are positively associated (.262) at the .05 level of significance using a two-tailed test (see Table 3). Those with a higher level of education experience, or at least perceive, more stigma (as measured by lack of understanding) compared with women with less education. This could be due to having a better understanding or consciousness of the expectations held by others, due to comparing oneself to a reference group that indeed holds a "higher standard" in regard to expectations, or due to the belief that she has more to lose than a woman with less education. Moreover, the White women in this sample are better educated than the Black women, which helps explain the difference between group means by race. Measured by either statistic—*t*-test or correlation—it appears the more advantaged group perceives more stigma than the potentially more disadvantaged group of women.

One other statistical finding of note is that those women ($N = 25$) who have completed all 12 steps report fewer stigmata and more understanding

TABLE 3 Correlations

		Education	Cumulative Stigma	Years in NA	Complete Steps
Education	Pearson Correlation	1	.262*	.270*	.112
	Sig. (2-tailed)		.015	.010	.289
	N	92	86	90	91
Cumulative Stigma	Pearson Correlation	.262*	1	−.117	−.231*
	Sig. (2-tailed)	.015		.291	.034
	N	86	86	84	85
Years in NA	Pearson Correlation	.270*	−.117	1	.645**
	Sig. (2-tailed)	.010	.291		.000
	N	90	84	90	90
Complete Steps	Pearson Correlation	.112	−.231*	.645**	1
	Sig. (2-tailed)	.289	.034	.000	
	N	91	85	90	91

*Correlation is significant at the .05 level (two-tailed).
**Correlation is significant at the .01 level (two-tailed).

by others compared with women who have not completed the 12 steps. This is not a surprising outcome because "working" the 12 steps is said to lead to long-term recovery and create other positive psychosocial effects. For instance, women in AA report higher levels of self-esteem once completing the 12 steps (Sanders, 2003). One last related statically significant finding is that time (years) in NA is positively correlated (.645 at the .01 level of significance using a two-tailed test) to having completed the 12 steps (see Table 3). This is intuitive—the longer time in the NA program, the more likely that a woman has completed the step work. Sanders (2003) found a similar relationship in her study of women in AA.

DISCUSSION

The women in this sample perceive stigma based on perceptions that they are bad mothers and promiscuous women, but these images are not as salient as the more generalized, gender-neutral characteristics associated with the addict. Moreover, women in NA interpret their inability to live up to traditional gender roles somewhat loosely compared with the middle-class, normative model. While their worth and public performance remain tied to their gendered body and gendered role expectations, allowance for error is observed. For instance, qualitative data expose that some of these women in NA believe it to be in the best interest of their children if others care for their children while they are active in the "lifestyle" of addiction. Similarly, although these same women will state that they are "not proud of it," sometimes the lifestyle led them to prostitute themselves. In either scenario, loss of children or engaging in prostitution, these women articulate the belief that they had limited options, that the compulsion to use took over their life, and that they could not stop. Once in recovery, these women seek support from each other and reassert more positive reproductive images of themselves.

The nature of stigma is more complicated than a universal blanket of negative perceptions experienced by all women as addicts. In fact, qualitative data comparing women who attend women-only AA meetings to women-only NA meetings revealed that women in AA, in some ways, experience more or at least articulate the experience of more stigma, than do women in NA (Sanders, 2011). In particular, reference to drinking and driving with children in the car and other direct parenting concerns as an alcoholic mother are mentioned in women-only AA meetings. Survey data, too, reinforce that in some instances, it is the guilt and shame associated with stigma related to reckless parenting that facilitates women to "hit their bottom." Conversely, women in NA will openly speak (even in mixed-gender meetings) about their inability to parent adequately. It stands to reason that women in a more privileged social position have more to protect and consequently more to lose in terms of reputation and a sense that they are being judged by others. Alternatively, NA is more diverse and the literature of this mutual-support group acknowledges, outright, the stigma related to the illicit nature of drug abuse and the lifestyle that accompanies it. NA is more deliberate in acknowledging stigma than even its predecessor AA. For women, acceptance of breaking with the expectations of traditional gender roles could be easier to negotiate within the subculture of NA than in the more mainstream groups of AA or WFS. This also helps to explain why there appears to be significant differences among the women in NA in regard to perceived stigma when comparing race and level of education. Those of the majority race and those with higher education could be more like those women in AA who perceive they have more to lose by breaking with gender expectations.

Strategies differ in how women across these mutual-support groups confront the stigma they perceive as either alcoholics or addicts. The perceived culture of the wider mutual-support community contributes to the strategies adopted. For instance, the double standard manifested in AA can still be heard in women's historical accounts of their own participation in the fellowship. Women recall being told not to share specifics of their gendered stories at the group level. This repression of women's stories advances a more conservative culture of discourse that reinforces the stigma women perceive. In recent years, AA has loosened up, but again, the history of keeping these specific gendered accounts outside of mixed-gender meetings can be heard. Also, compared with women's meetings (AA or NA) and some mixed-gender NA meetings, AA meetings continue to sound more conservative. To what extent integration of women into mixed-gender AA meetings has influenced the public discourse generally in AA is hard to determine. But gauging from women's stories, some have personally been trailblazers by continuing to share what they want even at mixed-gendered meetings in spite of receiving a "talking to" by male members early in their recovery. Alternatively, women may elect to attend women-only meetings of AA and NA or attend WFS.

Women with long-term sobriety who have experience negotiating the double standard in the 12-step fellowships simultaneously acknowledge that they get benefits from attending women-only meetings but do not necessarily prefer them (Sanders, 2003, 2009) and learn about recovery from all types of 12-step meetings. Similar to what Kaskutas finds in her studies of WFS, women do not exclude one meeting for another but rather learn to reconcile the differences between 12-step philosophy and the more secular approach of WFS. Kaskutas writes that women who attend both WFS and AA have "made their own peace" (1992, p. 646) in response to perceived differences. Similarly, Sanders (2010) finds that women construct their own gendered spaces, women-only meetings, in AA while remaining heavily involved and integrated into the larger male-dominated culture of AA. It could well be that the best strategy to overcome stigma requires both the acceptance of gender-specific needs and the determination to integrate and expose the patriarchal elements that persist in the 12-step recovery milieu. Women in NA, the socially most stigmatized, with their matter-of-fact stance toward disclosure, may already understand the therapeutic benefits of "telling all" even in mixed-gender meetings, and this alone helps to break down the double standard.

CONCLUSION

An alternative strategy could be that women in AA and WFS may "pass" easier than women in NA and so will take advantage of this privilege. Goffman (1963) differentiates between the discredited and the discreditable, and this can help to explain differences in perception of stigma found among women in recovery from addiction. According to Goffman, the discredited is someone whose deviance or stigma is known or apparent to others and tension in social interaction revolves around this identity. Alternatively, the discreditable can hide her deviance and focus in social interaction is concentrated on how to manage that which is not necessarily known to others. Goffman uses the word "passing" to suggest that the discreditable at least has the opportunity to declare no difference from others.

The recovering addict could, in fact, occupy both statuses—discreditable and discredited. While using, it could be obvious to others that she is deviant in her overconsumption, but in recovery as a member of NA, AA, or WFS, she has the option to remain anonymous to outsiders. Being discredited, known by others as an addict, can act as both a barrier to seeking treatment and also as a catalyst for hitting bottom and looking for help in mutual-support groups. Similarly, it is not clear whether anonymity or passing in recovery is only a positive development for long-term emotional growth. There remains the feminist argument that it is empowering to confront the double standard and talk out loud about one's deviance, and this, in turn, begins to reduce the stigma associated with that deviance. This is a costly proposal, however, for the vulnerable, and there is no guarantee that self-disclosure will contribute to a cultural softening of the stigma. Moreover, if the more privileged continue to opt for passing and adhere to the tradition of anonymity afforded them by 12-step participation (and to some extent membership in WFS), than this public claim has not been made.

In conclusion, the more privileged women in AA (as well as the women in this sample of NA that are better educated and White) perceive more stigma than their less privileged counterparts in NA but can simultaneously choose to protect their more anonymous discreditable status by passing. However, it is not clear which strategy, self-disclosure or anonymity, is the most empowering in terms of overall recovery sought via mutual-support groups. Ultimately, the strategies that addicted women employ to overcome stigma, especially that related to the double standard that women perceive, have potential impact on both individual therapeutic outcomes and mutual-support group outcomes.

REFERENCES

Belenko, S. (2000). *Drugs and drug policy in America: A documentary history.* Westport, CT: Greenwood.

Burton-Rose, D. (Ed.). (1998). *The celling of America: An inside look at the U.S. prison industry.* Monroe, ME: Common Courage.

Chavkin, W., & Breitbart, V. (1997). Substance abuse and maternity: The United States as a case study. *Addiction, 92*(9), 1201–1205.

Chavkin, W., Elman D., & Wise, P. H. (1998). National survey of the states: Policies and practices regarding drug-using pregnant women. *American Journal of Public Health, 88*(1), 117–119.

Downing, C. (1991). Sex role setups and alcoholism. In N. Van Den Bergh (Ed.), *Feminist perspectives on addictions* (pp. 47–60). New York, NY: Springer.

Goffman, E. (1963). *Stigma: Notes on the management of spoiled identity.* Englewood Cliffs, NJ: Prentice-Hall.

Johns, C. J. (1992). *Power, ideology, and the war on drugs: Nothing succeeds like failure.* New York, NY: Praeger.

Kaskutas, L. A. (1992). *An Analysis of "Women For Sobriety."* PhD dissertation, Department of Public Health, University of California, Berkeley.

Kaskutas, L. A. (1994). What do women get out of self-help? Their reasons for attending Women for Sobriety and Alcoholics Anonymous. *Journal of Substance Abuse Treatment, 11*(3), 185–195.

Kaskutas, L. A. (1996). A road less traveled: Choosing the 'Women for Sobriety' program. *Journal of Drug Issues, 26*(1), 77–94.

King, K., Dinos, S., Shaw, J., Watson, R., Stevens, S., Passetti, F., Weich, S., & Serfaty, M. (2007). The Stigma Scale: Development of a standardized measure of the stigma of mental illness. *British Journal of Psychiatry, 190,* 248–254. doi:0.1192/bjp.bp.06.024638

Link, B. G., Struening, E. L., Rahav, M., Phelan, J. C., & Nuttbrock, L. (1997). On stigma and its consequences: Evidence from a longitudinal study of men with dual diagnoses of mental illness and substance abuse. *Journal of Health and Social Behavior, 38*(2), 177–190.

Robinson, M. B., & Scherlen, R. G. (2007). *Lies, damned lies, and drug war statistics: A critical analysis of claims made by the Office of National Drug Control Policy.* Albany, NY: SUNY Press.

Sanders, J. M. (2003). *Twelve-step recovery and feminism: A study of empowerment among women in Alcoholics Anonymous (Unpublished doctoral dissertation).* Washington, DC: Department of Sociology, American University.

Sanders, J. M. (2009). *Women in Alcoholics Anonymous: Recovery and empowerment.* Boulder, CO: Lynne Rienner.

Sanders, J. M. (2010). Acknowledging gender in women-only meetings of Alcoholics Anonymous. *Journal of Groups in Addiction & Recovery*, *5*(1),17–33. doi:10.1080/15560350903543766

Sanders, J. M. (2011). Feminist perspectives on 12-step recovery: A comparative descriptive analysis of women in Alcoholics Anonymous and Narcotics Anonymous. *Alcoholism Treatment Quarterly*, *29*(4), 357–378.

Sandmaier, M. (1980). *The invisible alcoholics: Women and alcohol abuse in America*. New York, NY: McGraw-Hill.

Shoemaker, P. J. (1989). *Campaigns about drugs: Government, media, and the public*. Hillsdale, NJ: Lawrence Erlbaum.

Youth Participation in Mutual Support Groups: History, Current Knowledge, and Areas for Future Research

LORA L. PASSETTI, SUSAN H. GODLEY, and MARK D. GODLEY
Lighthouse Institute, Chestnut Health Systems, Normal, Illinois, USA

Mutual support groups have the potential to be a powerful support network for youth with substance use problems. There is a long history of youth being referred to and participating in these groups, yet research regarding the effectiveness of their participation is in its early stages. In recent years, a small but growing body of literature has been devoted to this topic. This article: (1) summarizes the history of youth involvement in mutual support groups; (2) reviews research on youth involvement in mutual support meetings and evidence of effectiveness; (3) describes implementation of and lessons learned from a pilot study that attempted to increase youth attendance and involvement with three types of 12-step groups; and (4) provides recommendations for future research related to mutual support groups and youth.

Significant decreases in substance use have been demonstrated for adolescents admitted to treatment for substance use problems (Dennis et al., 2004; Hser et al., 2001; Morral, McCaffrey, & Ridgeway, 2004). However, a large percentage of youth between the ages of 12 and 18 years old continue to struggle with periods of relapse and recovery after discharge, especially during the first 90 days (Brown, Vik, & Creamer, 1989; Dennis et al.; S. H. Godley,

This work was supported by funding from the National Institute on Drug Abuse, National Institutes of Health (NIH; 1 R01DA018183), and the National Institute on Alcohol Abuse and Alcoholism, NIH (R01AA010368-06A2). The content of this publication does not necessarily reflect the views or policies of the NIH. The authors wish to thank Stephanie Merkle for her assistance in preparing this manuscript.

Dennis, Godley, & Funk, 2004; S. H. Godley, Godley, & Dennis, 2001; Waldron, Slesnick, Brody, Turner, & Peterson, 2001). As a result, participation in continuing care (or "aftercare") services provided by professionals after an acute treatment stay has been recommended as standard practice (American Society of Addiction Medicine, 2001; Kaminer, 2001; McKay, 1999). Up to two thirds of youth, however, do not take advantage of these services unless assertive approaches to linkage and retention are used that rely on clinicians rather than clients to initiate care (M. D. Godley, Godley, Dennis, Funk, & Passetti, 2002, 2006; S. H. Godley et al., 2001). Such assertive approaches can be expensive to implement, and the cost of continuing care is not always reimbursable from traditional sources (Koyanagi, Alfano, & Stein, 2008).

Youth may enter peer-led community-based mutual support groups for substance use problems via multiple pathways. However, the most common pathway appears to be based on referrals made by treatment staff after a treatment episode (Drug Strategies, 2003; Humphreys et al., 2004; Jainchill, 2000). Many groups are free to interested individuals and hold meetings in communities throughout the United States and sometimes internationally. As technology advances, some groups are offering contact over the phone, through e-mail, or via online chats and recovery-oriented electronic social networks. Members share their experiences and encouragement, and they may be available for contact 24 hours a day. Additionally, meetings, group events, and one-on-one interactions can help provide increased opportunities for sober interactions and activities (Kaskutas, Bond, & Humphreys, 2002; Kelly, Myers, & Rodolico, 2008).

Mutual support groups have the potential to be a powerful support network for adolescents; however, research related to youth participation is in its early stages. The purposes of this article are to: (1) summarize the history of youth involvement in mutual support groups for their substance use problems (groups for other issues are beyond the scope of this article); (2) review research on youth involvement in mutual support meetings and evidence of their effectiveness; (3) describe implementation of and lessons learned from a pilot study that attempted to increase youth attendance and involvement with three groups: Alcoholics Anonymous (AA), Cocaine Anonymous (CA), and Narcotics Anonymous (NA); and (4) provide recommendations for future research. AA and NA receive the most attention in this article due to their longevity, large membership, accessibility, and the lack of published research about other groups. Additionally, identified published research regarding youth mutual support group participation only examines attendance *during and after treatment* for substance use problems.

HISTORY OF YOUTH INVOLVEMENT IN MUTUAL SUPPORT MEETINGS

Youth inclusion in mutual support groups for problems with substance use has been tied to patterns of substance use trends (White, 1999). In the 19th century, youth were admitted to professionally directed homes, asylums, and private institutes for alcohol or other substance use, but this treatment was adult-oriented and without specialized aftercare groups for young people (White, 1998). There were, however, "cadet" branches and "youth rescue" crusades that were part of early societies that encouraged abstinence through mutual support, such as the Washingtonian Temperance Society formed in 1840 and the Ribbon Reform Clubs that became active in the 1870s (White, 1998).

During the heroin epidemic in the early 20th century, more young people were arrested and more were admitted to methadone maintenance clinics between 1919 and 1924 (Terry & Pellens, 1928). Additionally, admissions increased to two federal "narcotics farms" in the late 1940s and to local hospitals in New York City in the early 1950s (New York Academy of Medicine, 1953). Despite this rise in contact with professional treatment organizations, there remained a lack of youth-oriented recovery supports until the mid-20th century.

The eventual growth in youth-focused activities of peer-based mutual support groups can be linked to several events. First, youth began seeking help in greater numbers at younger ages due to earlier alcohol and other drug use initiation, the use of multiple substances, and the more rapid development of significant substance-related problems. Second, public awareness of substance use problems and options for recovery support may have created more demand for these resources. Third, there was a growth of adolescent-specific treatment programs in the United States that referred young clients to mutual support groups, particularly AA. Finally, certain groups took specific steps to attract youth with substance use problems to their communities (Passetti & White, 2008).

AA is the primary example of a group that made early and ongoing efforts to draw youth to mutual support. For example, youth-oriented pamphlets (*Young People and AA*, *Too Young?*) and a film (*AA and Young People*) were created. The *AA Grapevine*, the international journal of AA, started publishing articles on young people in the late 1940s, and the number of these articles increased substantially in the 1960s and 1970s. Even though these practices were meant to attract young people to AA, youth who attended meetings often drew attention and reactions of surprise, suspicion, condescension, or criticism from adult members. As described in Passetti and White (2008), a review of *AA Grapevine* articles on young people published between 1948 and 1978 revealed responses from older members such as: "You're too young to be an alcoholic!"; "I've spilled more booze than you've drunk"; or "We don't want to hear about those other drugs." Subsequently, Young People's Groups in AA (then defined as being for AA members younger than the age of 35 years old) began appearing in Cleveland (1944), Los Angeles (1945), Philadelphia (1946), New York City (1947), and San Diego (1948), and the number of these groups has increased over time. These Young People's Groups were conferences rather than regular group meetings. In 1958, the International Conference of Young People in AA was formed, and their annual conventions are now attended by more than 3,000 young AA members (*Special Composition Groups in A.A.*, 2002). A review of similar *AA Grapevine* articles during the past 25 years revealed that attitudes described above have been weakening as the average age of AA members has been gradually declining (Passetti & White). In 1994, the journal established a regular feature called "Youth Enjoying Sobriety," and between 1948 and 2006, more than 100 articles have focused on young people recovering within AA (B. Weiner, personal communication, November 30, 2006).

In addition to AA, youth have become involved over time with other mutual support groups, although their availability differs across geographic regions and communities. Groups representing adaptations of AA's 12-step program include NA (late 1940s and early 1950s), Pot Smokers Anonymous (1968), Pills Anonymous (1975), Chemically Dependent Anonymous (1980), CA (1982), Crystal Meth Anonymous (1994), and Heroin Anonymous (2004). Alternatives to 12-step groups include Women for Sobriety (1975), Secular Organization for Sobriety (1985), Rational Recovery (1986), Self-Management and Recovery Training (1994), and LifeRing Secular Recovery (1999). Faith-based groups (e.g., Christian-based) include Alcoholics Victorious (1948), Alcoholics for Christ (1976), Overcomers Outreach (1977), Lion Tamers Anonymous (1980), and Celebrate Recovery (1991).

Because most of the groups listed above do not have their own versions of AA's Young People's Groups and offer few young people's meetings, it is common for youth to attend meetings with several adults who are 10 or more years older than they are. Table 1 summarizes the average age of mutual support group members and the percentage of young people in those groups according to available surveys (AA, 2007; CA World Services, 2011; LifeRing, 2005; NA World Services, 2009). No surveys from other groups

TABLE 1 Youth Membership in Mutual Support Groups by Age Category and Average Age of Members

Mutual Support Group	Age Category (%)	Average Age of Members
Alcoholics Anonymous	Younger than 21 (2.3%)	47 years old
Cocaine Anonymous	Younger than 18 (1%)	Average age not reported 18–24 years (10%) 25–34 years (38%) 35–44 years (40%) 45–65 years (10%) Older than 65 years (< 1%)
LifeRing[a]	Younger than 30 (5%)	48 years old
Narcotics Anonymous	Younger than 20 (2%)	43 years old

[a]LifeRing is a mutual support group for recovery from alcohol and other substances and is not based on the 12 steps.

were found for review. Teen-Anon (1999) is the first mutual support group specifically for adolescents. Today, there are about 20 meetings available across the United States (Teen-Anon, personal communication, December 17, 2011).

RESEARCH ON YOUTH INVOLVEMENT IN MUTUAL SUPPORT MEETINGS

In recent years, a small but growing body of literature has been devoted to youth participation in mutual support group meetings. Published studies focus exclusively on 12-step groups, and on AA and NA in particular. Investigations conducted thus far demonstrate that, like adults (Galaif & Sussman, 1995; Kelly & Moos, 2003), a significant percentage of youth who initiate attendance at 12-step meetings stop going over time. For example, Kelly, Myers, and Brown (2000) reported that attendance at one or more meetings after residential treatment declined from 75% at 3 months postdischarge to 59% at 6 months. Similarly, Kelly, Brown, and colleagues (2008) found that slightly more than 90% of youth attended at least one AA or NA meeting within the first 6 months following inpatient treatment, and this rate steadily declined to almost 60% between 6 and 12 months and to just more than 30% between 6 and 8 years after discharge. Weekly attendance rate averages provide a more detailed picture: 65% attended weekly in the first 6 months, 35% attended weekly between 6 and 12 months, and less than 10% attended weekly between 6 and 8 years after discharge. Recent research findings provide preliminary insight into factors that may influence patterns of attendance and these are reviewed in the following paragraphs.

Characteristics of Youth

A few characteristics have been identified that predict which youth will likely attend mutual support group meetings and which will stop going. One factor common to youth aged 12 to 18 years old is that most depend on other people (especially parents or other relatives) for transportation (Kelly, 2002). Therefore, transportation that is unavailable, inconsistent, or unreliable can impact one's ability to attend meetings. Moreover, at least two studies revealed that youth are more likely to go to meetings and/or become involved with 12-step groups if they present to inpatient treatment with more severe substance use problems (Kelly, Brown, et al., 2008; Kelly, Myers, & Brown, 2002). Additionally, increased attendance rates are often associated with the extent of substance use difficulties and other problems. For example, youth who believe that they cannot use substances in moderation and have a history of prior treatment are more likely to go to 12-step meetings (Hohman & LeCroy, 1996; Kelly, Brown, et al., 2008). Other research indicates that youth may be more likely to attend 12-step meetings if they experience more hopelessness and have less parental participation in treatment (Hohman & LeCroy). Conversely, youth have reported that they quit attending groups due to boredom, lack of fit with the group, relapse, low motivation, lack of perceived need, and the removal of external pressures to attend (Kelly, Myers, et al., 2008).

Characteristics of Treatment Programs and Clinician Referral Practices

Some evidence indicates that the philosophical orientation of adolescent treatment programs for substance use and how clinicians make referrals to mutual support groups influence attendance rates. Programs with a 12-step orientation frequently attempt to facilitate 12-step group participation during and following treatment. Strategies like requiring attendance at a certain number of meetings per week and recommending ongoing attendance in a discharge plan are used. As noted above, such efforts may be successful in the short term, because higher attendance rates tend to coincide with receipt of treatment services and/or the period immediately following their end. Long-term group involvement, however, often does not occur because attendance can and does drop dramatically as time passes after discharge (Kelly, Brown, et al., 2008; Passetti & Godley, 2008).

Adult studies and interviews with clinicians from adolescent treatment programs suggest that assertively linking youth to mutual support groups may help increase participation (Passetti & Godley, 2008; White & Kurtz, 2006). Assertive linkage procedures rely on actively connecting youth to meetings and shaping/reinforcing their attendance. Procedures may include early referral to support groups, education about the potential benefits and risks of meeting attendance, ongoing monitoring of involvement and obstacles, and discussion of each person's prior experiences with, responses to, and perceptions of participation (Laudet, 2003; Ogborne, 1989; White & Kurtz). One study with adults revealed that directly connecting individuals to someone from a 12-step group increased meeting attendance more than only providing meeting information and verbal encouragement (Sisson & Mallams, 1981). A different study with adults examined proactive connection to 12-step group volunteers, addressing concerns, setting attendance goals, and encouraging one find to a sponsor and a home group. These procedures did not increase attendance but were found to foster greater involvement in 12-step activities, such as providing a service (e.g., setting up/taking down tables and chairs for meetings) and obtaining a sponsor. Adults receiving this intervention had significantly higher abstinence rates from substances other than alcohol compared with those who did not, and those who had less 12-step group experience were more likely to attend a greater number of meetings (Timko, DeBenedetti, & Billow, 2006).

To learn how substance use treatment providers refer youth to mutual support groups, we investigated the relationship between the referral strategies of 28 clinicians working for eight programs across the United States and the rates of mutual support group meeting attendance. The clinicians' responses indicated that staff employed at sites with the highest overall rates of meeting attendance actively linked youth to the recovery community in one or more ways. One strategy was to transport youth to sober social activities sponsored by mutual support groups, such as conferences for young people, dances, and picnics. Some sites monitored attendance at mutual support groups after discharge from treatment through continuing care or case management services. Additional strategies involved: (a) working with service structures of support groups to host meetings on site and identify members willing to work with and serve as role models for youth; (b) creating networks of trusted people to go with youth to meetings, introduce them to groups, and facilitate familiarity with the program; and (c) helping youth identify, screen, and approach potential sponsors (Passetti & Godley, 2008). Given the results of adult studies, future research of assertive strategies to connect youth with mutual support groups has the potential to identify methods of influencing attendance rates both during active treatment and after discharge.

Characteristics of Mutual Support Groups and Meetings

A small number of studies combined with qualitative data from adolescents and clinicians suggest that characteristics of mutual support groups and meetings may affect attendance patterns. For example, research indicates that youth who attend 12-step meetings with at least a substantial proportion of people their age after inpatient treatment have better substance use outcomes (Kelly & Myers, 1997; Kelly, Myers, & Brown, 2005). These youth go to more meetings and perceive attendance as important. Surprisingly, these youth do not have a greater likelihood of having a sponsor or engaging in social activities with other 12-step group members (Kelly et al., 2005). Such results are consistent with the importance of peers in adolescent development. Peers can be a significant predictor of relapse to use of alcohol and/or other drugs, reduced substance use, or long-term recovery (Brown, Vik, & Creamer, 1989; Dishion & Owen, 2002; Garner, Godley, Funk, Dennis, & Godley, 2007; Garnier & Stein, 2002; Godley, Kahn, Dennis, Godley, & Funk, 2005; Kosterman, Hawkins, Guo, Catalano, & Abbott, 2000; Margolis, Kilpatrick, & Mooney, 2000; Preston & Goodfellow, 2006; Rai et al., 2003).

These findings are also important to consider in light of the widespread practice of referring youth to recovery support meetings that are mainly attended by adults (Drug Strategies, 2003; Jainchill, 2000). Recent membership surveys described in Table 1 reveal that less than 3% of members of common 12-step groups are younger than the age of 21 (AA, 2007; CA World Services, 2011; NA World Services, 2009). Even though published membership surveys for 12-step alternative groups are largely unavailable, a survey of LifeRing members (a newer non-12-step mutual support group for recovery from alcohol and other substances) shows a similar pattern with less than 1% identifying themselves as younger than the age of 20 (LifeRing, 2005). Kelly and Myers (1997) reported that 65% of 12-step meetings attended by youth in their study consisted mainly of older individuals. Although youth-oriented meetings are offered by some groups, they are not accessible to a large percentage of youth due to limited availability.

The age composition of groups may further influence meeting attendance rates because, due to their developmental level, adolescent substance use patterns and life experiences differ from those of adults. Youth may have trouble relating to issues they have little experience with, such as medical complications, withdrawal symptoms, using mainly one substance, and longer histories of substance-related difficulties (Brown, 1993; Stewart & Brown, 1995). Also, youth may have less interest in discussions of job loss and troubled relationships with spouses and children. Yet another difference is that youth often have less motivation for change and willingness to acknowledge substance use problems (Tims et al., 2002). Notably, our study of referral patterns revealed that clinicians thought the age composition of meetings was so important that it was one of their most common considerations when referring youth to 12-step meetings. Despite this concern, a few clinicians felt that some youth benefitted from adults at meetings for the wisdom and praise they received (Passetti & Godley, 2008).

In addition to the age composition of groups, clinicians expressed concerns that youth have difficulty understanding and "buying into" support group concepts that are framed in adult language and experiences. Adolescent brains are still in development, and the ability to think about abstract concepts, make deductions, and critically reflect on personal thoughts is often gradual and discontinuous (Piaget, 1969). Twelve-step concepts like "acceptance," "surrender," and "spirituality" have been identified as potentially too abstract for many adolescents to grasp (Deas & Thomas, 2001; Passetti & Godley, 2008). Clinicians further note that youth may not identify with feelings of powerlessness over substances or acknowledge a need to commit to lifelong abstinence (Passetti & Godley, 2008). Little research sheds light on the ability of adolescents to relate to these 12-step concepts. In qualitative interviews with adolescents in residential substance use treatment, we found that at least some young people acknowledge feeling powerless over alcohol or other drugs and that their lives are unmanageable. In contrast, some youth struggled with the concepts of "hitting bottom" and spirituality and with reading and understanding 12-step literature. Some also had reservations about making a fearless moral inventory and amends to people they had harmed (Passetti, 2006). Despite the idea that issues with spirituality may be one cause for youth to stop attending 12-step meetings, Kelly, Myers, and Rodolico (2008) did not find that the spiritual content of 12-step meetings was a main reason youth reported for discontinuing attendance.

Finally, youth may base their decisions on whether or not to participate in mutual support groups on their reactions to a specific meeting. Inevitably, there are differences between the many different meetings found within and between geographic areas (Montgomery, Miller, & Tonigan, 1993). For instance, one study of AA revealed that meetings can differ from one another in cohesiveness, independence, aggressiveness, expressiveness, and the perceived amount of focus on working the steps and the 12-step program (Tonigan, Ashcroft, & Miller, 1995). Clinicians also have expressed concerns about the safety of youth at a particular meeting or meetings in general. Worries range from the perception that older male members might prey on young females to the belief that members with criminal histories or gang involvement may threaten or intimidate youth. Although the majority of youth in one study reported feeling very safe at meetings, 22% of youth that attended AA or NA reported at least one negative experience at a meeting, such as feeling intimidated, threatened, or sexually harassed. Reports were more common among those who went to NA. However, youth did not report safety concerns as a reason for ceasing to attend groups (Kelly, Dow, Yeterian, & Myers, 2011). It is possible that youth who attend a meeting where they feel unsafe or where they feel they do not "fit in" may be reluctant to go back to that particular meeting or try another day, time, and location. Individual youth may prefer meetings based on particular characteristics of the group, such as: (a) a higher percentage of young members; (b) more members with long-term abstinence; (c) older members who are excited to work with young people; (d) smaller numbers of attendees; (e) members who primarily have the same substance of choice; (f) same-gender or same-sexual orientation groups; or (g) in the case of AA, more tolerance of individuals with substance problems other than alcohol (Forman, 2002; Passetti & Godley, 2008). Of course, the ability to try out different meetings depends on their availability and accessibility in a given geographical area. Overall, these findings suggest that it is best for clinicians and concerned others to attempt to match youth to particular meetings based on needs, preferences, and cultural background, and if there has already been an unsatisfactory experience at a particular meeting, encourage the youth to try another one (Caldwell, 1998; Humphreys et al., 2004; Laudet, 2003; Passetti & Godley).

EFFECTIVENESS OF YOUTH INVOLVEMENT IN MUTUAL SUPPORT MEETINGS

Most research regarding the effectiveness of mutual support groups has been conducted with adults and their involvement with 12-step meetings (see Connors, Tonigan, & Miller, 2001; Humphreys et al., 2004; Kissin, McLeod, & McKay, 2003; Moos & Moos, 2004). Initial research of youth participation in AA and NA revealed that attendance and involvement have the potential to yield benefits, but further studies are needed to provide more conclusive results. Table 2, which has been updated from an earlier paper (Passetti & White, 2008), summarizes published youth studies related to adolescent participation in mutual help groups. These studies suggest that youth who attend AA and/or NA after residential treatment for substance use are more likely to remain abstinent and use substances less frequently (Alford, Koehler, & Leonard, 1991; Hsieh, Hoffman, & Hollister, 1998; Kelly & Myers, 1997, 2007; Kelly et al., 2000, 2002; Kennedy & Minami, 1993).

Some of the most recent research in this area confirms and extends earlier findings. In the longest-term study of youth involvement in 12-step groups to date, Kelly, Brown, and colleagues (2008) examined substance use outcomes 8 years after discharge from inpatient treatment. Their results indicated that greater AA and NA attendance rates early after treatment were associated with better long-term outcomes as measured by percentage of days abstinent. Even with declining attendance over time, effects related to AA and NA remained significant and consistent.

Chi, Kaskutas, Sterling, Campbell, and Weisner (2009) followed 357 youth out to 3 years after intake to programs offering intensive outpatient treatment with referral to contracted residential services as needed. They found that 12-step meeting attendance measured at 1 year after intake predicted alcohol, but not drug, abstinence at Year 3. At 3 years after intake, youth who attended 10 or more 12-step meetings in the prior 6 months demonstrated abstinence rates from both alcohol and drugs that were significantly higher than those who reported attending fewer meetings, suggesting a minimum effective dosage. Furthermore, youth involvement in 12-step activities (e.g., considering oneself a member, having a sponsor, having sponsored someone, calling other members for help, or reading literature) was examined. Those youth who were involved in three or more 12-step activities showed significantly higher alcohol and drug abstinence rates than those reporting fewer activities.

Kelly, Dow, Yeterian, and Kahler (2010) analyzed data from 127 youth after intake into an outpatient treatment facility. Consistent with prior findings, attendance at 12-step meetings significantly and independently predicted the percentage of days abstinent both during and after treatment. While Chi et al. (2009) reported that attendance at 10 meetings over 6 months produced more beneficial outcomes, Kelly et al. (2010) found that an average of at least weekly attendance was associated with the most improvements.

Although this research base is expanding and evidence is accumulating that youth may benefit from participation in 12-step groups, the existing literature remains limited. The small number of studies conducted so far makes drawing firm conclusions about how to increase the effectiveness of youth participation in these groups difficult, especially because research designs have been observational and limit researchers' ability to make causal

TABLE 2 Studies of Youth Participation in Mutual Support Groups: Sample Characteristics, Settings, and Selected Outcomes[a]

Authors (Year)	*n*	Mean Age	Female	Race/Ethnicity	Setting[b]	Selected Outcomes
Alford, Koehler, & Leonard (1991)	157	16	38%	Not reported	Inpatient CD hospital unit	At 2 years postdischarge, youth who attended AA/NA at least weekly were significantly more likely to be abstinent or essentially abstinent than were those who attended less often or not at all.
Chi, Kaskutas, Sterling, Campbell, & Weisner (2009)	357	16	36%	49% Caucasian In overall sample of 419: 16% African American 6% Asian 50% Caucasian 19% Hispanic 9% Native American	Four CD recovery programs offering intensive outpatient treatment with referrals to contracted residential programs as needed	12-step meeting attendance at 1 year after intake predicted alcohol (but not drug) abstinence at Year 3. At 3 years after intake, those adolescents who attended 10 or more 12-step meetings in the past 6 months had alcohol and drug abstinence rates significantly higher than those reporting fewer meetings. Those involved in three or more 12-step activities had significantly higher abstinence rates from alcohol and drugs compared with those reporting fewer activities.
Hohman & LeCroy (1996)	70	15	60%	Not reported	Residential CD treatment program	Adolescents who were affiliated with AA postdischarge were more likely to have had prior treatment, friends who did not use drugs, less parental involvement in treatment, and more hopelessness.
Hsieh, Hoffman, & Hollister (1998)	2,317	Not reported	37%	2% African American 90% Caucasian 2% Hispanic 4% Other	24 residential CD treatment programs	Post-treatment variables, especially attendance at AA/NA or other self-help support groups, were the most powerful discriminators of substance abuse status at 6 and 12 months postdischarge.

(Continued on next page)

TABLE 2 Studies of Youth Participation in Mutual Support Groups: Sample Characteristics, Settings, and Selected Outcomes[a] *(continued)*

Authors (Year)	*n*	Mean Age	Female	Race/Ethnicity	Setting[b]	Selected Outcomes
Kelly, Brown, Abrantes, Kahler, & Myers (2008)	160	16	40%	5% African American 75% Caucasian 5% Hispanic 15% Other	Two inpatient substance use disorder treatment centers	Youth with greater addiction severity and those who believed they could not use substances in moderation were more likely to attend. Greater early participation was associated with better long-term outcomes (percentage of days abstinent). Even with declining attendance over time, effects related to AA/NA remained significant and consistent.
Kelly, Dow, Yeterian, & Kahler (2010)	127	17	24%	87% Caucasian	Outpatient substance use disorder treatment facility	AA/NA attendance was more likely among those with greater substance use severity, more extensive prior treatment experiences, and a goal of abstinence. Attendance significantly and independently predicted percentage of days abstinent both during (at 3 months postintake) and after outpatient treatment (at 6 months postintake). An average of at least once per week attendance was associated with the most marked improvements in outcomes.
Kelly, Dow, Yeterian, & Myers (2011)	127	17	24%	87% Caucasian	Outpatient substance use disorder treatment facility	At 12 months, 60% reported AA/NA attendance. Of these, 22% reported at least one negative experience (more commonly at NA, they reported feeling intimidated, threatened, or sexually harassed). Overall, youth reported feeling very safe, though NA generally rated lower than AA. Reasons for nonattendance were unrelated to safety or negative incidents

Kelly & Myers (1997)	43	15	61%	84% Caucasian 16% Other	Inpatient CD treatment program	More frequent AA/NA attendance was related to less frequent substance use at 3 months postdischarge. Those who attended groups with at least a substantial proportion of teens had significantly better substance use outcomes.
Kelly, Myers, & Brown (2000)	99	16	60%	4% African American 78% Caucasian 16% Hispanic 2% Other	Two inpatient CD treatment programs	After controlling for factors such as aftercare attendance and intake substance use levels, 12-step meeting attendance during the first 3 months postdischarge contributed uniquely to substance use outcome variance at 3 and 6 months postdischarge.
Kelly, Myers, & Brown (2002)	74	16	62%	8% African American 70% Caucasian 18% Hispanic 4% Other	Two inpatient CD treatment programs	Adolescents with greater substance use severity were more motivated for abstinence and more likely to attend meetings and to affiliate with 12-step groups in the first 3 months postdischarge. Higher frequency of attendance and greater affiliation were associated with better post-treatment substance use outcomes. Affiliation did not predict outcome over and above attendance.
Kelly, Myers, & Brown (2005)	74	16	62%	8% African American 70% Caucasian 18% Hispanic 4% Other	Two inpatient CD treatment programs	Greater age similarity to other meeting members was found to positively influence 12-step meeting attendance rates and the perceived importance of attendance. It was also marginally related to increased step-work and (at 6 months postdischarge) less substance use. Greater age similarity at meetings was not related to an increased likelihood of having a sponsor or engaging in social activities with 12-step members.

(continued on next page)

TABLE 2 Studies of Youth Participation in Mutual Support Groups: Sample Characteristics, Settings, and Selected Outcomes[a] *(continued)*

Authors (Year)	*n*	Mean Age	Female	Race/Ethnicity	Setting[b]	Selected Outcomes
Kelly, Myers, & Rodolico (2008)	Study 1: 74; Study 2: 377	Study 1: 16; Study 2: 17	Study 1: 62%; Study 2: 49%	Study 1: 8% African American 70% Caucasian 18% Hispanic 4% Other Study 2: 2% African American 81% Caucasian 5% Hispanic 12% Other	Inpatient CD treatment programs	Study 1: Aspects of AA/NA that youth liked best were general group dynamic processes related to universality, support, and instillation of hope. Study 2: The most common reason for discontinuing attendance was boredom/lack of fit, followed by relapse. Youths with prior AA/NA participation were significantly older and more likely to have had prior CD treatment, prior psychiatric treatment, and a parent who attended AA/NA.
Kennedy & Minami (1993)	91	17	21%	92% Caucasian 8% Other	Inpatient/wilderness CD treatment program	Compared with adolescents who participated in AA/NA, those who did not had fourfold higher odds of relapse during the first 12 months postdischarge. AA/NA attendance and severity of drug use problems were the two best predictors of relapse.
Passetti & Godley (2008)	1,889 youth; 28 clinicians	15–16 (youth within sites)	17%–33% (youth within sites)	2%–90% African American 1%–79% Caucasian 0%–45% Hispanic 3%–22% Multiracial 1%–4% Other (youth within sites)	Eight sites with different menus of outpatient, intensive-outpatient, day treatment, and inpatient services	Clinicians referred almost exclusively to 12-step groups. When making referrals, considerations included substance use severity and ability to understand 12-step concepts. Age composition of meetings and meeting availability influenced suggestions of specific meetings. Clinicians who described their programs as 12-step-based and those who actively linked adolescents to groups tended to be employed at sites with the highest rates of self-help attendance.

[a]This table is an updated version of one previously published in Passetti and White (2008).
[b]CD = chemical dependency.

judgments (Kelly & Myers, 2007). One of the logical next steps for research in this area is to progress to experiments that can help provide answers about how best to improve youth attendance and outcomes from participation in mutual support groups. In the next section of this article, we provide an example of how it might be possible to develop and study an intervention for increasing attendance. We describe a pilot study that evaluated linkage strategies, measured their implementation, and examined findings related to 12-step group participation. Although this project focused on attendance at AA, NA, and CA because of the availability of meetings where the study took place, many of the strategies used and challenges encountered are conceivably applicable to other mutual support groups.

PILOT STUDY TO INCREASE YOUTH LINKAGE TO 12-STEP GROUPS

Participants in the pilot study were 22 youth who had been admitted to either outpatient or residential treatment services for substance use problems. They were recruited between August 2007 and February 2008, and their demographic and clinical characteristics are summarized in Table 3. To be approached about participation, youth had to be 12 years of age or older, reside in the catchment area of the project, and meet *Diagnostic and Statistical Manual of Mental Disorders*-Fourth Edition (American Psychiatric Association, 2000) criteria for substance dependence when admitted to treatment. Youth were excluded if they were in a controlled environment or anticipated living in a controlled environment within 1 month of recruitment, had problems understanding study instruments or procedures, were deemed dangerous to themselves or others, were a ward of state child protective services, were in outpatient treatment for the first time without a history of residential treatment, were currently participating in another study, or were currently attending two or more 12-step meetings per week. Out of 29 youth approached about participation, 22 (76%) agreed to be enrolled in the pilot study.

All pilot study procedures were approved and monitored by Chestnut Health Systems' institutional review board. Youth were interviewed at the time of consent (baseline) and 60 days after the baseline interview. Among other questions, youth were asked about the number of mutual support group meetings they attended in the prior 60 days as well as items that asked whether or not they engaged in the activities listed in Table 4. Eighteen of the 22 participants (82%) completed the follow-up interview. Youth were also asked to have meeting chairs, sponsors, or parents sign papers that verified attendance. Implementation data were recorded by the project's linkage managers and included youth's weekly self-reported meeting attendance, completion of attendance verification forms, contacts with study-involved

TABLE 3 Pilot Study Participant Characteristics ($n = 22$)

	n	%
Female	7	32
Age		
14 years	1	5%
15 years	3	14%
16 years	5	23%
17 years	6	27%
18 years	3	14%
19 years	2	9%
20 years	2	9%
Race/Ethnicity		
African American	5	23%
Caucasian	11	50%
Multiracial	6	27%
Substance Use Diagnoses		
Alcohol Abuse	5	23%
Alcohol Dependence	5	23%
Cannabis Dependence	20	91%
Cocaine Abuse	1	5%
Cocaine Dependence	2	9%
Opioid Dependence	1	5%
Mental Health Diagnoses		
Acute Stress Disorder	1	5%
Anxiety Disorder	2	9%
Attention-Deficit Hyperactivity Disorder	5	23%
Bipolar Disorder	1	5%
Depressive Disorder	4	18%
Conduct Disorder	6	27%
Oppositional Defiant Disorder	2	9%
Treatment Level of Care		
Outpatient	5	23%
Residential	17	77%

volunteers from the 12-step community, and number of sessions completed with the linkage manager.

Every participant in the pilot study was assigned a linkage manager who attempted to complete four sessions with him/her during 60 days. Duties of the linkage manager included reviewing prior 12-step meeting experiences with youth, providing an orientation to meetings, assessing and enhancing motivation to attend, working with youth to agree on attendance goals, monitoring achievement of attendance goals and involvement, reviewing reactions to meetings and group members, encouraging attendance at 12-step group-sponsored activities, coaching youth in identifying and approaching sponsors, and providing transportation to meetings, if needed. They also distributed and collected attendance verification forms. Two other major duties of the linkage managers were to suggest particular meetings to youth from a Meeting Description Binder and to link youth with volunteers from

TABLE 4 Youth Involvement in Mutual Support Activities

Activity	Baseline ($n = 22$)	60-Day Follow-Up ($n = 18$)
Shared during a meeting	32%	44%
Had a sponsor	0%	22%
Talked to a sponsor at a meeting	0%	6%
Talked to a sponsor or another member outside of a meeting	5%	28%
Asked for help from sponsor or another member	9%	17%
Read recovery-related material	27%	33%
Actively worked the steps	23%	28%
Prayed or meditated for help from a higher power	36%	33%
Felt people in meetings understood them and their problems	27%	50%
Felt that they understood other people in meetings and their problems	32%	61%
Got ideas about how to handle problems better from meeting or meeting members	27%	44%
Agreed with those ideas	27%	44%
Considered themselves a member of a home group	9%	33%
Helped someone else from a meeting	9%	11%
Sponsored someone else	0%	6%
Performed a service, like setting up or serving as chair, treasurer, etc.	0%	17%
Participated in conferences, dances, picnics, or other social activities sponsored by a self-help group	5%	6%
Had a spiritual awakening through the meeting, working steps, or reading material	14%	6%
Considered participation in self-help meetings an important part of life	23%	33%

the 12-step community who were willing to connect with youth at or outside of meetings.

The Meeting Description Binder was developed by researching 12-step meetings in the project's catchment area to help match youth to meetings that might appeal the most to them. Many of the variables investigated about these meetings were chosen based on studies described in this article and on anecdotal stories from clinicians and youth about what could be important. To accomplish this, research staff attended all open meetings of AA, NA, and CA offered in the designated areas. While maintaining anonymity, they noted the percentage of young people in attendance at each meeting, the apparent age range and gender breakdown of those present, and the number of people in the room. They also noted general topics discussed and whether or not the meeting was smoking or nonsmoking, was focused on a particular step or tradition, or was open discussion versus speaker-based. At the close of the meeting, staff spoke with the chair and/or other attendees to find out if the meeting that just ended was typical for that day and time and what meetings they would recommend for young people, especially ones with higher percentages of youth or that were "youth-friendly." Information learned about all open meetings and closed meetings described by 12-step group members was summarized and placed in the Meeting Description Binder and was organized by day of the week.

The Meeting Description Binder was reviewed with youth to identify accessible meetings that interested them, and linkage managers asked youth to sign a release to link them with volunteer members from the 12-step community. The purpose of these volunteers was to foster a personal connection with each youth to 12-step groups, provide them with someone to attend meetings with if they felt awkward going alone, and give them a guide to the 12-step world and members in their area. Seven volunteers, five male and two female, were involved with the pilot study and were identified through personal relationships or after staff met them at open 12-step meetings for the Meeting Description Binder. All volunteers underwent a background check and were matched to youth based on gender. They were trained in the study's purpose as well as what was expected of them by the lead author. Desired characteristics were the ability to be enthusiastic, warm, positive, supportive, and nonjudgmental, and to work well with young people. Each volunteer was required to have a minimum of 1 year of sobriety and to have a sponsor. Volunteers were asked to answer youths' questions about 12-step meetings and 12-step ideas and to discuss whatever topics they would normally talk about with newcomers or other individuals who had not been to meetings in a while. Volunteers also were instructed to make youth aware of sober dances, picnics, or other 12-step group activities that may be available. When possible, volunteers met with youth during their first session with the linkage manager by phone or in person or on the treatment unit if the youth was recruited right before discharge from residential services. If that could not happen, volunteers attempted to initiate contact with the youth by the next day to schedule a time to meet at a 12-step meeting during the next week. If linkage managers learned that youth failed to keep appointments through weekly contacts with the volunteers, it was the linkage manager's responsibility to continue facilitating that connection throughout the duration of the intervention.

Eight participants (36%) completed all sessions with the linkage manager, and most ($n = 9$; 41%) attended between one and three sessions. Five youth (23%) never met with the linkage manager after recruitment. Volunteers made contact with nine youth (41%), and seven of these participants only met with the volunteer shortly before discharge in residential treatment or over the phone. Two participants (9%) met volunteers and attended meetings with them. Nine participants self-reported attending a total of 21 meetings to the linkage manager during their sessions. Of these nine participants, six turned in a least one meeting verification form. Attendance was thereby verified for 9 out of 21 (43%) reported meetings.

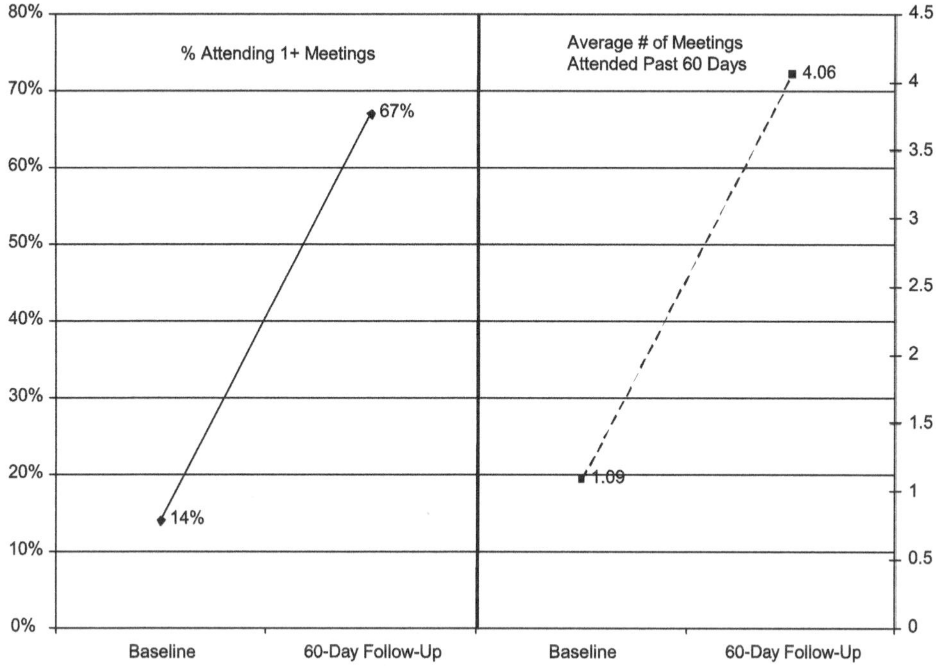

FIGURE 1 Percentage of Youth Attending One or More 12-Step Meetings and Average Number of Meetings Attended During the Past 60 Days.

The percentage of youth who attended one or more meetings in the prior 60 days increased substantially from baseline to the 60-day follow-up. There was also an increase in the average number of meetings attended during the same time period from 1.09 ($SD = 2.88$) to 4.06 ($SD = 6.28$; see Figure 1). Table 4 summarizes changes in involvement in nineteen 12-step activities from baseline to follow-up and shows that there were small to large increases in youths' self-report of participation in 17 of them (range = 1%–29%). Activities with increases of 20% or more were: having a sponsor; feeling that people in the meeting understood them and their problems; talking to a sponsor or another member outside of a meeting; considering themselves to be a member of a home group; and feeling like they understood other people in meetings and their problems.

DISCUSSION AND FUTURE DIRECTIONS

There is a long history of youth referrals to and participation in mutual support groups, yet there has been surprisingly little investigation into this practice and its effectiveness. Fortunately, this knowledge base is growing. Although early research shows promise that mutual support groups may benefit youth and the pilot study suggests that participation rates can be influenced, they also indicate that several barriers exist to designing interventions that aim to encourage the initiation and continuation of participation over time.

In the pilot study, for example, outcome data were encouraging, but it was difficult to convince youth to meet with volunteers from the 12-step community. The most common reasons youth gave for not meeting volunteers were that they: (a) were too busy; (b) did not have enough time because of other appointments; or (c) already had a sponsor so connecting with someone else was not important. Similarly, it was tricky to work with volunteers who were often well-meaning but could not always make their schedules match with the youths' availability for meetings. One struggled with lack of transportation, and one even did not show for a prearranged meeting with a youth. Given the small sample size for this pilot study, however, there was a limited pool of volunteers to work with across 10 or more communities, and some of these issues may have been alleviated by a larger selection of individuals with varied schedules and availability.

Another challenge was that even after training linkage managers in assertive methods of initiating intervention sessions with young people, youth were still difficult to contact and persuade to keep appointments for meetings. There were several missed and rescheduled sessions as well as youth who simply did not respond to repeated calls or home visits. A final implementation obstacle was obtaining verification of meeting attendance. Youth were provided with multiple verification forms and were reminded to complete them by the linkage manager, but more than half of the reported meetings attended could not be confirmed through this method.

Despite these challenges, data on meeting attendance and involvement were positive. We believe that the intervention's strength was in the ability of linkage managers to work with youth to agree to try out meetings, but the weakness was in convincing youth to connect with volunteers who may have been able to help increase ongoing attendance. There was also a lack of youth meetings in the target area, which limited the possibility of linking participants to group members who could have fostered more involvement.

In conclusion, the frequent referrals of youth to mutual support groups by treatment professionals, the prevalence of some groups in the United States, and the relatively small number of studies published on youth participation in these groups provide plentiful opportunities to address significant research questions. To date, research in this area has focused exclusively on youth participation in 12-step groups, particularly AA and NA. There is a severe lack of knowledge about the effectiveness of alternative groups and whether the results of 12-step group studies are generalizable to them. In their review of research on youth participation in 12-step groups, Kelly and Myers (2007) argued that there needs to be additional studies targeting youth treated in outpatient settings, because that is where most youth receive services. They also recommended that studies employ measures of mutual support group involvement beyond mere attendance rates. They advocated for more research that enhances understanding of developmentally specific barriers to participation and investigations into the optimal frequency, spacing, intensity, and duration of participation by youth. Such calls for further research apply to alternative groups as well.

Additional research needs to focus on testing of efforts to link youth to mutual support groups and barriers to those efforts. These studies could include a randomized clinical trial with youth randomly assigned to receive "assertive facilitation" strategies or "usual referral" strategies. Better methods of verifying meeting attendance will also need to be considered. The inclusion of text messaging and other technologies in such efforts may have the potential to increase youth engagement. Finally, more information is needed about which youth may be most appropriate for these services and which youth respond best to these services.

REFERENCES

Alcoholics Anonymous. (2007). *Alcoholics Anonymous 2007 membership survey*. New York, NY: AA World Services.

Alford, G. S., Koehler, R. A., & Leonard, J. (1991). Alcoholics Anonymous–Narcotics Anonymous and model inpatient treatment of chemically dependent adolescents: A 2-year outcome study. *Journal of Studies on Alcohol, 52*, 118–126.

American Psychiatric Association. (2000). *Diagnostic and statistical manual of mental disorders* (4th ed., text rev.). Washington, DC: Author.

American Society of Addiction Medicine. (2001). *Patient placement criteria for the treatment of substance-related disorders* (2nd ed., revised). Chevy Chase, MD: Author.

Brown, S. A. (1993). Recovery patterns in adolescent substance abuse. In J. S. Baer, G. A. Marlatt, & J. McMahon (Eds.), *Addictive behaviors across the life span: Prevention, treatment, and policy issues* (pp. 161–183). Newbury Park, CA: Sage.

Brown, S. A., Vik, P. W., & Creamer, V. A. (1989). Characteristics of relapse following adolescent substance abuse treatment. *Addictive Behaviors, 14*, 291–300. doi:10.1016/0306-4603(89)90060-9

Caldwell, P. E. (1998). Fostering client connections with Alcoholics Anonymous: A framework for social workers in various practice settings. *Social Work in Health Care, 28*, 45–61. doi:10.1300/J010v28n04_04

Chi, F. W., Kaskutas, L. A., Sterling, S., Campbell, C. I., & Weisner, C. (2009). Twelve-step affiliation and 3-year substance use outcomes among adolescents: Social support and religious service attendance as potential mediators. *Addiction, 104*, 927–939. doi:10.1111/j.1360-0443.2009.02524.x

Cocaine Anonymous World Services. (2011). *Membership survey*. Retrieved from http://www.ca.org/survey.html

Connors, G. J., Tonigan, J. S., & Miller, W. R. (2001). A longitudinal model of intake symptomatology, AA participation, and outcome: Retrospective study of the

Project MATCH outpatient and aftercare samples. *Journal of Studies on Alcohol, 62*, 817–825.

Deas, D., & Thomas, S. E. (2001). An overview of controlled studies of adolescent substance abuse treatment. *American Journal on Addictions, 10*, 178–189. doi:10.1080/105504901750227822

Dennis, M. L., Godley, S. H., Diamond, G., Tims, F. M., Babor, T., Donaldson, J., . . . Funk, R. R. (2004). The Cannabis Youth Treatment (CYT) Study: Main findings from two randomized trials. *Journal of Substance Abuse Treatment, 27*, 197–213. doi:10.1016/j.jsat.2003.09.005

Dishion, T. J., & Owen, L. D. (2002). A longitudinal analysis of friendships and substance use: Bidirectional influence from adolescence to adulthood. *Developmental Psychology, 38*, 480–491.

Drug Strategies. (2003). *Treating teens: A guide to adolescent drug programs*. Washington, DC: Author.

Forman, R. F. (2002). One AA meeting doesn't fit all: 6 keys to prescribing 12-step programs. *Current Psychiatry, 1*(10), 16–24.

Galaif, D. R., & Sussman, S. (1995). For whom does Alcoholics Anonymous work? *International Journal of the Addictions, 30*, 161–184.

Garner, B.R., Godley, M.D., Funk, R.R., Dennis, M.L., & Godley, S.H. (2007). The impact of continuing care adherence on environmental risks, substance use, and substance-related problems following adolescent residential treatment. *Psychology of Addictive Behaviors, 21*, 488–497.

Garnier, H. E., & Stein, J. A. (2002). An 18-year model of family and peer effects on adolescent drug use and delinquency. *Journal of Youth and Adolescence, 31*, 45–56.

Godley, M. D., Godley, S. H., Dennis, M. L., Funk, R., & Passetti, L. (2002). Preliminary outcomes from the assertive continuing care experiment for adolescents discharged from residential treatment. *Journal of Substance Abuse Treatment, 23*, 21–32. doi:10.1016/S0740-5472(02)00230-1

Godley, M. D., Godley, S. H., Dennis, M. L., Funk, R. R., & Passetti, L. L. (2006). The effect of Assertive Continuing Care (ACC) on continuing care linkage, adherence and abstinence following residential treatment for adolescents. *Addiction, 102*, 81–93. doi:10.1111/j.1360-0443.2006.01648.x

Godley, S. H., Dennis, M. L., Godley, M. D., & Funk, R. R. (2004). Thirty-month relapse trajectory cluster groups among adolescents discharged from outpatient treatment. *Addiction, 99*(Suppl. 2), 129–139. doi:10.1111/j.1360-0443.2004.00860.x

Godley, S. H., Godley, M. D., & Dennis, M. L. (2001). The Assertive Aftercare Protocol for adolescent substance abusers. In E. Wagner & H. Waldron (Eds.), *Innovations in adolescent substance abuse interventions* (pp. 311–329). New York, NY: Elsevier Science.

Godley, M.D., Kahn, J.H., Dennis, M.L., Godley, S.H., & Funk, R.R. (2005). The stability and impact of environmental factors on substance use and problems after adolescent outpatient treatment for cannabis abuse or dependence. *Psychology of Addictive Behaviors, 19*, 62–70.

Hohman, M., & LeCroy, C. W. (1996). Predictors of adolescent AA affiliation. *Adolescence, 31*, 339–352.

Hser, Y.-I., Grella, C. E., Hubbard, R. L., Hsieh, S.-C., Fletcher, B. W., Brown, B. S., & Anglin, M. D. (2001). An evaluation of drug treatments for adolescents in 4 U.S. cities. *Archives of General Psychiatry, 58*, 689–695.

Hsieh, S., Hoffman, N. G., & Hollister, C. D. (1998). The relationship between pre-, during-, post-treatment factors, and adolescent substance abuse behaviors. *Addictive Behaviors, 23*, 477–488. doi:10.1016/S0306-4603(98)00028-8

Humphreys, K., Wing, S., McCarty, D., Chappel, J., Gallant, L., Haberle, B., ... Weiss, R. (2004). Self-help organizations for alcohol and drug problems: Toward evidence-based practice and policy. *Journal of Substance Abuse Treatment, 26*, 151–158. doi:10.1016/S0740-5472(03)00212-5

Jainchill, N. (2000). Substance dependency treatment for adolescents: Practice and research. *Substance Use and Misuse, 35*, 2031–2060.

Kaminer, Y. (2001). Adolescent substance abuse treatment: Where do we go from here? *Psychiatric Services, 52*, 147–149.

Kaskutas, L. A., Bond, J., & Humphreys, K. (2002). Social networks as mediators of the effect of Alcoholics Anonymous. *Addiction, 97*, 891–900. doi:10.1046/j.1360-0443.2002.00118.x

Kelly, J. F. (2002). Do adolescents affiliate with 12-step groups? A multivariate process model of effects. *Journal of Studies on Alcohol, 63*, 293–304.

Kelly, J. F., Brown, S. A., Abrantes, A., Kahler, C. W., & Myers, M. (2008). Social recovery model: An 8-year investigation of adolescent 12-step group involvement following inpatient treatment. *Alcoholism: Clinical and Experimental Research, 32*, 1468–1478. doi:10.1111/j.1530-0277.2008.00712.x

Kelly, J. F., Dow, S. J., Yeterian, J. D., & Kahler, C. W. (2010). Can 12-step group participation strengthen and extend the benefits of adolescent addiction treatment? A prospective analysis. *Drug and Alcohol Dependence, 110*, 117–125. doi:10.1016/j.drugalcdep.2010.02.019

Kelly, J. F., Dow, S. J., Yeterian, J. D., & Myers, M. (2011). How safe are adolescents at Alcoholics Anonymous and Narcotics Anonymous meetings? A prospective investigation with outpatient youth. *Journal of Substance Abuse Treatment, 40*, 419–425. doi:10.1016/j.jsat.2011.01.004

Kelly, J. F., & Moos, R. (2003). Dropout from 12-step self-help groups: Prevalence, predictors, and counteracting treatment influences. *Journal of Substance Abuse Treatment, 24*, 241–250. doi:10.1016/S0740-5472(03)00021-7

Kelly, J. F., & Myers, M. G. (1997). Adolescent treatment outcome in relation to 12-step group attendance. *Alcoholism: Clinical and Experimental Research, 21*, 27A.

Kelly, J. F., & Myers, M. G. (2007). Adolescents' participation in Alcoholics Anonymous and Narcotics Anonymous: Review, implications, and future directions. *Journal of Psychoactive Drugs, 39*, 259–269.

Kelly, J. F., Myers, M. G., & Brown, S. A. (2000). A multivariate process model of adolescent 12-step attendance and substance use outcome following inpatient treatment. *Psychology of Addictive Behaviors, 14*, 376–389. doi:10.1037//0893-164X.14.4.376

Kelly, J. F., Myers, M. G., & Brown, S. A. (2002). Do adolescents affiliate with 12-step groups? A multivariate process model of effects. *Journal of Studies on Alcohol, 63*, 293–304.

Kelly, J. F., Myers, M. G., & Brown, S. A. (2005). The effects of age composition of 12-step groups on adolescent 12-step participation and substance use outcome. *Journal of Child and Adolescent Substance Abuse, 15*, 63–72. doi:10.1300/J029v15n01_05

Kelly, J. F., Myers, M. G., & Rodolico, J. (2008). What do adolescents exposed to Alcoholics Anonymous think about 12-step groups? *Substance Abuse, 29*, 53–62. doi:10.1080/08897070802093122

Kennedy, B. P., & Minami, M. (1993). The Beech Hill Hospital/Outward Bound adolescent chemical dependency treatment program. *Journal of Substance Abuse Treatment, 10*, 395–406. doi:10.1016/0740-5472(93)90025-W

Kissin, W., McLeod, C., & McKay, J. (2003). The longitudinal relationship between self-help group attendance and course of recovery. *Evaluation and Program Planning, 26*, 311–323. doi:10.1016/S0149-7189(03)00035-1

Kosterman, R., Hawkins, J. D., Guo, J., Catalano, R. F., & Abbott, R. D. (2000). The dynamics of alcohol and marijuana initiation: Patterns and predictors of first use in adolescence. *American Journal of Public Health, 90*, 360–366.

Koyanagi, C., Alfano, E., & Stein, L. (2008). *Following the rules: A report on federal rules and state actions to cover community mental health services under Medicaid*. Washington, DC: Bazelon Center for Mental Health Law.

Laudet, A. B. (2003). Attitudes and beliefs about 12-step groups among addiction treatment clients and clinicians: Towards identifying obstacles to participation. *Substance Use and Misuse, 38*, 2017–2047. doi:10.1081/JA-120025124

LifeRing. (2005). *2005 LifeRing participant survey: Results*. Retrieved from http://lifering.org/wp-content/uploads/Survey_Final.pdf

Margolis, R., Kilpatrick, A., & Mooney, B. (2000). A retrospective look at long-term adolescent recovery: Clinicians talk to researchers. *Journal of Psychoactive Drugs, 32*, 117–125.

McKay, J. R. (1999). Studies of factors in relapse to alcohol, drug and nicotine use: A critical review of methodologies and findings. *Journal of Studies on Alcohol, 60*, 566–576.

Montgomery, H. A., Miller, W., & Tonigan, J. S. (1993). Differences among AA groups: Implications for research. *Journal of Studies on Alcohol, 54*, 502–504.

Moos, R. H., & Moos, B. S. (2004). Long-term influence of duration and frequency of participation in Alcoholics Anonymous on individuals with alcohol use disorders. *Journal of Consulting and Clinical Psychology, 72*, 81–90. doi:10.1037/0022–006X.72.1.81

Morral, A. R., McCaffrey, D. F., & Ridgeway, G. (2004). Effectiveness of community-based treatment for substance abusing adolescents: 12-month outcomes of youths entering Phoenix Academy or alternative probation dispositions. *Psychology of Addictive Behaviors, 18*, 257–268. doi:10.1037/0893-164X.18.3.257

Narcotics Anonymous World Services. (2009). *Narcotics Anonymous 2009 membership survey*. Retrieved from http://www.na.org/admin/include/spaw2/uploads/pdf/NA_membership_survey.pdf

New York Academy of Medicine. (1953). *Conferences on drug addiction among adolescents*. New York, NY: The Blakiston Company.

Ogborne, A. C. (1989). Some limitations of Alcoholics Anonymous. *Recent Developments in Alcoholism, 7*, 55–65.

Passetti, L. L. (2006, March). *Adolescents' perceptions of the 12 steps and 12-step philosophy*. Paper presented at the Joint Meeting on Adolescent Treatment Effectiveness, Baltimore, MD.

Passetti, L. L., & Godley, S. H. (2008). Adolescent substance abuse treatment clinicians' self-help meeting referral practices and adolescent attendance rates. *Journal of Psychoactive Drugs, 40*, 29–40.

Passetti, L. L., & White, W. L. (2008). Recovery support meetings for youths: Considerations when referring young people to 12-step and alternative groups. *Journal of Groups in Addiction and Recovery, 2*(2–4), 97–121. doi:10.1080/15560350802081280

Piaget, J. (1969). The intellectual development of the adolescent. In G. Caplan & S. Lebovici (Eds.), *Adolescence: Psychosocial perspectives* (pp. 22–26). New York, NY: Basic Books.

Preston, P., & Goodfellow, M. (2006). Cohort comparisons: Social learning explanations for alcohol use among adolescents and older adults. *Addictive Behaviors, 31*, 2268–2283.

Rai, A. A., Stanton, B., Wu, Y., Li, X., Galbraith, J., Cottrell, L., . . . Burns, J. (2003). Relative influences of perceived parental monitoring and perceived peer involvement on adolescent risk behaviors: An analysis of six cross-sectional data sets. *Journal of Adolescent Health, 33*, 108–118.

Sisson, R. W., & Mallams, J. H. (1981). The use of systematic encouragement and community access procedures to increase attendance at Alcoholics Anonymous and Al-Anon meetings. *American Journal of Drug and Alcohol Abuse, 8*, 371–376.

Special composition groups in A.A. (2002). Retrieved from AAHistoryLovers@yahoo.groups

Stewart, D. G., & Brown, S. A. (1995). Withdrawal and dependency symptoms among adolescent alcohol and drug abusers. *Addiction, 90*, 627–635. doi:10.1046/j.1360-0443.1995.9056274.x

Terry, C. E., & Pellens, M. (1928). *The opium problem*. Montclair, NJ: Patterson Smith.

Timko, C., DeBenedetti, A., & Billow, R. (2006). Intensive referral to 12-step self-help groups and 6-month substance use disorder outcomes. *Addiction, 101*, 678–688. doi:10.1111/j.1360-0443.2006.01391.x

Tims, F. M., Dennis, M. L., Hamilton, N., Buchan, B. J., Diamond, G. S., Funk, R., & Brantley, L. B. (2002). Characteristics and problems of 600 adolescent cannabis abusers in outpatient treatment. *Addiction, 97*(Suppl. 1), S46–S57. doi:10.1046/j.1360-0443.97.s01.7.x

Tonigan, J. S., Ashcroft, F., & Miller, W. R. (1995). AA group dynamics and 12-step activity. *Journal of Studies on Alcohol, 56*, 616–621.

Waldron, H. B., Slesnick, N., Brody, J. L., Turner, C. W., & Peterson, T. R. (2001). Treatment outcomes for adolescent substance abuse at four- and seven-month assessments. *Journal of Consulting and Clinical Psychology, 69*, 802–813. doi:10.1037//0022-006X.69.5.802

White, W. L. (1998). *Slaying the dragon: The history of addiction treatment and recovery in America*. Bloomington, IL: Chestnut Health Systems.

White, W. L. (1999). A history of adolescent alcohol, tobacco and other drug use in America. *Student Assistance Journal, 11*(5), 16–22.

White, W. L., & Kurtz, E. (2006). *Linking addiction treatment and communities of recovery: A primer for addiction counselors and recovery coaches.* Pittsburgh, PA: Institute for Research, Education, and Training in Addictions/Northeast Technology Transfer Center.

Al-Anon Family Groups: Origins, Conceptual Basis, Outcomes, and Research Opportunities

CHRISTINE TIMKO

Center for Health Care Evaluation, Department of Veterans Affairs Health Care System; Department of Psychiatry and Behavioral Sciences, Stanford University Medical Center, Palo Alto, California, USA

L. BRENDAN YOUNG

Department of Communication Studies, The University of Iowa, Iowa City, Iowa, USA

RUDOLF H. MOOS

Center for Health Care Evaluation, Department of Veterans Affairs Health Care System; Department of Psychiatry and Behavioral Sciences, Stanford University Medical Center, Palo Alto, California, USA

Al-Anon Family Groups, commonly known as Al-Anon, is a mutual-help organization for relatives and friends of people misusing alcohol and other substances. We first summarize Al-Anon's history and current membership and then describe its theoretical basis and helping approach. We review evidence for Al-Anon's active ingredients and outcomes and present a conceptual model to guide future research. Research opportunities include understanding Al-Anon newcomers, specifying Al-Anon's active ingredients, and examining potential synergistic influences between Al-Anon participation and identified substance misusers' participation in mutual-help groups such as Alcoholics Anonymous. We suggest that mutual-help and professional communities work together to facilitate early participation in Al-Anon by shortening the time between problem recognition and seeking help from the fellowship.

This work was supported by the National Institute on Alcohol Abuse and Alcoholism (1R21AA019541-01) and the Department of Veterans Affairs Office of Research and Development (Health Services Research & Development Service, RCS 00-001). The views expressed here are the authors' and do not necessarily represent the views of the Department of Veterans Affairs.

INTRODUCTION

Alcohol and other drug use disorders have negative consequences not only for the drinking or using individual but also for his or her spouse or intimate partner and other family members. For example, the rate of divorce or separation is at least 4 times higher among couples with an alcoholic member compared with in the general population (Clarke-Stewart & Brentano, 2006). The purpose of Al-Anon Family Groups, a mutual-help organization more commonly known as "Al-Anon," is to help and support people who are affected by another person's drinking and/or drug use. Al-Anon is an international fellowship of relatives and friends of people misusing substances who share their experience, strength, and hope to solve their common problems. Alateen is the affiliate of Al-Anon that is for young people (mainly adolescents) who are affected by another's substance misuse. Al-Anon is the most widely used form of help for concerned family members and friends in the United States (Fernandez, Begley, & Marlatt, 2006; Miller, Meyers, & Tonigan, 1999; O'Farrell & Fals-Stewart, 2001).

In this article, we summarize Al-Anon's history and current membership and describe its theoretical basis and helping approach. We then review evidence for Al-Anon's active ingredients and outcomes. Although there are few empirical studies of Al-Anon, they span a wide time period, from the 1970s to the present. To address the need for studies on Al-Anon, we present a conceptual model to guide future research. The conceptual model (Finney & Moos, 1995; Moos, Finney, & Cronkite, 1990) considers life context, personal factors, and help obtained as determinants of outcomes. We discuss opportunities for research on Al-Anon using this framework, including understanding newcomers, specifying active ingredients, and examining the potential synergy between Al-Anon participation and the identified substance misuser's participation in mutual-help groups such as Alcoholics Anonymous (AA).

AL-ANON'S ORIGINS AND DEVELOPMENT

As documented by Al-Anon Family Groups World Service Office (http://www.al-anon.alateen.org/al-anon-history), the history of Al-Anon is intertwined with that of AA, which began in 1935. The 1939 publication of *Alcoholics Anonymous* (AA's "Big Book") included a chapter, *To Wives*, illustrating that concerned family members of AA members were primarily wives of alcoholic men and that they faced common challenges. During AA's early meetings, family members often gathered together nearby. As AA expanded, these informal meetings became sources of support, and family members came to believe that their own problems could be helped by applying AA principles and working the 12-step program.

Al-Anon is considered to have been founded in 1951 by Lois Wilson, the wife of Bill Wilson, a cofounder of AA, and Anne B, whose husband had chronic alcohol dependence. Lois Wilson and Anne B contacted groups of families who had written to the AA General Service Office and held a meeting of Family Group chairs and secretaries in New York. AA granted the Family Groups permission to adopt the 12 steps for Al-Anon. Only one word in the 12 steps was changed by Al-Anon: The 12th Step instructs members to carry the message of having had a spiritual awakening by working the steps to "others" rather than to "alcoholics." Al-Anon's first hardcover book, *The Al-Anon Family Groups*, was published in 1955.

The Al-Anon 12 traditions were accepted at Al-Anon's first World Service Conference in 1961, and Al-Anon's first International Convention was held in 1985 in Montreal, Quebec, Canada. Three legacies adopted from AA have served as guiding principles in Al-Anon: (1) recovery through the 12 steps, which encourage members to carry the Al-Anon message to others; (2) unity through the 12 traditions, which protect Al-Anon groups from influences that might distract or disrupt them from their common purpose; and (3) service through the 12 concepts of service, which provide a guide for broad-scale service within the Al-Anon program.

In the early days of AA and Al-Anon, teenagers often attended open AA meetings and Family Group meetings with their parents. Concern for the problems of children of parents with alcoholism emerged as early as 1955 at the AA International Convention, where a special session for teenage offspring was held. The first Alateen group took place in 1957 in Pasadena, CA; it was started by the teenage son of a father in AA and a mother in Al-Anon. In response to growing requests for help from teenagers, Al-Anon formed its Alateen affiliate. Al-Anon's 12 steps were adopted verbatim for Alateen, and the 12 traditions were modified to meet the needs of offspring. Alateen's guidelines require groups to have an adult Al-Anon member as a sponsor, although teens run their own meetings (Al-Anon Family Groups World Service Office, n.d.).

Although this article focuses on Al-Anon, which was developed to help people live better with another person's alcoholism, we note here that Nar-Anon was begun to help with another's addiction to drugs other than alcohol. Nar-Anon was originally founded by Alma B in Studio City, CA, but the initial launch of the program failed. It was later revived in 1968 by Robert Stewart Goodrich in the Palo Verdes Peninsula in Los Angeles County, CA. Nar-Anon filed articles of incorporation in 1971 and established the Nar-Anon World Service Office in 1986 in Torrance, CA. Currently, Nar-Anon Family Groups is a worldwide fellowship that is adapted from Narcotics Anonymous and uses its own 12 steps, 12 traditions, and 12 concepts. There are Nar-Anon face-to-face meetings as well as online meetings, forums, and chat rooms.

AL-ANON'S MEMBERSHIP

Currently, there are more than 28,000 Al-Anon Family Groups and more than 24,000 Alateen groups in 115 countries. Al-Anon Family Groups have an average of 16 members per group, involving more than 384,000 individuals worldwide. Each month in the United States, almost 57,000 people go to a meeting for the first time (Al-Anon Family Groups World Service Office, n.d.).

The best source of data on Al-Anon members is the World Service Office's triennial membership survey. A convenience sample of 1,775 members with an average of 13 years of Al-Anon membership was surveyed in 2009. Of these members, 84% were women, and 93% were White; on average, they were 56 years old. In addition, 58% of members were married, 56% had a college degree, and 60% were employed. On average, members attended 1.8 in-person meetings per week; 6% of members participated in an online meeting weekly. One fifth of Al-Anon members were also members of AA. The person whose substance misuse had the most negative effect on the Al-Anon member was most commonly identified as the husband (23% of members) or son (11%); 49% of identified substance misusers were still actively using.

Al-Anon members are encouraged to attend face-to-face meetings, work the 12 steps, obtain a sponsor, read Al-Anon literature, and develop spiritual practices such as prayer and meditation. Some meetings are open to attendance by anyone, and others are closed—that is, only for members or prospective members who have a relative or friend with substance use problems. Increasingly, support from the Al-Anon fellowship is available through online meetings and email listservs. In a typical meeting, participants share and listen to each other's experiences, strengths, and hopes on a confidential basis. Often, meetings begin with a reading of the 12 steps and one or more of the 12 traditions, and then they focus on a topic initially addressed by a lead-off speaker. Attendees are not required to speak, but when they do, they are encouraged to share of themselves without giving direct advice—that is, telling another person what to think or do or how to act—and without questioning or interrupting others. Many meetings close with the Serenity Prayer.

A sponsor is an Al-Anon member who provides personal support to another individual, whether the sponsee is new or has been in Al-Anon for a longer period of time. Sponsors share their experience, strength, and hope, explain the Al-Anon program, guide sponsees in using tools of the program, and help sponsees work and apply the 12 steps. One of the main Al-Anon tools of recovery is service to the group (e.g., set up, welcome newcomers, handle literature) or district (e.g., serve as group representative to the district or on committees such as those for public outreach or hospitals and institutions). Al-Anon's view is that members help themselves by helping others, as captured by the saying, *To keep it, you have to give it away.*

AL-ANON'S THEORETICAL BASIS AND HELPING APPROACH

In the view of Al-Anon, alcoholism and addiction to other substances is a disease, and family members are often codependent. Much like the substance misuser, the family member develops a preoccupation with controlling the substance use and its consequences. In this way, the identified misuser and family members become simultaneously dependent on substances to define their behavior toward each other.

Family members are helped separately from the loved one who is addicted to alcohol or other drugs. Such separation is emblematic of the detachment prescribed by Al-Anon. The family member's help seeking implicitly acknowledges that previous attempts to intervene and control the identified substance misuser have failed. In Al-Anon, family members are discouraged from actively trying to change the loved one's drinking or other drug use. Instead, family members are advised to detach from the loved one, focus on themselves, and obtain help for their own emotional distress to increase the skills they need to cope with the difficulties of living with someone misusing substances. Al-Anon encourages the spouse and other family members to reach outside the family for help.

The focus of Al-Anon is relief from the pain and suffering that result from living with an alcohol- or drug-dependent person. Al-Anon and Alateen direct members' attention away from the identified person misusing substances and refocus their attention toward their own behaviors and emotions. People concerned about a loved one's addiction typically try to control the loved one's behaviors. Thus, the concerned family member often becomes codependent—that is, as obsessed with the identified substance misuser's behavior as misusers are with their substance of choice. Al-Anon makes available the 12 steps for members as a way to reduce the controlling behaviors and resentments they often display (Cermak, 1989).

Al-Anon's view that alcoholism and other addictions are a disease helps to relieve the family member's guilt that he or she is responsible for the loved one's addiction and increases the family member's self-worth. As family members learn to assign responsibility for family problems to the disease rather than to themselves, they begin to forgive themselves, accept that they have been adversely affected by the addicted individual's shortcomings, and begin to improve their functioning. Al-Anon's focus on the family member indicates that the Al-Anon member should work toward personal peace and serenity, rather than toward controlling the identified substance misuser. The Al-Anon program suggests that that the member engages in a completely honest self-examination to take responsibility for his or her own behaviors. Although this can be quite difficult, the member is supported and directed by the caring and concerned Al-Anon fellowship (Anthony M., 1977).

As noted, Al-Anon uses the 12 steps to help people recover from codependence. In part because the term "codependence" became intertwined with the term "enabling" (the idea that the codependent family member enables the drinking or drugging habits of the addicted person), its use is sometimes controversial. (For more discussion of this controversy, see Rotunda & Doman, 2001; Rotunda, West, & O'Farrell, 2004.) As suggested by its link with the concept of enabling, codependence has many facets, but one often cited by the Al-Anon community is the investment of self-esteem in the effort and success of trying to control the feelings and behaviors of the substance-misusing family member or friend and sometimes of other people (Cermak, 1989). In the Al-Anon context, codependence involves trying to take care of and change the identified substance misuser at the expense of one's own physical, emotional, and spiritual well-being. Essentially, codependence includes engaging in self-defeating behaviors, such as taking responsibility for regulating the substance misuser's actions and trying to rescue or fix the damage caused by that individual's irresponsible behavior, combined with the tendency to put others' needs ahead of one's own and an excessive reliance on other people for approval and identity (Dear, 2002).

Al-Anon emphasizes personal responsibility and encourages members to let go of controlling the behaviors of the loved one by accepting that they are powerless to do so. A key component is surrender, the process of increasingly accepting the need for external help, such as from a higher power and the fellowship of Al-Anon (Roth & Tan, 2007).

The apparent contradiction between emphases on personal responsibility and surrender is one of many paradoxes in Al-Anon's helping approach and the approach of 12-step groups more generally. Herndon (2001) described the paradox of asking the group to admit powerlessness when the ultimate purpose is empowerment. She noted that Al-Anon's Step 1 ("We admitted we were powerless over alcohol—that our lives had become unmanageable") encourages members to understand that by admitting powerlessness over "the facts of our situation and the other people involved," they will discover that they "are not helpless." (Al-Anon Family Group Headquarters, Inc, 1990). That is, admitting powerlessness leads to feelings of empowerment, and surrender produces self-responsibility. Herndon suggests defining self-responsibility as being autonomous and acting in a caring and respectful way toward others.

As explained more specifically by Eastland (1995), the empowering aspects of surrender emerge from the realization that the family member cannot control other people (the drinker) but can control him or herself. With this new view, the Al-Anon member is not responsible for others' behavior, but for his or her own. This shift from reactor to actor provides the possibility of choice, and the interaction in Al-Anon meetings provides a collective experience of choice making and action.

EVIDENCE FOR AL-ANON'S ACTIVE INGREDIENTS AND OUTCOMES

As noted, the few existing empirical studies of Al-Anon cover a wide time span. They also used different methods to obtain their samples, such as recruitment of concerned family members through media advertisements, through substance use disorder or medical treatment programs for addicted individuals, or through the researcher's personal acquaintance with individuals in Al-Anon.

Active Ingredients

The therapeutic processes that likely underlie the benefits of Al-Anon are described in Moos's (2008) model of the active ingredients of substance use-related mutual-help groups. The active ingredients include: (a) bonding (the group is cohesive and supportive), goal direction (the group encourages personal growth, such as responsibility, self-discovery, and spirituality), and structure (the group embodies clear expectations); (b) the provision of norms and role models; (c) involvement in rewarding activities; and (d) bolstering self-efficacy and coping skills. These active ingredients are hypothesized to be effective in diverse mutual-help group and cultural contexts, although the specific goals, norms, activities, and coping methods emphasized will vary (Moos, 2008).

Research on the active ingredients of Al-Anon suggests that this model of therapeutic processes is a useful way to examine how Al-Anon works (Ablon, 1974; Barber & Gilbertson, 1997; Roth & Tan, 2007, 2008). Al-Anon clearly provides the active ingredient of interpersonal bonding and support, as well as structure via embracing positive social values. In this regard, Al-Anon members reported great relief in finding others who shared their problems and understood them (Ablon, 1974). An essential dynamic of Al-Anon is the candid sharing of experiences and reactions (Barber & Gilbertson, 1997). Al-Anon also provides the active ingredient of positive norms and role models. For example, Al-Anon exposes members to other people who have created satisfying lives despite having a loved one who is drinking excessively (Barber & Gilbertson, 1997).

Qualitative findings also highlight the importance of pre- and post-Al-Anon meeting social interactions that encourage member bonding (Roth & Tan, 2007, 2008). These informal social opportunities facilitate exposure to positive role models (e.g., potential sponsors who help with working the steps) and participation in rewarding activities. In addition, Al-Anon meetings display healthy group functioning for members—that is, clear roles that allow group meetings to proceed well despite miscommunications.

Outcomes

Relatively few empirical studies have been conducted to examine Al-Anon's benefits and how they are achieved. Some studies have surveyed members with a broad range of membership duration (1 month to more than 20 years) or those who have been long-term, stable members. As we review in this section, domains in which Al-Anon participation has been associated with positive outcomes are physical and mental health, substance use, personal functioning (e.g., coping, self-esteem, social functioning), well-being and quality of life, and couple and family functioning. For example, in the most recent Al-Anon survey in 2009 (Al-Anon Family Groups World Service Office, n.d.), members reported that their physical and mental health symptoms declined after attending Al-Anon meetings.

Among wives of husbands who misused substances, those attending Al-Anon for at least a year reported less vulnerability to stress, less stress in family situations, and less maladaptive coping compared with wives who did not attend Al-Anon (McGregor, 1990). A review of family-based interventions for alcoholism concluded that Al-Anon helps family members cope more adaptively with the loved one's drinking and with life stressors that are related or unrelated to the drinking (O'Farrell & Fals-Stewart, 2001). Moreover, wives of alcoholic husbands who attended Al-Anon longer reported greater decreases in negative coping; in turn, decreases in negative coping were associated with a longer duration of the husband's abstinence. Possibly, the greatest improvements in coping occur early in Al-Anon membership, such as within the 1st year (Gorman & Rooney, 1979).

Family members in Al-Anon benefit from participation not only in terms of coping, but also by experiencing less depression, anger, and family conflict, and more family cohesion and relationship satisfaction (Cutter & Cutter, 1987; Dittrich & Trapold, 1984; Miller et al., 1999). Other often-cited positive outcomes of Al-Anon participation, especially when it is sustained for longer periods, are increased self-esteem (Ablon, 1974; Cutter & Cutter; Dittrich & Trapold; Anthony M., 1977) and declines in isolation and the concerned family member's own problem drinking (Cutter & Cutter). In particular, a longer duration of Al-Anon participation was related to members having better marital adjustment and higher self-esteem (Keinz, Schwartz, Trench, & Houlihan, 1995).

One study suggests that the benefits of Al-Anon reported in naturalistic, observational studies may be conferred to individuals in randomized trials. Specifically, partners of heavy drinkers who were randomly assigned to attend Al-Anon groups instead of treatment showed greater reductions in personal problems (e.g., loneliness, irritability, money shortages, feeling to blame for partner's drinking) compared with partners assigned to a treatment wait list (Barber & Gilbertson, 1996). These benefits were measured 5 weeks after beginning meeting attendance.

Qualitative analyses of online Al-Anon meetings with 9 to 11 members per meeting have both reinforced and broadened prior literature on Al-Anon outcomes (Roth, 2004; Roth & Tan, 2007, 2008). These analyses indicate that positive outcomes of Al-Anon may include better job functioning, relief from isolation and anger, and gaining strength and hope. They also describe relief from a depth and intensity of negative feelings that include fear, hurt, shame, frustration, and worry, as well as thoughts of perpetrating violence and suicide.

OPPORTUNITIES FOR RESEARCH

Because the empirical base is limited, there is a need for research on the outcomes of Al-Anon participation. Needed research foci include specification of active ingredients of Al-Anon, Al-Anon's outcomes, better understanding of newcomers to Al-Anon, and examination of the potential synergy between the concerned family member's participation in Al-Anon and the identified substance misuser's participation in AA. Possibly, participation in Al-Anon and AA may positively influence each other, in that a family member's involvement in Al-Anon may motivate the identified substance misuser to try AA and continue active and sustained AA participation.

A conceptual framework is helpful to guide examination of these different areas of research (Finney & Moos, 1995; Moos et al., 1990). As shown in Figure 1, life context at baseline (Panel I) consists of the life stressors that bring the family member to Al-Anon and the severity of the identified substance misuser's problems. Personal factors at baseline (Panel II) include the family member's sociodemographic characteristics (e.g., gender, race, and ethnicity) and personal characteristics (e.g., coping, self-esteem) and medical, psychological, and social functioning. Panel III encompasses the family member's participation in Al-Anon and professional treatment, including the timing, amount, and duration of participation. The model specifies that the family member's outcomes (Panel V) are influenced by personal characteristics at baseline (Panel II), life context factors at baseline (Panel I) and those that occur during the follow-up interval (Panel IV), and mutual-help and treatment experiences (Panel III).

Active Ingredients of Al-Anon

More information is needed about the active ingredients or social processes that may account for the positive effects of Al-Anon. One research opportunity is to formulate conceptually integrated measures of the active ingredients of Al-Anon. An inventory of the active ingredients would encompass the emphasis on social control processes (support, goal direction, and structure),

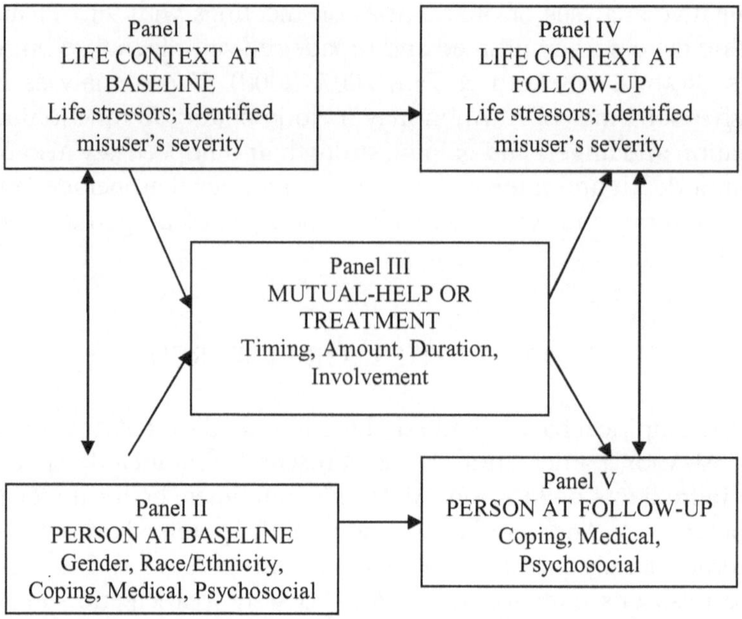

FIGURE 1 A Model of Personal, Life Context, and Mutual-Help or Treatment Factors That Affect Al-Anon Members.

social learning processes (norms and role models), behavioral choice processes (rewards for desired behaviors and participation in rewarding activities), and aspects of stress and coping theory (identifying high-risk situations and stressors, building self-efficacy, and developing effective coping skills).

The development of an integrated inventory to assess these areas is a complex undertaking, but initial models are available, such as the Group Environment Scale (GES; Moos, 2004), the 12-Step Participation and Expectancies Questionnaire (Kahler, Kelly, Strong, Stuart, & Brown, 2006), and the Addiction Treatment Attitudes Questionnaire (Morgenstern, Bux, Labouvie, Blanchard, & Morgan, 2002). In this regard, a study that used the GES found that four AA groups had moderate-to-high emphasis on support (cohesion and expressiveness), goal direction (independence, self-discovery, and spirituality), and organization (Montgomery, Miller, & Tonigan, 1993).

When the active ingredients of Al-Anon can be measured, it will be possible to examine how well and consistently different groups "deliver" them and the extent to which they are associated with specific outcomes for individuals with different characteristics. Such an inventory could be used to examine the consistency in active ingredients in different Al-Anon groups, such as groups targeted to newcomers, adult children, or Latino or African American families. It could also be used to examine the extent to which members are more satisfied and obtain more benefits in groups that are relatively supportive, goal-directed, and structured.

Another research opportunity focuses on personal factors that moderate the effects of the active ingredients of Al-Anon. That is, some individuals may be especially open to the influence of specific active ingredients, whereas others may either resist or not benefit from them. For example, individuals who are high in reactance and/or anger may be less likely to respond positively to highly directive interventions that rely heavily on confrontation (Karno & Longabaugh, 2005). Also, compared with men, women, who tend to be more codependent (Fuller & Warner, 2000) but may be more responsive to support, goal direction, and structure, may benefit more from well-functioning role models, an emphasis on rewarding social activities, and building self-esteem and coping skills. Spirituality may also be associated with enhanced awareness of feelings and, in turn, more involvement in mutual-support groups such as Al-Anon (Carrico, Gifford, & Moos, 2007).

We need to examine links between active ingredients of Al-Anon, treatment, and aspects of the life contexts of people living with loved ones experiencing substance addiction. That is, the active ingredients or social processes that characterize Al-Anon are closely related to those in other social contexts in the recovery environment, such as family, friends, and the workplace (Moos, 2007). In this vein, family members and friends who strengthen social bonds and goal direction by maintaining a cohesive and well-organized family, espouse traditional norms and role models, promote engagement in rewarding social and recreational pursuits, and build recovering individuals' self-efficacy and coping skills tend to have a positive influence on well-being and quality of life.

These ideas point to the need for integrative studies to find out how much the influence of Al-Anon depends on the same social processes that underlie the beneficial effects of families and social networks (Moos, 2008). How much synergy and value is added when recovering individuals obtain support and structure from both Al-Anon and family members? Alternatively, how well can support and structure obtained in Al-Anon compensate for a lack of cohesion and monitoring in other aspects of an individual's social network? Comparable questions arise with respect to norms and role models, engagement in rewarding activities, and building self-confidence and coping skills.

Al-Anon's Outcomes

To fully examine the outcomes of participation in Al-Anon, we need better measures of the constructs contained in the model's panels, as well as a better understanding of how these constructs are associated with one another. A specific need is for more comprehensive measures of involvement in Al-Anon (Panel III). Meeting attendance (that is, number, duration, and frequency of meeting attendance) is an important indicator of participation, but it may not adequately reflect an individual's level of group involvement, as shown by such indexes as number of steps completed, acceptance of 12-step ideology, and obtaining and becoming a sponsor. The AA Involvement Scale (Tonigan, Connors, & Miller, 1996) or AA Affiliation Scale (Humphreys, Kaskutas, & Weisner, 1998) would be a starting point for adaptation for measuring Al-Anon involvement.

Moreover, regarding Panel III, many individuals attend both Al-Anon and professional treatment. In the most recent Al-Anon survey of 1,775 members (Al-Anon Family Groups World Service Office, n.d.), 58% of respondents had received treatment, counseling, or therapy (mainly mental health, marriage, or family counseling) prior to attending Al-Anon meetings, and of these, 79% viewed the counseling as having a positive effect on their lives. The same proportion (58%) of respondents received treatment subsequent to initiating Al-Anon attendance, and 91% said the counseling affected their lives for the better. In principle, these two sources of help could contribute independently to better outcomes or they could either bolster or detract from each other; in addition, their effect on one another could depend on when each occurs with regard to the other. For example, involvement in Al-Anon could enhance the effectiveness of concurrent treatment for psychological, marital, and family problems.

Regarding Panel V, success in Al-Anon is not straightforward to measure. (This is in contrast to AA, in which success is measured primarily by remaining clean and sober.) More research is needed on whether or how Al-Anon is helpful to members and even what "helpful" means in the context of Al-Anon membership. In what life areas do Al-Anon attendees experience improvements early on? How do positive outcomes evolve over time as the duration of membership lengthens? Why do individuals drop out of Al-Anon (does dropout signal recovery, or failed recovery, on the part of the Al-Anon member and/or the identified substance misuser?), and are there any detrimental effects of participation?

Another research opportunity is to examine the potential detrimental effects of Al-Anon. There have been some criticisms of Al-Anon, such as enforced group cohesion that encourages conformity, psychological harm due to the emotional intensity of group discussions, encouragement of a sick-role identity by convincing individuals that they have the lifelong condition of codependence, and problems associated with the emphasis on powerlessness, especially for women (Herndon, 2001). Another criticism is that the length of time it takes to achieve stable recovery may discourage a newcomer's sustained participation.

Newcomers to Al-Anon

Even though the most positive changes may occur in the first few weeks or months of membership (Gorman & Rooney, 1979), the experiences of newcomers to Al-Anon have not been studied. Existing studies suggest that the main reason for initiating Al-Anon participation is the accumulation of acute and chronic life stressors (Ablon, 1974). Such problems may include family violence: 33% of a sample of wives in Al-Anon had been beaten by their husbands, and 63% had witnessed him engage in violent and destructive acts (Gorman & Rooney). Compared with spouses of people dependent on alcohol or other drugs who did not participate in a mutual-help group such as Al-Anon, spouses who chose to participate were older, more educated, more concerned about their family life, had a higher prevalence of health problems and a longer period of exposure to the other's substance use, and believed that they needed help for themselves, not just for the identified substance misuser (Cormier, 1995). However, more information is needed about the characteristics of newcomers to Al-Anon, reasons for and patterns of early participation, and factors associated with dropout or sustained participation.

Another important finding is that seeking help from Al-Anon is often delayed. Wives in Al-Anon waited an average of almost 9 years after the first occurrence of problems due to the husband's problem drinking before going to Al-Anon (Gorman & Rooney, 1979). We need to know more about why family members delay help seeking until their problems have become numerous and burdensome and how the mutual-help and professional treatment community may facilitate relief by motivating individuals to seek help more quickly.

Following the model shown in Figure 1, newcomers to Al-Anon meetings could be asked about their personal characteristics (Panel II), life stressors (Panel I), and use of Al-Anon and treatment (Panel III), including reasons for trying, and expectations about, Al-Anon. Then, at one or more follow-ups, these individuals would again be asked about their use of Al-Anon and treatment (Panel III), life stressors (Panel IV), and personal functioning (Panel V) to examine associations between help obtained and outcomes.

An example to illustrate the model concerns Al-Anon newcomers' victimization by partner violence (Panel I). In particular, White women (Panel II), who are often victims of partner violence when the partner is drinking (Caetano, Cunradi, Schafer, & Clark, 2000), may be more likely to initiate and sustain Al-Anon participation (Panel III). As noted, Al-Anon's membership is mainly White women, and individuals who share the predominant characteristics of members are more likely to initiate mutual-help group attendance (Humphreys & Woods, 1993). In turn, Al-Anon participation may be associated with a reduction in victimization from the drinking partner (Panel IV) and better medical and psychosocial outcomes (Panel V).

Synergy Between Al-Anon and AA Membership

Very little is known about the potential synergistic influences between a family member's participation in Al-Anon and the identified substance misuser's participation in AA (or other mutual-help group). Literature from both AA and Al-Anon acknowledges that relationship difficulties often arise when the identified substance misuser and/or the concerned family member seek recovery. For example, the family member may resent AA's success in what he or she has been unable to accomplish in terms of the loved one's sobriety, or the family member may feel neglected as the identified misuser spends time and emotional investment on other AA members and the fellowship. Al-Anon may offer increased understanding of new relationship dynamics such that the family member is able to continue to support the misuser's AA participation and sobriety.

When concerned family members or friends participate more in Al-Anon (i.e., have a longer duration of meeting attendance, more involvement in group practices), the identified substance misuser may become more involved in AA. In this regard, qualitative analyses of online Al-Anon meetings suggest reciprocity between the concerned family member's Al-Anon participation and outcomes and the identified misuser's AA participation (Roth & Tan, 2007, 2008). For example, a family member's participation in Al-Anon may facilitate a drinker's initiation of AA attendance.

In addition, when the concerned person benefits from Al-Anon, positive outcomes may accrue for the identified substance user. Among married couples, when the nonalcoholic wife was active in Al-Anon, her alcoholic husband was more likely to be abstinent (Wright & Scott, 1978). The combination of the wife's participation in Al-Anon and the husband's participation in AA was associated with the highest rate of abstinence. Also, among AA members, longer duration of a family member's Al-Anon attendance was associated with less family stress reported by the AA member and the family member. A family member's Al-Anon attendance was related to the drinker's continuous AA attendance (McBride, 1992). These findings suggest a family member's active Al-Anon membership can facilitate a drinker's AA participation and recovery.

This suggestion is strengthened by findings that family members attending Al-Anon were less angry and resentful and thus had better communication with the drinker's treatment staff (Huppert, 1976). At a 3-month follow-up of treatment in a substance use disorder residential program, clients whose family members were in Al-Anon had a 69% remission rate, compared with a 39% rate for clients who did not have a family member in Al-Anon. Clients and family members in the Al-Anon group perceived their families as more effective than did clients and family members with no Al-Anon participation (Friedemann, 1996). Among women with partners who were untreated for alcohol problems, those who received Al-Anon facilitation decreased in depression, and the partner drank less, at a 1-year follow-up (Rychtarik & McGillicuddy, 2005).

SUMMARY, CONCLUSIONS, AND FUTURE DIRECTIONS

In this article, we reviewed possible active ingredients and positive outcomes of Al-Anon participation and presented a conceptual model to guide research on these potential mechanisms and benefits. We conclude by noting that this model may also guide efforts to facilitate participation in Al-Anon. In particular, methods are needed to facilitate earlier attendance of Al-Anon (Panel III), before the accumulation of life stressors due to the identified substance misuser's problems becomes too burdensome (Panel I). That is, it would be helpful for the mutual-help, professional treatment, and research communities to work together to help individual family members shorten the delay between recognizing the problems of living with a substance misuser and obtaining help.

The idea would be to facilitate help seeking before the family member hits bottom, viewing life as unmanageable, hopeless, and full of despair. Effective strategies might parallel those that have been found to be effective to facilitate help seeking by people with addictions—namely, motivational interviewing and arranging contact with people already in 12-step recovery (Timko & DeBenedetti, 2007; Young, 2011). Relatedly, the mutual-help, professional, and research communities might join together to aid Al-Anon in increasing the diversity of its membership (Panel II). Although Al-Anon is open to everyone, the pattern of mainly White women seeking help because of the alcoholic men they live with has persisted over decades (Al-Anon Family Groups World Service Office, n.d.; Rosenqvist, 1991).

To accomplish these goals of earlier help seeking from Al-Anon and increased diversity of Al-Anon membership, it will be helpful to continue to build strong alliances among professional treatment providers, researchers, and mutual-help group leaders. For example, to increase referrals to Al-Anon, many providers may prefer to have available research findings, as well as anecdotal evidence, for Al-Anon's effectiveness. However, research is a source of controversy in the Al-Anon community, which likely contributes to the relative lack of empirical studies. Because Al-Anon has traditions of nonaffiliation with outside organizations, some members may believe that they are prohibited from participation in research studies. However, in our experience conducting research on Al-Anon, most members do not see the traditions and participation in research as incompatible. In fact, they perceive a value in research to demonstrate, to the professional community but even more so to those in need of help, the benefits of Al-Anon participation, how they are achieved, and what aspects of participation are most helpful to whom. Our hope is to continue to increase cooperation and collaboration among mutual-help group members, treatment providers, and researchers to benefit people living in hardship due to a loved one's drinking and other drug use.

REFERENCES

Ablon, J. (1974). Al-Anon Family Groups: Impetus for learning and change through the presentation of alternatives. *American Journal of Psychotherapy*, *28*(1), 30–45.

Al-Anon Family Groups World Service Office. (n.d.). *Welcome to Al-Anon Family Groups*. Retrieved from http://www.al-anon.alateen.org

Al-Anon Family Group Headquarters, Inc. (1990). In all our affairs: Making crises work far you. New York: Al-Anon Family Group Headquarters, Inc. p. 31.

Barber, J. G., & Gilbertson, R. (1996). An experimental study of brief unilateral intervention for the partners of heavy drinkers. *Research on Social Work Practice*, *6*(3), 325–336.

Barber, J. G., & Gilbertson, R. (1997). Unilateral interventions for women living with heavy drinkers. *Social Work*, *42*(1), 69–78.

Caetano, R., Cunradi, C., Schafer, J., & Clark, C. (2000). Intimate partner violence and drinking patterns among White, Black, and Hispanic couples in the US. *Journal of Substance Abuse*, *11*, 123–138.

Carrico, A. W., Gifford, E. V., & Moos, R. (2007). Spirituality/religiosity promotes acceptance-based responding and twelve-step involvement. *Drug and Alcohol Dependence*, *89*, 66–73.

Cermak, T. L. (1989). Al-Anon and recovery. *Recent Developments in Alcoholism*, *7*, 91–104.

Clarke-Stewart, A., & Brentano, C. (2006). *Divorce: Causes and consequences*. New Haven, CT: Yale University Press.

Cormier, P. (1995). Decision to join a mutual aid group. *Canadian Nurse*, *91*(5), 41–45.

Cutter, C. G., & Cutter, H. S. (1987). Experience and change in Al-Anon Family Groups: Adult children of alcoholics. *Journal of Studies on Alcohol*, *48*(1), 29–32.

Dear, G. E. (2002). The Holyoake Codependency Index: Further evidence of the factorial validity. *Drug and Alcohol Review*, *21*, 59–64.

Dittrich, J. E., & Trapold, M. (1984). A treatment program for the wives of alcoholics: An evaluation. *Bulletin of the Society of Psychologists in Addictive Behaviors*, *3*, 91–102.

Eastland, L. S. (1995). Recovery as an interactive process: Examination and empowerment in 12-step programs. *Qualitative Health Research*, *5*(3), 292–314.

Fernandez, A. C., Begley, E. A., & Marlatt, A. (2006). Family and peer interventions for adults: Past approaches and future directions. *Psychology of Addictive Behaviors*, *20*(2), 207–213.

Finney, J. W., & Moos, R. H. (1995). Entering treatment for alcohol abuse: A stress and coping model. *Addiction*, *90*, 1223–1240.

Friedemann, M. L. (1996). Effects of Al-Anon attendance on family perception of inner-city indigents. *The American Journal of Drug and Alcohol Abuse*, *22*(1), 123–134.

Fuller, J. A., & Warner, R. M. (2000). Family stressors as predictors of codependency. *Genetic, Social, and General Psychology Monographs*, *126*(1), 5–22.

Gorman, J. M., & Rooney, J. F. (1979). Delay in seeking help and onset of crisis among Al-Anon wives. *American Journal of Drug and Alcohol Abuse*, *6*(2), 223–233.

Herndon, S. (2001). The paradox of powerlessness: Gender, sex, and power in 12-step groups. *Women and Language*, *24*(2), 7–12.

Humphreys, K. N., Kaskutas, L., & Weisner, C. (1998). The Alcoholics Anonymous Affiliation Scale (AAAS). *Alcoholism: Clinical and Experimental Research, 22*, 974–978.

Humphreys, K., & Woods, M. (1993). Researching mutual-help group affiliation in a segregated society. *Journal of Applied Behavioral Science, 29*, 181–201.

Huppert, S. (1976). The role of Al-Anon groups in the treatment program of a VA alcoholism unit. *Hospital & Community Psychiatry, 27*(10), 693–697.

Kahler, C. W., Kelly, J. F., Strong, D. R., Stuart, G. L., & Brown, R. A. (2006). Development and initial validation of a 12-step participation expectancies questionnaire. *Journal of Studies on Alcohol, 67*(4), 538–542.

Karno, M. P., & Longabaugh, R. (2005). An examination of how therapist directiveness interacts with patient anger and reactance to predict alcohol use. *Journal of Studies on Alcohol, 66*, 825–832.

Keinz, L. A., Schwartz, C., Trench, B. M., & Houlihan, D. D. (1995). An assessment of membership benefits in the Al-Anon program. *Alcoholism Treatment Quarterly, 12*(4), 31–38.

Anthony, M. (1977). Al-Anon. *Journal of the American Medical Association, 238*(10), 1062–1063.

McBride, J. L. (1992). Assessing the Al-Anon component of Alcoholics Anonymous. *Alcoholism Treatment Quarterly, 8*(4), 57–65.

McGregor, P. (1990, March). *The influence of Al-Anon on stress of wives of alcoholics.* Cincinnati, OH: Paper presented at the Annual Meeting of the American Association for Counseling and Development

Miller, W. R., Meyers, R. J., & Tonigan, J. S. (1999). Engaging the unmotivated in treatment for alcohol problems: A comparison of three strategies for intervention through family members. *Journal of Consulting and Clinical Psychology, 67*(5), 688–697.

Montgomery, H. A., Miller W. R., & Tonigan J. S. (1993). Differences among AA groups: Implications for research. *Journal of Studies on Alcohol, 54*, 502–504.

Moos, R. (2004). *Group Environment Scale manual (3rd ed.).* Redwood City, CA: Mind Garden.

Moos, R. (2007). Theory-based processes that promote remission of substance use disorders. *Clinical Psychology Review, 27*, 537–551.

Moos, R. H. (2008). Active ingredients of substance use-focused self-help groups. *Addiction, 103*(3), 387–396.

Moos, R. H., Finney, J. W., & Cronkite, R. C. (1990). *Alcoholism treatment: Context, process, and outcome.* New York, NY: Oxford University Press.

Morgenstern, J., Bux, D., Labouvie, E., Blanchard, K. A., & Morgan, T. I. (2002). Examining mechanisms of action in 12-step treatment: The role of 12-step cognitions. *Journal of Studies on Alcohol, 63*, 665–672.

O'Farrell, T. J., & Fals-Stewart, W. (2001). Family-involved alcoholism treatment: An update. *Recent Developments in Alcoholism, 15*, 329–356.

Rosenqvist, P. (1991). AA, Al-Anon, and gender. *Contemporary Drug Problems, 18*(4), 687–705.

Roth, J. D. (2004). *Group psychotherapy and recovery from addiction: Carrying the message.* New York, NY: Haworth.

Roth, J. D., & Tan, E. M. (2007). Analysis of an online Al-Anon meeting. *Journal of Groups in Addiction & Recovery, 2*(1), 5–39.

Roth, J. E., & Tan, E. M. (2008). Spirituality and recovery from familial aspects of alcohol and other drug problems: Analysis of an online Al-Anon meeting. *Alcoholism Treatment Quarterly, 26*(4), 399–426.

Rotunda, R., & Doman, K. (2001). Partner enabling of alcoholics: Critical review and future directions. *American Journal of Family Therapy, 29*, 257–270.

Rotunda, R., West, L., & O'Farrell, T. J. (2004). Enabling behavior in a clinical sample of alcohol-dependent clients and their partners. *Journal of Substance Abuse Treatment, 26*, 269–276.

Rychtarik, R. G., & McGillicuddy, N. B. (2005). Coping skills training and 12-step facilitation for women whose partner has alcoholism: Effects on depression, the partner's drinking, and partner physical violence. *Journal of Consulting and Clinical Psychology, 73*(2), 249–261.

Timko, C., & DeBenedetti, A. (2007). A randomized controlled trial of intensive referral to 12-step self-help groups: One year outcomes. *Drug and Alcohol Dependence, 90*(2/3), 270–279.

Tonigan, J. S., Connors, G. J., & Miller, W. R. (1996). Alcoholics Anonymous Involvement (AAI) Scale: Reliability and norms. *Psychology of Addictive Behaviors, 10*(2), 75–80.

Wright, K. E., & Scott, T. B. (1978). The relationship of wives' treatment to the drinking status of alcoholics. *Journal of Studies on Alcohol, 39*(9), 1577–1581.

Young, L. B. (2011). Hitting bottom: Help seeking among Alcoholics Anonymous members. *Journal of Social Work Practice in the Addictions, 11*, 321–335.

New Addiction-Recovery Support Institutions: Mobilizing Support Beyond Professional Addiction Treatment and Recovery Mutual Aid

WILLIAM L. WHITE
Research Division, Chestnut Health Systems, Punta Gorda, Florida, USA

JOHN F. KELLY
Harvard Medical School, Department of Psychiatry, Massachusetts General Hospital-Harvard Center for Addiction Medicine, and Addiction Recovery Management Service, Boston, Massachusetts, USA

JEFFREY D. ROTH
Private Practice, Chicago, Illinois, USA

For more than 150 years, support for the personal resolution of severe and persistent alcohol and other drug problems in the United States has been provided through three mechanisms: family, kinship, and informal social networks; peer-based recovery mutual-aid societies; and professionally directed addiction treatment. This article: (1) briefly reviews the history of these traditional recovery supports, (2) describes the recent emergence of new recovery support institutions and a distinctive, all-inclusive culture of recovery, and (3) discusses the implications of these recent developments for the future of addiction treatment and recovery in the United States.

INTRODUCTION

There is growing evidence that the central organizing construct guiding addiction treatment and the larger alcohol and other drug (AOD) problems

---

The authors would like to thank Pat Taylor of Faces and Voices of Recovery for her assistance in identifying resources identified in Table 2. This article was prepared as a briefing paper for the 2012 Betty Ford Institute/UCLA Annual Conference on Recovery.

arena is shifting from longstanding pathology and intervention paradigms toward a solution-focused recovery paradigm (El-Guebaly, 2012; Laudet, 2008; White, 2008b). Calls are increasing to extend the prevailing acute care (AC) model of addiction treatment to a model of sustained recovery management (Dennis & Scott, 2007; McLellan, Lewis, O'Brien, & Kleber, 2000) and to nest these expanded treatment and support models within larger recovery-oriented systems of care (Kelly & White, 2011; White, 2008a). Related trends include increased interests in defining recovery (Betty Ford Institute Consensus Panel, 2007); evaluating the effects of participation in recovery mutual-aid societies on long-term personal recovery and social cost outcomes (Humphreys et al., 2004; Kelly & Yeterian, 2008); identifying effective linkage procedures between addiction treatment and recovery mutual-aid societies (Kaskutas, Subbaraman, Witbrodt, & Zemore, 2009; White & Kurtz, 2006); and expanding access to new forms of peer-based recovery support services (White, 2009b). There is also heightened interest in posttreatment recovery support mechanisms (McKay, 2009) for adults (Dennis & Scott, 2012) and for adolescents (Godley, Godley, Dennis, Funk, & Passetti, 2007). This latter trend is encouraging, particularly in light of the contention that recovery-focused "systems transformation" efforts that only focus on professional treatment and mutual aid miss opportunities to develop and mobilize broader addiction-recovery support resources within the community (White, 2009b).

Cloud and Granfield (2008) introduced the term *recovery capital* to designate the collective internal and external resources that can be mobilized to initiate and sustain the resolution of AOD problems at a personal level. Traditionally, recovery capital exists as a continuum of assets within three distinct spheres: (1) support from family, kinship, and social networks; (2) generalized support from indigenous cultural institutions (e.g., the arenas of medicine, business, education, religion, and social welfare); and (3) the more specialized support provided by addiction-recovery mutual-aid groups and professionally directed addiction treatment. For more than 150 years, these latter specialized addiction-recovery resources have provided the major help for persons with the most severe, complex, and prolonged AOD problems. There are, however, newly emerging addiction-recovery support institutions that do not fit within the addiction-recovery mutual-aid or addiction treatment dichotomy.

This article is an exercise in "connecting the dots" between what have been viewed as discreet developments to tell a larger story with potentially profound historical significance. The authors will: (1) briefly review the history of traditional recovery support structures in the United States, (2) describe the recent emergence of new recovery support institutions and an increasingly vibrant culture of recovery beyond the arenas of addiction treatment and recovery mutual aid, and (3) discuss how these developments could affect the future of addiction treatment and recovery.[1]

THE HISTORY OF TRADITIONAL RECOVERY SUPPORT STRUCTURES

Sophisticated epidemiological surveys and large-scale clinical studies have triggered debates on whether AOD problems are self-regulating and self-limiting (as suggested by the former) or whether they require professional intervention and long-term care (as suggested by the latter). There is an extensive body of research on the phenomenon of "natural recovery"—the resolution of AOD problems without participation in addiction treatment or recovery mutual-aid groups (Cunningham, 1999; Roizen, Cahalan, & Shanks, 1978; Sobell, Cunningham, & Sobell, 1996). This style of recovery is also reflected in a literary tradition of recovery memoirs within which people cast off AOD problems through a spectrum of religious, spiritual, and secular experiences outside the context of professional treatment or organized recovery support societies (for a review of early U.S. memoirs, see White, 2000). Even today, one does not have to travel far to find individuals who claim to have shed these problems without doing "rehab" or "meetings."

Recent community surveys revealing that most people (as many as 75%) who resolve AOD-related problems do so without formal treatment or mutual-aid involvement (Dawson, 1996; Lopez-Quintero et al., 2010; Schutte, Moos, & Brennan, 2006). This finding may be disconcerting to addiction professionals who spend their lives caring for those with the most severe, complex, and chronic AOD problems and who tend to see all AOD problems as progressive, chronically relapsing disorders resolved only through professional treatment and/or sustained involvement in a recovery mutual-aid society. In contrast, those who study the trajectory of AOD problems in larger community populations have come to expect that such problems are self-limiting (rather than progressive) and resolvable through one's natural resources. The former perspective has been referred to as the "clinician's illusion" (Cohen & Cohen, 1984) and the latter as the "epidemiologist's illusion" (Moos & Finney, 2011).

Neither perspective, in isolation, fully encompasses the two overlapping worlds of AOD problems or adequately explains the marked differences between the course of AOD problems in clinical and community populations (Storbjork & Room, 2008). The ability to resolve AOD problems across these populations seems to depend on the interaction between differing levels of personal/family/community recovery capital and different degrees of personal vulnerability and problem severity/complexity/chronicity (see White, 2008a, for review).

The role external resources play in the resolution of AOD problems in clinical and community populations raises two interesting questions that set the stage for our continued discussions:

1. Within the general population, could focused and sustained efforts to expand recovery support resources beyond addiction treatment and recovery mutual aid increase the prevalence of natural recovery from a broad spectrum of AOD problems?
2. Within clinical populations, could development of an expanded menu of community-based recovery support services be combined with addiction treatment and/or participation in recovery mutual aid to increase rates of successful recovery initiation and maintenance—particularly among those with the most severe substance use disorders?

A BRIEF HISTORY OF U.S. ADDICTION-RECOVERY TREATMENT AND MUTUAL AID

The story of addiction-recovery mutual aid in the United States begins with the rise of abstinence-based religious and cultural revitalization movements among Native American tribes (e.g., the Handsome Lake Movement [1799], the Shawnee Prophet Movement [1805]). This tradition of culturally nuanced mutual support organized by and for people in addiction recovery continued in Native American communities through subsequent religious and cultural revitalization movements, including the subsequent "Indianization of AA," the Red Road, and the contemporary Wellbriety Movement (Coyhis & White, 2006).

Organized mutual support for recovery in Euro-American communities began with people with alcohol problems seeking sanctuary within newly forming temperance societies (1830s) and extended through the more exclusive recovery-focused groups such as the Washingtonians (1840), recovery-focused temperance societies (1840s–1850s), Dashaway Association (1859), the Ribbon Reform Clubs (1870s), and the Drunkard's Club (1871). These early efforts encompassed both secular and explicitly religious as well as abstinence-based and moderation-based frameworks of recovery (White, 1998, 2001a).

Following the collapse of the first wave of alcoholism-recovery mutual-aid groups, new transition groups, such as the Brotherhood of St. Luke (1904), the Jacoby Club (1910), and the United Order of Ex-Boozers (1914), set the stage for the founding of Alcoholics Anonymous (AA [1935]), the first efforts to adapt AA for narcotic addicts (Addicts Anonymous [1947], Habit Forming Drugs [1951], Hypes and Alcoholics [early 1950s]), the founding of Narcotics Anonymous (NA) in New York City (1948), and the birth of NA as it is known today on the West Coast (1953; White, 2011).

In the years that followed, specialty groups branched from AA (e.g., the Calix Society [1947], Al-Anon [1951], Alateen [1957]), and AA's 12 steps were adapted for people dependent on other drugs—Pot Smokers Anonymous (1968), Pills Anonymous (1975), Marijuana Anonymous (1989), Cocaine

Anonymous (1982), Nicotine Anonymous (1985)—and for persons with co-occurring disorders (e.g., Dual Disorders Anonymous [1982], Dual Recovery Anonymous [1989], and Double Trouble in Recovery, [1993]; White, 2011).

The latest phase in this history is the diversification of recovery mutual aid with the growth of secular and religious alternatives to 12-step programs (e.g., Women for Sobriety [1975], American Atheists Alcohol Recovery Group [1980], Secular Organization for Sobriety/Save Our Selves [1985], Rational Recovery [1986], Smart Recovery [1994], Moderation Management [1994], and LifeRing Secular Recovery [1999]). Explicitly religious recovery support groups also emerged (e.g., Alcoholics Victorious [1948], Alcoholics for Christ [1977], Overcomers Outreach [1977], Liontamers Anonymous [1980], Millati Islami [1989], and the Buddhist Recovery Network [2008]; White, 1998, 2011).

Most recovery mutual-aid organizations, perhaps because of the stigma attached to AOD problems, have operated as closed, self-contained organizations, but there are exceptions. There is a long history of social clubhouses spawned by mutual-aid members. Clubhouses operate independently but in close tandem with their mutual-aid organizations. Mutual-aid organizations have also been involved in creating treatment organizations—from detoxification beds set up in the upstairs of Washingtonian Hall (in the 1840s) to AA cofounder Bill Wilson's vision of AA hospitals and AA missionaries. Recovery organizations have also been spawned inside addiction treatment organizations, including the Ollapod Club (1868), the Godwin Association (1872), and the Keeley Leagues (1891). The boundary between mutual aid and treatment has not always been a clear one.

Marking the early roots of today's specialty sector treatment system, an elaborate network of inebriate homes, medically directed inebriate asylums, private for-profit addiction cure institutes, and proprietary home cures for addiction flourished in the second half of the 19th century. These treatments, along with their mutual-aid counterparts, collapsed in the opening decades of the 20th century in the wake of alcohol and drug prohibition movements. Following this collapse, cultural authority for the control of those with severe AOD problems passed to the criminal justice system (e.g., inebriate penal colonies, federal prisons), to the emergency rooms and "foul wards" of large public hospitals, and to the back wards of aging state psychiatric asylums. Compassion and care gave way to sequestration, punishment, and control (White, 1998).

The resurgence of a vibrant, specialized addiction treatment field required decades of assertive advocacy and the development of replicable models of treatment between 1940 and 1965 (e.g., social setting detoxification, outpatient alcoholism clinics, residential models of alcoholism treatment, therapeutic communities, methadone maintenance, outpatient drug-free counseling clinics). Landmark legislation in the early 1970s set the stage for the rise of modern addiction treatment as a specialized health care field. The federal, state, and local partnership framed within this legislation and the subsequent extension of insurance coverage for the treatment of addiction led to the growth of specialized addiction treatment from a few hundred small programs to more than 15,000 institutions with a daily treatment capacity of more than 1.75 million patients served by a workforce of 130,000 full-time and 67,000 part-time and contractual workers (Kaplan, 2003; McLellan, Carise, & Kleber, 2003; Substance Abuse and Mental Health Services Administration, 2011).

This history has been presented elsewhere in far greater detail (White, 1998), but four themes within this history are pertinent to the current discussion. First, in spite of divergent philosophies and methods of care, the primary and almost exclusive unit of intervention within addiction treatment has been the *individual*—not the family, kinship network, or the larger natural environment in which recovery is sustained or extinguished.

Second, the primary model of addiction treatment delivery mimics the AC hospital with its functions of screening, admission, assessment, brief (and ever-briefer) treatment, discharge, and termination of the service relationship. Early critics of this AC model of addiction treatment characterized it as a mechanistic, expensive illusion, disconnected from the processes of long-term recovery (Dodd, 1997). Later critiques focused on weaknesses of the AC model related to attraction, access, retention, inadequate service dose, low utilization of evidence-based clinical practices, weak linkage to communities of recovery, the absence of posttreatment monitoring and support, and high rates of readdiction and readmission (Kelly & White, 2011; White, 2008a).

Third, the methods of treatment were distinctly clinical in their orientation (e.g., professional roles and interventions adapted from the fields of psychiatry, psychology, and psychiatric social work), with a particular focus on biopsychosocial stabilization. Intervention models that focused on recovery community resource development and assertive linkage to community recovery support systems were briefly considered in the 1960s and early 1970s but rapidly gave way to more medicalized models of care and the subsequent professionalization and commercialization of addiction treatment (White, 2002). As a result, nonprofessional recovery resources in the local community came to be seen as an adjunct to treatment—an afterthought to the more important intrapersonal clinical work—as opposed to treatment being viewed as an adjunct to more accessible and enduring recovery maintenance resources in the community. Few modern programs defined their role as a catalyst for the development of nonclinical recovery support resources in the communities they served, in great part because such activities were not reimbursable within prevailing AC models of care.

There have been efforts to break out of these encapsulated categories of recovery mutual aid and clinically directed addiction treatment. The halfway house movement of the 1950s sought a connecting bridge between these two worlds and to the larger process of community reintegration (Rubington, 1967); the Minnesota Model programs sought to blend these worlds within a treatment milieu (Spicer, 1993); the social model of recovery pioneered in California provided a distinct alternative to clinical treatment (Borkman, Kaskutas, Room, Bryan, & Barrows, 1998; Shaw & Borkman, 1990/1991); and early therapeutic communities existed as cultures of their own isolated from both mainstream addiction treatment and mainstream recovery mutual-aid groups (Janzen, 2001). In spite of such exceptions, professionally directed addiction treatment and recovery mutual-aid groups have remained, until recently, the primary specialized recovery support institutions.

NEW ADDICTION-RECOVERY SUPPORT INSTITUTIONS

The self-containment of recovery mutual-aid organizations and the similar self-containment and isolation of the addiction treatment enterprise has created a void of unmet need in the larger community for a broader spectrum of recovery support resources. That need is being filled in part by the rise of new recovery support institutions and a broader culture of recovery.

New Addiction-Recovery Advocacy Movement

In the late 1990s, new grassroots recovery community organizations (RCOs) began dotting the American landscape, stimulated in part by the Center for Substance Abuse Treatment's Recovery Community Support Program that in 1998 began providing seed money for such organizations (Kaplan, Nugent, Baker, & Clark, 2010). RCOs are organized by and on behalf of people in recovery and participate in a wide variety of recovery advocacy and peer recovery support activities. In 2004, the White House-initiated Access to Recovery program also began providing grants to states and tribal organizations for peer and other recovery support services.

In 2001, RCO representatives from around the country met in St. Paul, MN, to launch what has since been christened the new addiction-recovery advocacy movement. The 2001 meeting brought together local RCOs and existing national advocacy organizations such as the National Council on Alcoholism and Drug Dependence, the Johnson Institute's Alliance Project, and the Legal Action Center. A new organization, Faces and Voices of Recovery, was created at the summit and has since provided the connecting tissue for RCOs across the United States and beyond. In 2011, these RCOs formed the Association of Recovery Community Organizations (White, 2006).

The goals of what is rapidly becoming an international recovery advocacy movement (Roth, 2010) include: (1) the political and cultural mobilization of communities of recovery, (2) recovery-focused public and professional education, (3) advocacy of prorecovery laws and social policies, (4) advocacy for a recovery-focused redesign of addiction treatment, (5) promotion of peer-based recovery support services, (6) support for international, national, state, and local recovery celebration events, and (7) promotion of a recovery research agenda (White, 2007). The movement's core organizing themes are displayed in Table 1.

TABLE 1 Kinetic Ideas of the New Addiction-Recovery Advocacy Movement.

1. Addiction recovery is a reality in the lives of millions of individuals, families, and communities.
2. 2. There are many paths to recovery—and all are cause for celebration.
3. Recovery flourishes in supportive communities.
4. Recovery is a voluntary process.
5. Recovering and recovered people are part of the solution; recovery gives back what addiction has taken—from individuals, families, and communities (White, 2006).

As a point of perspective, in 1976, 52 prominent Americans publicly announced their long-term recovery from alcoholism as part of the National Council of Alcoholism's Operation Understanding—an antistigma campaign aimed at challenging stereotypes about alcoholism. It was the largest public "coming out" of people in recovery in the 20th century. In September 2011, more than 100,000 people in recovery and their families, friends, and allies participated in more than 200 public Recovery Month celebration events across the United States. That magnitude of cultural and political mobilization of people in recovery is historically unprecedented. The present recovery advocacy movement is distinctive in its explicit focus on eliminating policy barriers to addiction recovery and promoting a policy environment in which addiction recovery can flourish.

Recovery Community Centers

Many RCOs are creating local recovery community centers (RCCs), and some states (e.g., Connecticut, Vermont, Rhode Island) have created regional networks of RCCs. RCCs host recovery support meetings; provide recovery coaching; provide linkage to a wide spectrum of resources including recovery housing and recovery-conducive education and employment; serve as a site for recovery-focused social networking; and serve as a central hub for advocacy, peer support, and community service activities. In a recent year, for example, Vermont's nine RCCs, with just 15 part-time staff and 150 volunteers (30,000 hours of volunteer support per year), were open 70 hours per week, hosted 127 recovery support meetings per week, and had a total of 143,903 visits—25% of whom had less than a year of recovery, and 33% of whom had never participated in addiction treatment (White, 2009b).

Recovery Homes

Recovery residences are distinguished from addiction treatment by their homelike environment, self-determined lengths of stay, democratic self-governance, and their reliance on experiential rather than professional authority—no paid professional staff. The majority of recovery homes are financially self-supported by the residents. Most visible among the recovery residence network is Oxford House. Founded in 1975, Oxford House has grown to include more than 1,500 recovery homes in 48 states (432 cities) with a collective annual occupancy of more than 24,000 recovering people (Molloy & White, 2009; *Oxford House Inc. Annual Report*, 2011).

Jason and colleagues have conducted extensive studies of Oxford House and have found that the prospects of long-term recovery increase with length of stay (Jason, Davis, & Ferrari, 2007; Jason, Olson, Ferrari, & Lo Sasso, 2006; Jason, Olson, et al., 2007). These outcomes extend to women, racial and ethnic minorities, and people with co-occurring psychiatric disorders (d'Arlach, Olson, Jason, & Ferrari, 2006; Ferrari, Curtin-Davis, Dvorchak, & Jason, 1997; Majer et al., 2008).

Indicative of the spread of recovery homes, a recent survey in Philadelphia, PA, identified 21 city-funded recovery residences (primarily for persons re-entering the community from the criminal justice system) and a larger network of 250 financially self-supported recovery homes (Johnson, Martin, Sheahan, Way, & White, 2009). In 2011, representatives from the growing national network of recovery homes founded the National Association of Recovery Residences with the aims of assuring the quality of recovery residences and linking them into a more integrated network of long-term recovery support.

Recovery Schools

People in recovery face great obstacles in entering or returning to secondary and postsecondary schools—settings that have been characterized as "abstinence-hostile environments" (Cleveland, Harris, Baker, Herbert, & Dean, 2007). A broad spectrum of programs, collectively embraced within the rubric of the "recovery school movement," has emerged to provide recovery support within the academic environment (Roth & Finch, 2010). Beginning with Brown University, Rutgers University, Texas Tech University, and Augsburg College, specialized campus-based recovery support programs have provided an array of recovery supports ranging from scholarships for students in recovery, sober housing, on-campus recovery support groups, recovery coaching, academic mentoring, study groups, sober social activities, and community service projects. Since Ecole Nouvelle (now Sobriety High) in Minnesota was opened in 1986, there has been a similar growth in the development of recovery high schools. Twenty-five recovery high schools opened across the United States between 1999 and 2005 (White & Finch, 2006).

Studies to date of school-based recovery support programs confirm high rates of uninterrupted abstinence (70%–80%), early intervention and retention of students following any AOD use, excellent academic performance, high class attendance rates (90%–95%), high graduation rates, and high rates (65%) of college attendance among students in recovery high schools (Botzet,

Winters, & Fahnhorst, 2007; Cleveland et al., 2007; Gibson, 1991; Harris, Baker, Kimball, & Shumway, 2007; Moberg & Finch, 2007; White, 2001b). The growth of school-based programs led to the formation in 2002 of the Association of Recovery Schools.

Recovery Industries

Although obtaining meaningful, recovery-conducive work is a significant challenge for many people entering recovery within the current economic climate, vocational counseling/training, assertive linkage to recovery-supportive employment, and job coaching are not standard components of modern specialty-sector addiction treatment in the United States (Magura, 2003; Room, 1998). Several recent community responses to employment needs of people in recovery are worthy of note. First, RCOs, often through their RCCs or recovery coaching projects, are establishing employment clearinghouses and incorporating work-related support into the recovery coaching process. Second, two specialized types of employment resources are emerging specifically for people in recovery entering or re-entering the workforce. The first consists of recovery-friendly employers who have had good experiences hiring people in recovery and who remain receptive to such hiring, particularly those in a structured recovery support process. Examples of such employers range from small businesses like Zingerman's Deli in Ann Arbor, MI, to large businesses such as Venturetech—a manufacturer of hydraulic pumps in Houston, TX (see http://www.recoveryatwork.org). The second type of specialized employment resource involves businesses established by people in recovery who exclusively employ people in recovery (e.g., Recovery at Work in Atlanta, GA; Business Enterprises in Portland, OR). In these settings, people in recovery have the opportunity to acquire work skills, establish a recent employment history, and work with and be supervised by other people in recovery as a pathway to continued employment at these sites or to develop a work history that increases opportunities for alternative employment opportunities (White, 2009b).

Recovery Ministries

Churches, mosques, synagogues, and temples have become increasingly involved in providing addiction-recovery support services through the sponsorship of their respective faith communities. These efforts include recovery-friendly churches (e.g., Mercy Street in Houston, TX), megachurches with one or more "recovery pastors" (e.g., Saddleback Church in Southern California), lay leaders of church-sponsored recovery support groups (e.g., the spread of Celebrate Recovery in more than 10,000 churches), recovery-focused worship services and workshops, recovery churches (e.g., Central Park Recovery Church in St. Paul, MN), and faith-based recovery colonies (e.g., Dunklin

Memorial Camp in Okeechobee, FL; Swanson & McBean, 2011). One of the most well-known and enduring recovery ministries is that led by Reverend Cecil Williams at Glide Memorial Methodist Church in the Tenderloin District of San Francisco, CA (Williams, 1992). Many of the Christian recovery ministries are linked and mutually supported through the National Association for Christian Recovery founded in 1989. The growth of recovery ministries has also spawned a support industry of which mission is to spread recovery ministries nationally and internationally (e.g., NorthEast Treatment Centers Institute; White, 2009b).

RCOs, RCCs, recovery residences, recovery schools, recovery industries, and recovery ministries share several distinctive features. First, these new recovery support institutions fit neither the designation of addiction treatment nor designation as a recovery mutual-aid fellowship. Second, they provide recovery support needs not directly addressed through addiction treatment or recovery mutual-aid societies. Third, their target of support extends beyond the individual. Where addiction treatment and mutual aid provide personal guidance during the recovery process, these new recovery support institutions seek to create a physical and social world, including a policy environment, in which personal and family recovery can flourish. Fourth, these new institutions reflect, and are in turn being shaped by, a larger culture of recovery that transcends association with any treatment or recovery mutual-aid organization.

THE COMING OF AGE OF AN AMERICAN CULTURE OF RECOVERY

The transition from addiction to recovery is a personal journey, but it can also involve a journey between two physical and social worlds—from a culture of addiction to a culture of recovery (White, 1996). Historically, this transition has been marked by shedding the trappings and folkways of the culture of addiction (language, values, symbols, rituals, relationships, dress, etc.) and replacing these with the cultural folkways of a particular treatment institution or recovery mutual-aid society. What is significant today is the rise of a culture of recovery in the United States through a process of mutual identification that transcends where one's recovery started and the meetings one may or may not attend.

A broader cultural and political mobilization of people in recovery across diverse pathways and styles of recovery is emerging—a broader consciousness as *people in recovery*. People within particular recovery clans have been meeting in large numbers since the mass Washingtonian meetings of the 1840s, but people walking arm-in-arm on public streets in the United States representing an array of secular, spiritual, and recovery pathways and walking not as AA, NA, Women for Sobriety, Secular Organizations for Sobriety, LifeRing, or Celebrate Recovery members but as "people in recovery" is historically unprecedented. With that breakthrough has come the rapid rise and maturation of what might be thought of as a "nondenominational" culture of recovery.

With this broadened sense of identity, previously marginalized individuals are undergoing processes of consciousness raising, mobilization, and culture making. This culture is providing a diverse menu of words, ideas, metaphors, rituals, support institutions, support roles, and recovery support services to ease the process of recovery initiation, recovery maintenance, and enhanced quality of life in long-term recovery. What recovering people historically experienced inside treatment or a recovery fellowship—connection, mutual identification, and community—is now being extended beyond the walls of these institutions and meeting rooms.

The extent to which a culture of recovery in the United States is emerging beyond the arenas of addiction treatment and recovery mutual aid is illustrated in Table 2.

This brief description does not adequately capture the growing sense of community experienced by people across pathways of recovery and the potential importance of this trend to the future of recovery. The community-building process that is currently underway is comparable to that experienced at the height of the civil rights movement, the women's rights movement, and the lesbian, gay, bisexual, and transgender rights movement. What remains to be seen are the limits of mutual identification and the boundaries of inclusion/exclusion within this emerging culture of recovery.

IMPLICATIONS OF THE NEW SUPPORT INSTITUTIONS FOR TREATMENT, MUTUAL AID, AND THE ENHANCEMENT OF RECOVERY

For more than 150 years, addiction-recovery support beyond the natural resources of family, extended family, and social networks and general support from mainstream social institutions, has been provided by two specialized cultural institutions: addiction-recovery mutual-aid societies and professionally directed addiction treatment. In this article, we have documented the emergence of new recovery support institutions (RCOs, RCCs, recovery homes, recovery schools, recovery industries, recovery ministries) and a broader culture of recovery in the United States.

With the exception of the growing body of research on recovery residences, particularly the Oxford House network, and preliminary studies on collegiate recovery programs, little scientific attention has been directed toward investigating these new support mechanisms for addiction recovery. These new recovery supports also exist beyond the consciousness of the fields' clinical and policy leaders. The questions we pose below underscore our belief that the changes outlined in this article constitute a significant

TABLE 2 The Culture of Recovery in the United States: Emerging Elements and Representative Activities.

Recovery Cultural Element	Representative Activities
Values	RCO identification of "recovery values" (e.g., primacy of personal recovery, singleness of purpose/mission fidelity, organizational transparency, honesty, humility, simplicity, respect, tolerance, inclusion, stewardship); Recovery Bill of Rights—Faces and Voices of Recovery.
History	History clubs (e.g., AA History Lovers); groups working on state/local recovery group histories; growing archivist movement within mutual-aid groups; a book on the history of addiction recovery has gone through 10+ printings since 1998.
Language	Recovery-focused language audits; multiple advocacy papers on language challenging prevailing words and ideas (e.g., challenging the pervasive use of "abuse" within the AOD problems arena that has received recent research support; Kelly, Dow, & Westerhoff, 2011; Kelly & Westerhoff, 2010; White, 2006); Faces & Voices of Recovery Messaging Training.
Iconic Symbols	Recovery-themed posters, greeting cards, jewelry; the color amethyst (purple) used in T-shirts, posters, buttons, etc. from the Greek *amethystos*, meaning "not intoxicated"; and the butterfly, which symbolizes transition and rebirth.
Television	Recovery Television Network; increased recovery-themed cable television programming; heightened recovery-themed programming by the national networks; broader corporate sponsorship of recovery programming and activities.
Film	Recovery-themed documentaries and independent films (e.g., *The Secret World of Recovery*, *The Healing Power of Recovery*, *The Wellbriety Movement: Journey of Forgiveness*, *Lost in Woonsocket*, *Bill W*); growth in recovery film festivals.
Radio	Increased presence of recovery on conventional and Internet radio; Recovery Radio Network; Recovery 101 Radio; Recovery Coast-to Coast; Boston Recovery Radio; Afflicted and Affected; Recovery Matters; Steppin' Out Radio.
Theatre	Improbable Players in Watertown Square, MA; San Francisco Recovery Theatre; Phoenix Theatre Group (Helping Recovering Addicts via Art); The Vision Troupe (Bob LoBue's play *Visions*).
Music	Major recording artists expressing their recovery through music (e.g., Eminem, Mary J. Blige); Recovery Idol in Philadelphia, PA; the growing network of recovery music festivals—Sober in the Sun, Half Moon Sober Fest; Rockstar Superstar Project (Rebranding Sobriety).
Art	Recovery Murals in Philadelphia; growth of Recovery Fine Arts Festivals.
Literature	Recovery memoirs replacing drink/drug memoirs (Oksanen, 2012); papers and pamphlets related to recovery advocacy; annual recovery essay contests; recovery support for writers (e.g., Writers in Treatment).

(Continued on next page)

TABLE 2 The Culture of Recovery in the United States: Emerging Elements and Representative Activities. *(Continued)*

Recovery Cultural Element	Representative Activities
Media Communications	Recovery lifestyle magazines—*Journey: A Magazine of Recovery*; *Recovery Living, Renew Magazine, Serene Scene Magazine*—and books; *Addictions and Answers: Dr. Dave and Bill*; *New York Daily News* column; growth in recovery blogs and sober lifestyle Web sites (e.g., http://www.thefix.com/content/blogs).
Comedy	Recovery comedians (e.g., Mark Lundholm, Tara Handron, Jessie Joyce); Laughs without Liquor—Recovery Comedy Tour.
Sports	Philadelphia's Clean Machine and Milwaukee's Rebound Basketball teams; Colorado-based Phoenix Multisport.
Social Clubs	Recovery clubhouses, Recovery Coffee Shop, in Wichita, KS, and other coffee shops/cafes owned and operated by recovering people as recovery gathering sites; recovery dances; social events at RCCs.
Internet-Based Social Networking	Recovery-focused social networking on My Space, Facebook, and Twitter; www.intherooms.com; www.addictiontribe.com; www.soberrecovery.com; www.sobercircle.com; http://www.cyberrecovery.net/forums
Travel	Recovery-focused travel (e.g., www.TravelSober.com; www.SoberCelebrations.com; www.SoberCruises.com; www.SoberTravelers.com).
Recovery Community Leadership Development	Faces & Voices of Recovery Leadership Academy; Recovery Corps, Baltimore, MD; training programs to prepare people to serve as recovery coaches (e.g., Connecticut Community of Addiction Recovery); McShin Foundation; recovering people participating in mapping community recovery resources (e.g., Philadelphia).
Community Service	Community Volunteer Corps, Portland, OR; Missouri Recovery Network's community cleanup projects.
Science	Participation in recovery-focused scientific research (e.g., National Quit and Recovery Registry); people in recovery participating in development of recovery measures with research scientist Lee Ann Kaskutas, Ph.D.; people in recovery pursuing advanced education toward goal of conducting recovery research.
Recovery Advocacy Web sites	www.facesandvoicesofrecovery.org (see for listing of RCOs across the country); www.recoveryiseverywhere.com; www.recoverymonth.gov
National Recovery Celebration Events	Annual Rally for Recovery; Recovery Month events; America Honors Recovery Awards.
International Exchanges	UK recovery advocates visiting U.S. RCOs via Winston Churchill Scholarships; U.S. recovery advocates speaking at public recovery rallies in Europe, Asia, Africa, and South America.

milestone in the history of addiction recovery—a milestone that will have profound implications to the future study and treatment of AOD problems.

Historical Identity and Cultural Status

How will new recovery support institutions affect the identities and cultural status of addiction-recovery mutual-aid groups and addiction treatment institutions and their respective claims of cultural ownership of AOD problems?

Utilization and Effectiveness of Existing Institutions

Will the spread of these new recovery support structures serve to increase rates of entrance, early retention, and continued participation in addiction treatment and formal recovery mutual-aid groups? Will recovery rates within local addiction treatment and recovery mutual-aid groups rise in tandem with the development of these broader recovery support institutions? Could addiction treatment organizations increase the long-term recovery outcomes of those they serve by taking a more assertive role in the development, support, and mobilization of indigenous community recovery support resources?

Natural Recovery

Will the prevalence of natural recovery—the resolution of AOD problems without participation in recovery mutual-aid groups or professional treatment—increase under the influence and heightened accessibility of these new recovery support structures? Will new recovery support structures serve primarily as adjuncts or alternatives to addiction treatment and recovery mutual-aid groups?

Active Ingredients

What are the similarities and differences in the active ingredients (elements that elevate long-term recovery outcomes) within new recovery support institutions compared with those within addiction treatment and recovery mutual-aid groups?

Potent Combinations/Sequences

Are there particularly potent combinations or sequences of addiction treatment, recovery mutual aid, and participation in broader recovery support institutions that generate significantly higher rates of long-term recovery than could have been achieved through the use of each in isolation (e.g., combining outpatient treatment, mutual aid, and sober housing; Polcin, Korcha, Bond, & Galloway, 2010)?

Responses Across Diverse Populations

Are there particular populations for whom participation in these broader recovery support institutions are indicated or contraindicated? Will new recovery support institutions reach ethnic group members with severe substance use disorders who currently underutilize addiction treatment and mainstream recovery mutual-aid resources (Chartier & Caetano, 2011)?

The cultural management of AOD problems has historically focused on two targets: the individual and the community environment, with the activities of traditional recovery support institutions (i.e., professionally directed treatment and mutual-aid organizations) focused almost exclusively on the individual. The trends outlined in this article mark a movement into the chasm between the individual and the community. It is our expectation that greater attention will be given to improving recovery outcomes through strategies aimed at increasing *community recovery capital* (White & Cloud, 2008). This will involve a blending of traditional clinical strategies of intervention with strategies of cultural revitalization and community development. With that will come studies of the role of community recovery capital (including the emerging resources described in this article), as distinguished from the role of personal vulnerabilities and assets, in predicting long-term recovery outcomes.

Already rising from these new recovery support institutions is the concept of *community recovery*—the idea that broader social systems beyond the individual have been significantly wounded by severe and prolonged AOD dependence and related problems that may require a process of consciousness raising and sustained healing. Coyhis (Coyhis & White, 2002) has referred to this community recovery process as a "healing forest" within which the individual, family, community, and culture are healed simultaneously.

It is incumbent on addiction professionals to become students of and participants within this national and international transformation of the ecology of recovery (White, 2009a). The goal of the new recovery advocacy movement is to create a world in which recovery can flourish. It appears the construction of that world is well under way.

NOTE

1. All historical events and trends not otherwise cited are abstracted from White (1998)

REFERENCES

Betty Ford Institute Consensus Panel. (2007). What is recovery? A working definition from the Betty Ford Institute. *Journal of Substance Abuse Treatment, 33*, 221–228. doi:10.1016/j.jsat.2007.06.001

Borkman, T. J., Kaskutas, L. A., Room, J., Bryan, K., & Barrows, D. (1998). An historical review and developmental analysis of social model programs. *Journal of Substance Abuse Treatment, 15*(1), 7–17. doi:10.1016/S0740-5472(97)00244-4

Botzet, A. M., Winters, K., & Fahnhorst, T. (2007). An exploratory assessment of a college substance abuse recovery program: Augsburg College's StepUP Program. *Journal of Groups in Addiction & Recovery, 2*(2–4), 257–270. doi:10.1080/15560350802081173

Chartier, K. G., & Caetano, R. (2011). Trends in alcohol services utilization from 1991–1992 to 2001–2002: Ethnic group differences in the U.S. population. *Alcoholism: Clinical & Experimental Research, 35*(8), 1485–1497. doi:10.1111/j.1530-0277.2011.01485.x

Cleveland, H. H., Harris, K. S., Baker, A. K., Herbert, R., & Dean, L. R. (2007). Characteristics of a collegiate recovery community: Maintaining recovery in an abstinence-hostile environment. *Journal of Substance Abuse Treatment, 33*(1), 13–23. doi:10.1016/j.jsat.2006.11.005

Cloud, W., & Granfield, R. (2008). Conceptualizing recovery capital: Expansion of a theoretical concept. *Substance Use and Misuse, 43*(12/13), 1971–1986. doi:10.1080/10826080802289762

Cohen, P., & Cohen, J. (1984). The clinician's illusion. *Archives of General Psychiatry, 41*, 1178–1182.

Coyhis, D., & White, W. (2002). Addiction and recovery in Native America: Lost history, enduring lessons. *Counselor, 3*(5), 16–20.

Coyhis, D., & White, W. (2006). *Alcohol problems in Native America: The untold story of resistance and recovery—The truth about the lie*. Colorado Springs, CO: White Bison.

Cunningham, J. (1999). Untreated remission from drug use: The predominant pathway. *Addictive Behaviors, 24*(2), 267–270. doi:10.1016/S0306-4603(98)00045-8

d'Arlach, L., Olson, B. D., Jason, L. A., & Ferrari, J. R. (2006). Children, women, and substance abuse: A look at recovery in a communal setting. *Journal of Prevention & Intervention in the Community, 31*(1/2), 121–131. doi:10.1300/J005v31n01_11

Dawson, D. A. (1996). Correlates of past-year status among treated and untreated persons with former alcohol dependence: United States, 1992. *Alcoholism: Clinical and Experimental Research, 20*(4), 771–779. doi:10.1111/j.1530-0277.1996.tb01685.x

Dennis, M. L., & Scott, C. K. (2007). Managing addiction as a chronic condition. *Addiction Science & Clinical Practice, 4*(1), 45–55.

Dennis, M. L., & Scott, C. K. (2012). Four-year outcomes from the Early Re-Intervention (ERI) experiment using recovery management checkups (RMCs). *Drug and Alcohol Dependence, 121*, 10–17. doi: 10.1016/j.drugalcdep.2011.07.026

Dodd, M. H. (1997). Social model of recovery: Origin, early features, changes and future. *Journal of Psychoactive Drugs, 29*(2), 133–139.

El-Guebaly, N. (2012). The meanings of recovery from addiction: Evolution and promises. *Journal of Addiction Medicine, 6*, 1–9. doi:10.1097/ADM.0b013e31823ae540

Ferrari, J. R., Curtin-Davis, M., Dvorchak, P., & Jason, L. A. (1997). Recovering from alcoholism in communal-living settings: Exploring the characteristics of

African American men and women. *Journal of Substance Abuse, 9*, 77–87. doi:10.1016/S0899-3289(97)90007-9

Gibson, R. L. (1991, April). *School-based recovery support: The time is now.* Reno, NV: Paper presented at the annual convention of the American Association of Counseling and Development, Reno, NV.

Godley, M. D., Godley, S. H., Dennis, M. L., Funk, R. R., & Passetti, L. L. (2007). The effect of assertive continuing care on continuing care linkage, adherence, and abstinence following residential treatment for adolescents with substance use disorders. *Addiction, 102*, 81–93. doi:10.1111/j.1360-0443.2006.01648.x

Harris, K. S., Baker, A. K., Kimball, T. G., & Shumway, S. T. (2007). Achieving systems-based sustained recovery: A comprehensive model for collegiate recovery communities. *Journal of Groups in Addiction and Recovery, 2*(2–4), 220–237. doi:10.1080/15560350802080951

Humphreys, K., Wing, S., McCarty, D., Chappel, J., Galant, L., Haberle, B., Weiss, R. (2004). Self-help organizations for alcohol and drug problems: Toward evidence-based practice and policy. *Journal of Substance Abuse Treatment, 26*(3), 151–158. doi:10.1016/S0740-5472(03)00212-5

Janzen, R. (2001). *The rise and fall of Synanon: A California utopia.* Baltimore, MD: Johns Hopkins University Press.

Jason, L., Davis, M., & Ferrari, J. (2007). The need for substance abuse aftercare: Longitudinal analysis of Oxford House. *Addictive Behaviors, 32*, 803–818. doi:10.1016/j.addbeh.2006.06.014

Jason, L. A., Olson, B. D., Ferrari, J. R., & Lo Sasso, A. T. (2006). Communal housing settings enhance substance abuse recovery. *American Journal of Public Health, 96*, 1727–1729. doi:10.2105/AJPH.2005.070839

Jason, L. A., Olson, B. D., Ferrari, J. R., Majer, J. M., Alvarez, J., & Stout, J. (2007). An examination of main and interactive effects of substance abuse recovery housing on multiple indicators of adjustment. *Addiction, 102*, 1114–1121. doi:10.1111/j.1360-0443.2007.01846.x

Johnson, R., Martin, N., Sheahan, T., Way, F., & White, W. (2009). *Recovery resource mapping: Results of a Philadelphia Recovery Home Survey.* Philadelphia, PA: Philadelphia Department of Behavioral Health and Mental Retardation Services. Retrieved from http://www.facesandvoicesofrecovery.org

Kaplan, L. (2003). *Substance abuse treatment workforce environmental scan.* Rockville, MD: Center for Substance Abuse Treatment.

Kaplan, L., Nugent, C., Baker, M., & Clark, H. W. (2010). Introduction: The Recovery Community Services Program. *Alcoholism Treatment Quarterly, 28*, 244–255. doi:10.1080/07347324.2010.488522

Kaskutas, L. A., Subbaraman, M. S., Witbrodt, J., & Zemore, S. E. (2009). Effectiveness of Making Alcoholics Anonymous Easier (MAAEZ): A group format 12-step facilitation approach. *Journal of Substance Abuse Treatment, 37*(3), 228–239. doi:10.1016/j.jsat.2009.01.004

Kelly, J. F., Dow, S. J., & Westerhoff, C. (2011). Does our choice of substance-related terms influence perceptions of treatment need? An empirical investigation with two commonly used terms. *Journal of Drug Issues, 40*, 805–818. doi:10.1177/002204261004000403

Kelly, J. F., & Westerhoff, C. (2010). Does it matter how we refer to individuals with substance-related conditions? A randomized study of two commonly used terms. *International Journal of Drug Policy, 21*, 202–207. doi:10.1016/j.drugpo.2009.10.010

Kelly, J. F., & White, W. L. (2011). *Addiction recovery management: Theory, research and practice*. New York, NY: Springer.

Kelly, J. F., & Yeterian, J. (2008). Mutual-help groups. In W. O'Donohue & J. R. Cunningham (Eds.), *Evidence-based adjunctive treatments* (pp. 61–106). New York, NY: Elsevier.

Laudet, A. B. (2008). The road to recovery: Where are we going and how do we get there? Empirically driven conclusions and future directions for service development and resarch. *Substance Use & Misuse, 43*, 2001–2020. doi:10.1080/10826080802293459

Lopez-Quintero, C., Hason, D. J., de los Cobas, J. P., Pines, A., Wang, S., Grant, B. F., & Blanco, C. (2010). Probability and predictors of remission from life-time nicotine, alcohol, cannabis or cocaine dependence: Results from the National Epidemiologic Survey on Alcohol and Related Conditions. *Addiction, 106*(3), 657–669. doi:10.1111/j.1360-0443.2010.03194.x

Magura, S. (2003). The role of work in substance dependency treatment: A preliminary overview. *Substance Use and Misuse, 38*(11–13), 1865–1876.

Majer, J. M., Jason, L. A., North, C. S., Ferrari, J. R., Porter, N. S., Olson, B., Molloy, P. (2008). A longitudinal analysis of psychiatric severity upon outcomes among substance abusers residing in self-help settings. *American Journal of Community Psychology, 42*(1/2), 145–153. doi:10.1007/s10464-008-9190-z

McKay, J. R. (2009). *Treating substance use disorders with adaptive continuing care*. Washington, DC: American Psychological Association.

McLellan, A. T., Carise, D., & Kleber, H. D. (2003). Can the national addiction treatment infrastructure support the public's demand for quality care? *Journal of Substance Abuse Treatment, 25*, 117–121. doi:10.1016/S0740-5472(03)00156-9

McLellan, A. T., Lewis, D. C., O'Brien, C. P., & Kleber, H. D. (2000). Drug dependence, a chronic medical illness: Implications for treatment, insurance, and outcomes evaluation. *Journal of the American Medical Association, 284*(13), 1689–1695.

Moberg, D. P., & Finch, A. J. (2007). Recovery high schools: A descriptive study of school programs and students. *Journal of Groups in Addiction & Recovery, 2*(2–4), 128–161. doi: 10.1080/15560350802081314

Molloy, P., & White, W. L. (2009). Oxford Houses: Support for recovery without relapse. *Counselor, 11*(2), 28–33.

Moos, R. H., & Finney, J. W. (2011). Commentary on Lopez-Quintero et al. (2011): Remission and relapse—the yin-yang of addictive disorders. *Addiction, 106*, 670–671. doi:10.1111/j.1360-0443.2010.00003284.x

Oksanen, A. (2012). To hell and back: Excessive drug use, addiction, and the process of recovery in mainstream rock autobiographies. *Substance Use & Misuse, 47*, 143–154. doi: 10.3109/10826084.2012.637441

Oxford House, Inc. annual report. (2011). Silver Springs, MD: Oxford House.

Polcin, D. L., Korcha, R., Bond, J., & Galloway, G. (2010). Eighteen month outcomes for clients receiving combined outpatient treatment and sober living houses. *Journal of Substance Use, 15*(5), 352–366. doi:10.3109/14659890903531279

Roizen, R., Cahalan, D., & Shanks, P. (1978). 'Spontaneous remission' among untreated problem drinkers. In D. B. Kandel (Ed.), *Longitudinal research on drug use, empirical findings and the methodological issues* (pp. 197–221). New York, NY: John Wiley & Sons.

Room, J. (1998). Work and identity in substance abuse recovery. *Journal of Substance Abuse Treatment, 15*(1), 65–74. doi:10.1016/S0740-5472(97)00250-X

Roth, J. D. (2010). Crossing international boundaries in recovery from addiction. *Journal of Groups in Addiction & Recovery, 5*(3/4), 179–182. doi:10.1080/1556035X.2010.523335

Roth, J., & Finch, A. (2010). *Approaches to substance abuse and addiction in education communities: A guide to practices that support recovery in adolescents and young*. Philadelphia, PA: Taylor & Francis.

Rubington, E. (1967). The halfway house for the alcoholic. *Mental Hygiene, 51*, 552–560.

Schutte, K. K., Moos, R. H., & Brennan, P. L. (2006). Predictors of untreated remission from late-life drinking problems. *Journal of Studies on Alcohol, 67*, 354–362.

Shaw, S., & Borkman, T. (1990/1991). *Social model alcohol recovery: An environmental approach*. Burbank, CA: Bridge Focus.

Sobell, L. C., Cunningham, J. A., & Sobell, M. B. (1996). Recovery from alcohol problems with and without treatment: Prevalence in two population surveys. *American Journal of Public Health, 86*(7), 966–972.

Spicer, J. (1993). *The Minnesota Model: The evolution of the interdisciplinary approach to addiction recovery*. Center City, MN: Hazelden Educational Materials.

Storbjork, J., & Room, R. (2008). The two worlds of alcohol problems: Who is in treatment and who is not? *Addiction Research and Theory, 16*(1), 67–84. doi:10.1080/16066350701578136

Substance Abuse and Mental Health Services Administration. (2011). *National Survey of Substance Abuse Treatment Services (N-SSATS): 2010. Data on substance abuse treatment facilities* (DASIS Series S-59, HHS Publication No. [SMA] 11–4665). Rockville, MD: Author.

Swanson, L., & McBean, T. (2011). *Bridges to grace: Innovative approaches to recovery ministry*. Grand Rapids, MI: Zendervan.

White, W. L. (1996). *Pathways from the culture of addiction to the culture of recovery*. Center City, MN: Hazelden.

White, W. L. (1998). *Slaying the dragon: The history of addiction treatment and recovery in America*. Bloomington, IL: Chestnut Health Systems.

White, W. L. (2000). Listening to Lazarus: The voices of America's first 'reformed drunkards.' *Contemporary Drug Problems, 26*, 533–542.

White, W. L. (2001a). Pre-AA alcoholic mutual aid societies. *Alcoholism Treatment Quarterly, 19*(1), 1–21. doi:10.1300/J020v19n02_01

White, W. L. (2001b). Recovery university: The campus as a recovering community. *Student Assistance Journal, 13*(2), 24–26.

White, W. L. (2002). A lost vision: Addiction counseling as community organization. *Alcoholism Treatment Quarterly, 19*(4), 1–32. doi:10.1300/J020v19n04_01

White, W. L. (2006). *Let's go make some history: Chronicles of the new addiction recovery advocacy movement*. Washington, DC: Johnson Institute and Faces and Voices of Recovery.

White, W. L. (2007). The new recovery advocacy movement in America. *Addiction, 102*, 696–703. doi:10.1111/j.1360-0443.2007.01808.x

White, W. L. (2008a). *Recovery management and recovery-oriented systems of care: Scientific rationale and promising practices.* Pittsburgh, PA: Northeast Addiction Technology Transfer Center, Great Lakes Addiction Technology Transfer Center, Philadelphia Department of Behavioral Health & Mental Retardation Services.

White, W. L. (2008b). Recovery: Old wine, flavor of the month or new organizing paradigm? *Substance Use and Misuse, 43*(12/13), 1987–2000. doi:10.1080/10826080802297518

White, W. L. (2009a). The mobilization of community resources to support long-term addiction recovery. *Journal of Substance Abuse Treatment, 36*, 146–158. doi:10.1016/j.jsat.2008.10.006

White, W. L. (2009b). *Peer-based addiction recovery support: History, theory, practice, and scientific evaluation.* Chicago, IL: Great Lakes Addiction Technology Transfer Center and Philadelphia Department of Behavioral Health and Mental Retardation Services.

White, W. L. (2011). *A chronology of recovery mutual aid groups in the United States.* Retrieved from http://www.williamwhitepapers.com

White, W. L., & Cloud, W. (2008). Recovery capital: A primer for addictions professionals. *Counselor, 9*(5), 22–27.

White, W. L., & Finch, A. (2006). The recovery school movement: Its history and future. *Counselor, 7*(2), 54–58.

White, W., & Kurtz, E. (2006). *Linking addiction treatment and communities of recovery: A primer for addiction counselors and recovery coaches.* Pittsburgh, PA: Institute for Research, Education, and Training in Addictions/Northeast Technology Transfer Center.

Williams, C., with Laird, R. (1992). *No hiding place: Empowerment and recovery for troubled communities.* New York, NY: Harper San Francisco.

Index

Page numbers in *italics* represent tables